Nutrition Balance for Athletic Performance and Recovery

Supaprawat Siripipatthanakul
https://orcid.org/0000-0001-6671-2682
Bangkokthonburi University, Thailand

Astri Dwi Andriani
https://orcid.org/0000-0003-3951-4829
Universitas Putra Indonesia, Indonesia

Tamonwan Sitthipon
https://orcid.org/0009-0008-9939-5546
GlobalNxt University, Malaysia

IGI Global
Scientific Publishing
Publishing Tomorrow's Research Today

Vice President of Editorial	Melissa Wagner
Director of Acquisitions	Mikaela Felty
Director of Book Development	Jocelynn Hessler
Production Manager	Mike Brehm
Cover Design	Jose Rosado

Published in the United States of America by
IGI Global Scientific Publishing
701 East Chocolate Avenue
Hershey, PA, 17033, USA
Tel: 717-533-8845 | Fax: 717-533-7115
Website: https://www.igi-global.com E-mail: cust@igi-global.com

Library of Congress Cataloging-in-Publication Data

LCCN: 2026011387 (CIP Data Pending)
ISBN13: 979-8-3373-9544-9
Isbn13Softcover: 979-8-3373-9545-6
EISBN13: 979-8-3373-9546-3
British Cataloguing in Publication Data
A Cataloguing in Publication record for this book is available from the British Library.

Table of Contents

Detailed Table of Contents

thus having sufficient energy available is crucial to avoid fatigue and decreased ability to recover from exercise and perform at a high level. Finally, the chapter will discuss how the use of plant-based foods has become increasingly important for those who lead active lifestyles, as these foods provide proteins, carbohydrates, and micronutrients as well as contain bioactive compounds to aid in recovery and decreasing the inflammatory process.

This chapter examines the concept of periodized nutrition as a strategic approach to aligning dietary intake with different phases of athletic training. It highlights how carbohydrate manipulation supports glycogen depletion and restoration, including "train low, compete high" strategies and glycogen supercompensation for endurance performance. The role of protein timing and distribution in maximizing muscle protein synthesis and recovery is discussed, alongside optimal daily intake recommendations. Emphasis is placed on maintaining adequate energy availability to prevent Relative Energy Deficiency in Sport (RED-S), particularly among female and adolescent athletes. The chapter integrates macronutrient planning, micronutrient sufficiency, supplementation, and recovery strategies into a practical framework designed to enhance long-term adaptation, performance, and athlete health.

Nutrition balance for female athletes is a specialized, data-driven approach focusing on maintaining high energy availability to support training, hormonal health, and menstrual cycle variations. This chapter utilizes a systematic review of literature indexed in Scopus, WOS, and Google Scholar from 2024 to 2026. The findings highlight that AI assistants and wearable technology are transforming the field by providing personalized, real-time insights for optimization. To maximize performance, nutritional balance is essential, ensuring adequate intake of carbohydrates for energy, protein for muscle repair, healthy fats for hormone regulation, and micronutrients like iron and calcium to prevent common deficiencies. AI assistants play a significant role by offering individualized recommendations, monitoring hydration, and providing evidence-based guidance tailored to specific training regimens. With these tools, female athletes can maintain optimal nutrition, improving overall performance and facilitating more efficient recovery.

Khoiruddin Muchtar, Universitas Islam Negeri, Indonesia
Denny Aditya Dwiwarman, Universitas Putra Indonesia, Indonesia
Chirapat Kaewnaknaew, City University, Petaling Jaya, Malaysia
Asep Iwan Setiawan, Universitas Islam Negeri Gunung Djati Bandung, Indonesia

Post-exercise nutrition and electrolyte harmony are essential for tissue healing, energy restoration, and injury prevention for athletes. Consuming carbohydrates and protein during the “anabolic window” is recommended for 30 minutes to two hours post-workout to maximize muscle protein synthesis and replenish glycogen stores for rapid recovery, especially when training schedules allow less than 24 hours between sessions. In particular, 1–1.2 g/kg of carbs and protein promote insulin release, increasing glycogen repletion and mending muscle fiber microtears, reducing muscular discomfort and long-term injury. Hydration and electrolytes, such as sodium, potassium, and magnesium, could replace sweat losses, maintain blood volume and muscular function, and prevent cramps. Electrolyte-rich liquids or beverages are indicated for fluid retention and good physiological function during recuperation.

Sohom Saha, Lakshmibai National Institute of Physical Education, India
Mahendra Kumar Singh, Lakshmibai National Institute of Physical Education, India
Sachin Shekhawat, Lakshmibai National Institute of Physical Education, India
Prashant Kumar Choudhary, Lakshmibai National Institute of Physical Education, India
Patcharavadee Sriboonruang, Kasetsart University, Thailand

Training depends not only on an athlete's performance but also on recovery. This chapter employs a systematic review to describe the benefits of nutrition for

Foreword

Attaining optimal athletic performance and facilitating effective recovery require a balanced nutritional approach that provides the body with a consistent supply of high-quality macronutrients and micronutrients to meet energy requirements and support tissue repair. Carbohydrates serve as the principal energy source, crucial for sustaining glycogen reserves to support vigorous, prolonged exercise, and should be derived from complex, slow-digesting foods such as whole grains, fruits, and vegetables to avert energy fluctuations. Protein consumption is essential for muscle protein synthesis, repair, and growth, requiring consistent intake throughout the day to optimize recovery and mitigate muscle degradation. A balanced approach incorporates healthy fats to meet energy requirements, along with sufficient water and electrolyte replacement to prevent muscle fatigue and injury. Nutrient timing is crucial; pre-workout meals should emphasize carbs, but post-workout diet should include carbohydrates and protein to replenish glycogen stores and repair tissue, ideally ingested within a few hours after the activity. A food-first strategy, rather than forward relying on supplements, is typically advised to enhance overall nutrition, bolster immune function, and maintain long-term sports fitness.

Penpim Phuangsuwan
College of Management, University of Phayao, Thailand

Preface

AN OVERVIEW OF THE SUBJECT MATTER

Nutrition balance for athletic performance and recovery involves a strategic, personalized approach to food intake, aimed at maximizing energy, repairing muscle damage, and enhancing adaptation to training. Key areas include managing macronutrient ratios, optimizing micronutrient intake, ensuring precise hydration, and strategically timing nutrient consumption before, during, and after activity, often summarized by the 4Rs: Rehydrate, Refuel, Repair, and Rest.

A DESCRIPTION OF THIS TOPIC FITS IN THE WORLD TODAY

In today's world, athletes need to eat a balanced diet to perform well and recover. Eating the right mix of carbohydrates, proteins, fats, vitamins, and minerals gives athletes the energy they need, helps them build and repair muscle, and lowers their risk of injury. Sports science and technology help athletes create personalized nutrition plans that fit their sport, the intensity of their training, and their recuperation needs. This focus on balanced nutrition, coupled with drinking enough water and eating at the right times, helps not only peak performance but also speedier recovery. It is a key part of modern athletic success and long-term health.

A DESCRIPTION OF THE TARGET AUDIENCE

The target audience for "Nutrition Balance for Athletic Performance and Recovery" includes athletes, coaches, and physically active individuals seeking to optimize performance, accelerate recovery, and support overall health through proper nutrition. This group spans a broad age range, from adolescents participating in school sports to adults involved in recreational, collegiate, or professional athletics. They are motivated to learn about the roles of macronutrients, micronutrients, hydration, and meal timing in enhancing endurance, strength, and recovery. Additionally, this audience may include fitness enthusiasts, sports nutritionists, personal trainers, and healthcare professionals who support athletes. They value evidence-based, practical strategies and may have varying levels of nutrition knowledge, but all share the goal of achieving peak physical performance and minimizing injury or fatigue through balanced nutrition.

THE IMPORTANCE OF EACH OF THE CHAPTER SUBMISSIONS

Chapter 1: The Integration between Nutrition Balance and AI-Supported Fitness Training for Athletes' Performance and Recovery

The integration of nutrition and AI-supported fitness training represents a paradigm shift in healthcare and athletic performance, moving from generic, one-size-fits-all recommendations to highly personalized, real-time, and adaptive strategies. By leveraging data from wearable devices, genetic profiling, and metabolic assessments, AI enables the creation of tailored nutrition and training plans that optimize performance, accelerate recovery, and prevent injury. This chapter employs a systematic review with thematic content analysis. The findings show that integrating nutrition and AI-supported fitness training is transforming healthcare and physical activity for athletes by providing highly personalized, data-driven approaches to performance and wellness. With AI, athletes can receive tailored training programs that adapt in real time based on their biometrics, training responses, and specific goals.

Chapter 2: Health Applications and E-Commerce Strategies for Promoting Nutritional Balance and Athletic Performance: A Social Return on Investment Perspective in Thailand

This chapter explores how health applications integrated with electronic commerce (e-commerce) strategies support nutritional balance and athletic performance in Thailand and examines their perceived social return on investment (SROI). Using a qualitative approach, in-depth interviews were conducted with key stakeholders, including healthcare professionals, digital health developers, administrators, and end-users. The findings indicate that such applications enhance nutritional awareness, facilitate behavioral change, and translate dietary guidance into practical action through convenient access to health-related products and services, thereby supporting improved athletic performance. Beyond individual health benefits, stakeholders perceive broader social value in terms of improved quality of life, reduced caregiver burden, and potential long-term efficiency gains for the healthcare system.

Chapter 3: The Role of User Experiences and Technology Adoption in Digital Business–Driven Nutrition Platforms for Athletic Performance

The integration of artificial intelligence (AI) and digital business models is transforming sports nutrition from a product-oriented industry into a platform-based, intelligence-driven ecosystem. This chapter explores user experiences and examines how AI-enabled, digital business–driven nutrition platforms are adopted and valued in sport contexts. Drawing on qualitative interviews with athletes, performance nutritionists, coaches, and sports administrators, the study demonstrates that these platforms function as socio-technical systems rather than simple technological tools. Their effectiveness depends on the alignment of technological capabilities with user experience design and organizational context. The findings reveal a clear shift from traditional product-based sports nutrition toward intelligence-driven, platform-based value creation, while also identifying institutional barriers—including digital literacy gaps, professional trust, and data governance concerns—that influence adoption and long-term use.

Chapter 4: Building Trust in Sports' Nutrition & Supplementation for a Strategic Marketing Perspective in Athletic Performance and Recovery

The sports supplement market has been booming globally, and there has been a growing acceptance of a performance-based lifestyle. This chapter employs a systematic thematic content analysis. The findings show that building trust in the sports nutrition and supplementation market is essential to engaging athletes who increasingly seek evidence-based products to improve performance and recovery, while navigating the risks of contamination and misinformation. Strategic marketing in this space requires moving beyond hype to demonstrate safety, efficacy, and individualization, particularly as the market matures beyond elite sports into general wellness and active lifestyles.

Chapter 5: Strategic Nutritional Interventions for Enhancing Recovery and Reducing Exercise-Induced Inflammation

Exercise-induced inflammation is an essential yet tightly regulated component of physiological adaptation. While acute inflammatory signaling supports tissue remodeling and performance gains, excessive or prolonged responses may impair recovery and increase susceptibility to overtraining. This chapter synthesizes contemporary evidence on strategic nutritional interventions to enhance recovery while preserving adaptive mechanisms. Current literature indicates that omega-3 fatty acids modulate membrane composition and promote the resolution of inflammation, whereas curcumin and polyphenol-rich foods attenuate cytokine amplification and oxidative stress. Probiotics contribute to gut-mediated immune stability, and adequate protein, whether plant-based or dairy-derived, supports structural repair and systemic inflammatory balance. Carbohydrate availability further influences metabolic–inflammatory interactions. Emphasis is placed on periodized and individualized implementation, recognizing inter-individual variability in inflammatory phenotype and training demands.

Chapter 6: Balancing Natural Nutrition for Athletic Performance, Recovery, and Well-Being

An effective and well-balanced nutritional plan is essential for optimum athletic performance and recovery. This chapter will evaluate the concept of dietary balance from a functional perspective to support athletes by increasing energy availability, enhancing muscle tissue regeneration, reducing oxidative damage, and promoting long-term sustenance. The demands on an athlete's body are greater than those of a non-athlete due to excessive training and competition; thus, having sufficient energy is crucial for avoiding fatigue, improving exercise recovery, and performing at a high level. Finally, the chapter will discuss how the use of plant-based foods has become increasingly important for those who lead active lifestyles, as these foods provide protein, carbohydrates, and micronutrients, and contain bioactive compounds that aid recovery and reduce inflammation.

Chapter 7: Periodized Nutrition Strategies for Optimizing Glycogen Restoration, Muscle Protein Synthesis, and Long-Term Athletic Adaptation

This chapter examines the concept of periodized nutrition as a strategic approach to aligning dietary intake with different phases of athletic training. It highlights how carbohydrate manipulation supports glycogen depletion and restoration, including "train low, compete high" strategies and glycogen supercompensation for endurance performance. The role of protein timing and distribution in maximizing muscle protein synthesis and recovery is discussed, alongside optimal daily intake recommendations. Emphasis is placed on maintaining adequate energy availability to prevent Relative Energy Deficiency in Sport (RED-S), particularly among female and adolescent athletes. The chapter integrates macronutrient planning, micronutrient sufficiency, supplementation, and recovery strategies into a practical framework designed to enhance long-term adaptation, performance, and athlete health.

Chapter 8: Nutrition Balance for Females' Athletic Performance and Recovery Using AI Assistants

Nutrition balance for female athletes is a specialized, data-driven approach that focuses on maintaining high energy availability to support training, hormonal health, and menstrual cycle variability. This chapter utilizes a systematic review of literature indexed in Scopus, WOS, and Google Scholar from 2024 to 2026. The findings highlight that AI assistants and wearable technology are transforming the field by providing personalized, real-time insights for optimization. To maximize performance, nutritional balance is essential, ensuring adequate intake of carbohydrates for energy, protein for muscle repair, healthy fats for hormone regulation, and micronutrients like iron and calcium to prevent common deficiencies. AI assistants play a significant role by offering individualized recommendations, monitoring hydration, and providing evidence-based guidance tailored to specific training regimens. With these tools, female athletes can maintain optimal nutrition, improving overall performance and facilitating more efficient recovery.

Chapter 9: Nutrition Balance and Electrolyte Synergy in Post-Exercised Athletes for Rapid Recovery and Injury Prevention

Post-exercise nutrition and electrolyte harmony are essential for tissue healing, energy restoration, and injury prevention for athletes. Consuming carbohydrates and protein during the "anabolic window" is recommended for 30 minutes to two hours post-workout to maximize muscle protein synthesis and replenish glycogen stores for rapid recovery, especially when training schedules allow less than 24 hours between sessions. In particular, 1–1.2 g/kg of carbs and protein promote insulin release, increasing glycogen repletion and mending muscle fiber microtears, reducing muscular discomfort and long-term injury. Hydration and electrolytes, such as sodium, potassium, and magnesium, could replace sweat losses, maintain blood volume and muscular function, and prevent cramps. Electrolyte-rich liquids or beverages are indicated for fluid retention and good physiological function during recuperation.

Chapter 10: Functional Recovery Evidence-Based Nutritional Strategies for Athletes' Performance Enhancement and Injury Prevention

Training depends not only on an athlete's performance but also on recovery. This chapter employs a systematic review to describe the benefits of nutrition for helping athletes recover quickly, preventing injuries, and achieving high levels of performance. It discusses the roles of carbohydrates in energy restoration, protein in muscle rejuvenation, and healthy fats in managing inflammation. Significant nutrients include omega-3 fatty acids, vitamin D, iron, and antioxidants, as well as appropriate hydration and electrolyte balance. Other evidence-based supplements, such as creatine and collagen peptides, have also been reviewed in the chapter. Adolescent and master's athletes with unique recovery needs receive special attention. In general, this chapter presents evidence-based, practical nutritional interventions that coaches, athletes, and sport practitioners can find very easy to implement to enhance recovery and long-term performance.

Chapter 11: Anti-Inflammatory Nutrition Strategy for Athletes' Performance and Recovery

Athletes everywhere are looking for more anti-inflammatory foods to crush their performance and recovery. This chapter aims to highlight and systematically review the hypothesized implications of an anti-inflammatory dietary pattern for diet adequacy and for performance during peak exercise training and recovery after endurance or strength exertion. The review provides an overview of the biology of post-acute and chronic inflammation induced by exercise, with a special focus on redox-sensitive elements believed to act as trigger pathways, as well as those associated with immune function and musculoskeletal repair. This chapter summarizes recent knowledge about anti-inflammatory nutritional factors, i.e., omega-3 fatty acids, and single micronutrients, that adjust central pathways of inflammation and immune-metabolism. It also offers applied, periodized practicalities for incorporating these foods into athlete-specific sport nutrition plans during training, competition, and injury, in relation to energy-balance perspectives, including complementary micro- and macronutrient balance.

CONCLUSIONS

The integration of advanced nutrition strategies and AI-supported technologies is significantly transforming the field of sports performance and recovery. By enabling highly personalized, data-driven approaches, these innovations move beyond traditional, generic recommendations to deliver tailored solutions that optimize performance, accelerate recovery, and reduce injury risk for athletes. The use of digital platforms, evidence-based supplementation, and real-time monitoring not only enhances individual outcomes but also contributes to broader health improvements and more efficient healthcare systems. Collectively, these advancements elevate the standard of care in sports science, drive innovation in athlete management, and set new benchmarks for performance, recovery, and well-being in both elite and general athletic populations.

Supaprawat Siripipatthanakul
Bangkokthonburi University, Thailand

Astri Andriani
Universitas Putra Indonesia, Indonesia

Tamonwan Sitthipon
GlobalNxt University, Malaysia

Chapter 1
The Integration Between Nutrition Balance and AI-Supported Fitness Training for Athletes' Performance and Recovery

Supaprawat Siripipatthanakul
http://orcid.org/0000-0001-6671-2682
Bangkokthonburi University, Thailand

Pichakoon Auttawechasakoon
http://orcid.org/0000-0002-2247-6750
Sukhothai Thammathirat Open University, Thailand

ABSTRACT

The integration of nutrition and AI-supported fitness training represents a paradigm shift in healthcare and athletic performance, moving from generic, one-size-fits-all recommendations to highly personalized, real-time, and adaptive strategies. By leveraging data from wearable devices, genetic profiling, and metabolic assessments, AI enables the creation of tailored nutrition and training plans that optimize performance, accelerate recovery, and prevent injury. This chapter employs a systematic review with thematic content analysis. The findings show that integrating nutrition and AI-supported fitness training is transforming healthcare and physical activity

DOI: 10.4018/979-8-3373-9544-9.ch001

for athletes by providing highly personalized, data-driven approaches to performance and wellness. With AI, athletes can receive tailored training programs that adapt in real time based on their biometrics, training responses, and specific goals.

1. INTRODUCTION

The future paths and new developments highlight the use of artificial intelligence (AI) to create customized nutritional plans, the growing significance of holistic approaches that incorporate physical activity, sleep hygiene, and mental health, and the expected evolution of nutrition's role in the competitive esports landscape. Nutritional practices may change in response to current research findings and industry projections, guiding esports players, teams, and professionals toward long-term performance and health outcomes (Arslan, 2025).

With significant effects on performance and health, AI is transforming a wide range of industries, including sports and corporate management. The function of AI in managing athletic and corporate health, improving decision-making in business and sports organizations, and optimizing sports performance. AI-driven technologies such as wearables, biometric monitoring, predictive analytics, and machine learning algorithms are being used to increase organizational and individual productivity through a multidisciplinary approach. AI applications in professional sports teams and health-oriented business plans. When combined with efficient management techniques, AI has the potential to revolutionize the convergence of sports, business, and health, resulting in enhanced performance, reduced risk, and strategic advantage (Okon, 2025).

AI is transforming modern healthcare through innovative diagnosis, treatment, and rehabilitation. Artificial intelligence in physiotherapy and oncology, emphasizing its potential to enhance diagnosis, tailor therapies, and maximize rehabilitation. It investigates the application of AI in healthcare, specifically in early cancer detection with AI imaging and customized rehabilitation programs for mobility restoration. Ethical considerations, including data privacy and algorithmic bias, as well as future outlooks on AI technology, such as robotics and wearables in predictive medicine. Artificial intelligence is transforming various medical disciplines by enhancing precision, treatment strategies, and patient management. The significant effects of AI in cancer include early identification and screening, histopathological analysis, optimization of meal delivery services, personalized treatment planning, and AI-driven drug discovery. Integrating AI into physiotherapy enables medical professionals to deliver tailored rehabilitation programs, improve patient recovery, and enhance treatment efficiency (Mamta, 2025).

Conventional sports nutrition is based on standardized formulas that don't account for individual physiological and metabolic variations. An AI-driven system integrates physiological response modeling, ingredient attributes, and biochemical data to support customized sports nutrition. While Genetic Algorithms and Bayesian Optimization optimize ingredient ratios, machine learning approaches such as Random Forest, XGBoost, and Artificial Neural Networks are used to predict nutrient-performance associations.

Data integrity, model interpretability, and compliance with food safety regulations are prioritized. The findings show how precise, AI-based supplement design can improve overall athletic performance, endurance, and recovery (Pandya et al., 2026).

By offering individualized, data-driven, and real-time modifications to training loads and nutritional requirements, the combination of Nutrition Balance and AI-Supported Fitness Training is revolutionizing athletic performance. In addition to improving performance by up to 20% compared with traditional training, this synergistic method accelerates recovery, reduces injury risk, and enables round-the-clock monitoring.

2. LITERATURE REVIEW

2.1 Nutrition Balance and Recovery for Athletes

Nutrition is fundamental to an athlete's existence, significantly influencing their performance and overall health. Athletes must follow a well-balanced diet customized to their individual nutritional requirements to realize their best potential. This method not only enables optimal performance but also promotes rapid recovery and minimizes injury risk. Alongside a balanced diet, many athletes use nutritional supplements to enhance their nutrition and support their training goals. These supplements encompass a broad spectrum of benefits, addressing dietary deficiencies, facilitating recovery, increasing muscle protein synthesis, elevating energy levels, and optimizing performance in certain sports or activities. The various nutritional needs of athletes are to enhance their performance, recovery, and overall health. The optimal daily intakes of carbohydrates, proteins, fats, and micronutrients, as well as hydration strategies, ergogenic aids, nutritional supplements, and nutrient timing, are crucial. To eliminate prevalent myths about sports nutrition, it is also important to equip athletes with precise knowledge and enable informed nutritional decisions (Amawi et al., 2024).

A proper and balanced diet is crucial for recovery and rehabilitation. "Rehabilitation nutrition" for athlete injury recovery is comparable to sports nutrition, but it also helps prevent sarcopenia, malnutrition, and dysphagia. Rehabilitation nutrition and training aim to improve the athlete's long-term nutritional status, endurance, and resistance. The optimum nutrition for athletes to speed their return to sports following surgery or injury. Sarcopenia prevention requires 25–30 kcal/kg of body weight more energy than the objective. Metabolism, energy, hemoglobin, lean mass, bone mass, immunity, health, and prevention of oxidative damage depend on macro- and micronutrients. Supplementing with leucine to address poor protein intake can overcome anabolic resistance. Thus, wounded athletes struggle to maintain muscular mass without accumulating fat. An athlete's diet should include the quantity, frequency, and types of food, and, most importantly, the quality of protein. Consuming carbs and protein during rehabilitation can help prevent muscle breakdown and atrophy. Long-term omega-3 fatty acid intake increases anabolic sensitivity to amino acids, potentially benefiting injured athletes. Adequate macronutrient intakes support athletes' anabolism (Papadopoulou, 2020).

After physical training, replenishing glycogen, regenerating muscle tissue, normalizing hormonal balance, and restoring electrolyte balance are needed for recovery. Nutrition helps maintain and accelerate these processes, making it essential to rehabilitation programs. Combining proteins and carbohydrates in a 3:1 or 4:1 ratio and replenishing fluids and electrolytes to prevent dehydration can speed recovery. BCAAs (leucine, isoleucine, and valine), EAAs (lysine, methionine, threonine, phenylalanine, tryptophan, and histidine), and creatine are also thought to improve recovery and strength performance. Vitamin C and E, powerful antioxidants, protect cells from oxidative damage, speeding recovery. The sports nutrition overview current research on proteins, carbs, vitamins, and minerals. Sports nutrition and supplementation are crucial to post-workout recovery (Shlykov et al., 2025).

The intricate relationship among sport, nutrition, and sustainable foods highlights how a sustainability-oriented diet can enhance athletic performance, facilitate swift post-training recovery, and aid in injury prevention. The enduring effects of these dietary choices on athletes' health and the environment are crucial in providing a comprehensive perspective that links human well-being to global health. The prospective advantages of a sustainable diet for athletes. It emphasizes that specific nutritional choices can enhance physical performance while fostering a more ethical and responsible lifestyle, amid the growing demand for global sustainability. Practitioners, especially those specializing in sports, play a crucial role in early diagnosis and in educating and advising on optimal choices (Grosso & Turco, 2026).

Recent research has highlighted hydration and dietary optimization, while low energy availability, polyphenols, anthropometry, and recovery techniques have been studied. The conceptual framework emphasized terms such as sports, nutrition, energy consumption, dietary intake, performance, soccer, and training load. Peripheral terminology, including fluid balance and sweat rate. The co-occurrence analysis identified insufficiently examined subjects, including oxidative stress, lipid peroxidation, beta-alanine supplementation, and antioxidant indicators. Progressing these study domains is crucial to integrating nutritional methods that directly impact the performance and health of soccer players (de Oliveira et al., 2025).

Nutrition boosts athlete performance. Nutrition affects sports performance. Given the growing body of research, the expanding range of dietary options, and the increased publicity surrounding professional athletes, nutrition affects sports performance. The Mediterranean diet reduces inflammation and improves power, muscle endurance, and body composition. Ketogenic diets limit carbs and protein. Both exhibit no weight loss decreases, but ketogenic diets, a more rigorous low-carbohydrate diet, are harder to follow. Athletic performance is also improved by high-protein, protein-paced, low-carb diets. Plant-based diets vary. Vegans may experience nutritional deficiencies and lower leucine levels, which can reduce muscle protein synthesis. Many kinds of intermittent fasting may not suit persons with comorbidities or specific needs and may slow sprint performance and increase fatigue. Diet affects athletic performance and highlights key concerns to watch for. No diet is universally recommended for athletes, but this article provides information to help athletes assess their diet with medical guidance and consider sustainable modifications to achieve performance and body-habitual goals (Kaufman et al., 2023).

Coaches in most sports have used periodization for decades to improve athletic adaptation and performance by planning and sequencing training blocks throughout macro, meso, and micro cycles of training and racing. Nutrition should be periodized to support training and racing goals. Endurance athletes' diets may range from low to high energy availability (EA) or carbohydrate (CHO) availability (e.g., body composition management with brief periods of low EA or CHO vs optimized adherence to sports nutrition guidelines via high EA and CHO). Despite strong data supporting current guidelines, knowledge and use of periodized nutrition regimens among world-class endurance athletes across training and racing levels are seldom documented. Some athletes and scientists use a chronic, long-term ketogenic, low-CHO, high-fat (LCHF) diet to improve endurance and health. Notably, it is not a claim of better performance, and most evidence for the latter comes from clinical groups, including obesity, cancer, and epilepsy. This is an important topic that has been largely unexplored in the literature because endurance athletes are at high risk for low bone mineral density (BMD) and stress fractures, and evidence suggests that both acute low EA and CHO availability may negatively affect bone modeling in active individuals. Thus, dietary periodization in elite endurance athletes and the effects of low energy and low CHO availability on bone modeling and bone health markers (Heikura, 2020).

The pivotal role of nutrition in the rehabilitation of sports injuries underscores the importance of energy balance and specific nutrients in the recovery process. Essential recommendations encompass sustaining energy equilibrium to avert muscle atrophy, emphasizing protein consumption for muscular repair, ingesting complex carbohydrates for energy provision, supplementing with omega-3 fatty acids to mitigate inflammation, employing creatine monohydrate to augment muscle recuperation, ensuring adequate vitamin D levels for skeletal and muscular well-being, supplementing with gelatin and vitamin C for tendon and ligament integrity, contemplating HMB (Beta-Hydroxy Beta-Methylbutyrate) to safeguard muscle mass, integrating antioxidants to facilitate recovery, and modifying nutritional approaches according to the nature of the injury. Adhering to this advice enables athletes to enhance their recovery, expedite their return to training, and realize their full athletic potential (Buceta, 2025).

Endurance athletes may benefit from low-carbohydrate (CHO) diets for metabolic adaptation and body composition. Diets may harm bone health due to insufficient availability of calories or CHO. Low-CHO diets in elite endurance athletes may affect bone injuries and remodeling, according to this thesis. 28% of athletes consumed low-CHO diets; their comprehension varied. Fasting exercise 38% more often and had a significant link with bone damage. Fasted training users were 1.61 times as likely to have a career bone injury as non-users. A gap in nutrition and sports nutrition knowledge. Many athletes ignored sports nutrition guidelines, underestimating CHO and overeating protein, which could lead to energy deficiencies. Pre-exercise CHO-rich or low-CHO diets did not affect indicators of bone resorption or formation. Low-CHO diets are controversial and may confuse athletes and coaches. Periodize nutrient consumption for training and competition. Nutrition requirements must be communicated well in the online media age. The high injury rate and poor bone health among endurance athletes warrant inquiry into the effects of reduced CHO intake on bone health and remodeling. Short-term low-CHO diets did not affect bone remodeling, but sustained low-CHO or low-energy availability (LEA) may impair bone mass and health (Raleigh, 2025)

Health-oriented objectives were crucial, tailored to the athlete's sport, position, gender, age, and competitive phase, incorporating incremental modifications (e.g., 0.5–1.0 kg/week fat reduction) to optimize performance. Common tactics for modifying body mass and composition involve establishing an energy surplus (500–1000 kcal/day) or deficit (250–1000 kcal/day), ensuring energy availability exceeds 30 kcal/kg of fat-free mass per day, and periodizing carbohydrate consumption (3–12 g/kg/day) according to training requirements. Protein consumption (1.6–2.4 g/kg/day) was advised throughout 4–6 meals from premium sources, in conjunction with specific supplements including creatine, whey protein, and a multivitamin and mineral complex. Recommendations emphasized scant attention to nutrients such as lipids, fiber, and micronutrients, and the terminology used was frequently ambiguous, allowing considerable scope for interpretation (Delany et al., 2025).

Thus, optimal nutrition for athletes necessitates a balanced consumption of macronutrients—approximately 45 kcal/kg of fat-free mass daily—emphasizing carbs for energy, 1.2–1.7 g/kg of protein for muscle repair, and healthy fats. Recovery is optimized by ingesting protein and carbohydrates within 30-60 minutes following exercise, utilizing nutrient-dense foods, and maintaining hydration. Thus, AI could benefit in these tasks.

2.2 AI-Supported Smart HIIT Program on Cardiovascular Fitness and Physical Performance

In recent years, fitness and wellness training programs have gained popularity. One of the most popular is High-Intensity Interval Training (HIIT), which quickly improves cardiovascular efficiency and physical performance. With significant advances in artificial intelligence (AI), smart training systems that analyze biometric and physiological data to create personalized programs are possible. AI algorithms may assess users' biological and physical data and design physiologically based training routines, thereby enhancing exercise efficacy and reducing injury risk. The effects of an AI-supported smart HIIT program on cardiovascular fitness and physical performance in 20-to-40-year-olds. In a trial, 60 participants were randomly assigned to two groups: 30 who followed the smart HIIT program and an equal number who followed a traditional program. AI-driven HIIT program and standardized cardiovascular capacity and physical performance tests. The experimental group outperformed the control group on cardiovascular and performance parameters. These data demonstrate the program's efficacy and the usefulness of technology-enhanced training for cardiovascular fitness. AI-supported technology in improving health and performance (Ghanem, 2025).

The prospective function of wearable and digital technology in the interaction between health and fitness professionals and customers. A favorable relationship could potentially alter the industry's Business-to-Consumer (B2C) dynamics. Offer information to help users in the subsequent areas: A) applications of wearable technologies and digital resources in the daily practices of health and fitness professionals, B) the potential of these tools for holistic client and patient monitoring, regardless of age or digital literacy, and C) optimizing the use of these resources to augment consumer engagement in health and fitness initiatives. Wearable technologies, fitness applications, and data-driven tools. Practical insights into the applicability and usability of prevalent artificial intelligence systems are detailed, covering various health and fitness user objectives, including technological empowerment, improved professional-client connectivity, optimized industry dynamics, and the potential for ongoing evolution (Addolorato, 2025).

Demand for healthcare and long-term care has increased, especially for mental health. AI has shown potential for health management, but its effects on physical activity, mental health, and their relationship remain unknown. AI promotes physical exercise among adults to improve mental health and elucidate the underlying mechanisms. Personalized psychological support, cognitive rehabilitation, and cardiovascular and musculoskeletal therapies were key. This improved cognitive function, emotional stability, and physical resilience. Biomarkers of BDNF, serotonin, and increased physical activity supported these therapies. AI, physical activity, and mental health insights to enable new research and applications. For personalized fitness programs, sophisticated health monitoring, and cognitive and emotional rehabilitation, AI is crucial. crucial suggestions for scientists and practitioners to better use artificial intelligence to meet the mental health requirements of aging societies. This work advances the use of AI-assisted physical activity to boost mental health in aging populations by comprehensively detailing AI's possible roles in future interventions (Fang et al., 2025).

Static rules and protocols are common in traditional exercise and health management systems. These methods make it difficult to integrate heterogeneous multisource data and adapt to individual demands. User engagement and intervention efficacy remain low. A Generative Artificial Intelligence (GAI)-driven personalized management system was created to address these difficulties. The technology dynamically generates exercise, nutritional, and risk alerts. It uses a Transformer-based Large Language Model (LLM) for semantic profiling, a Generative Adversarial Network (GAN) for synthetic data augmentation, and a Graph Neural Network (GNN) to capture complex correlations among health factors. Optimize adaptive decision-making with Deep Reinforcement Learning (DRL). Performance was strong empirically. The system has 92.7% workout-type suggestion accuracy, 7.9% calorie prediction error, and a 4.7/5 personalized recommendation rating. User satisfaction rose 35.3%, and BMI and resting heart rate improved. An efficient and scalable technology platform for intelligent health management. GAI can enable accurate and effective health interventions (Wang et al., 2026).

Obesity is a global health issue with large inter-individual food and lifestyle effects. Traditional weight-loss methods disregard genetics, metabolic profiles, and gut flora composition, leading to poor adherence and inconsistent results. There are essential biological and behavioral factors relevant to precision medicine for weight control, with an emphasis on nutrition, and addressing their existing and potential integration into digital health platforms. The key precision medicine elements (e.g., genetic, metabolic, and microbiome characteristics) and how they are integrated into digital health technologies. Nutrigenomics, nutritional metabolomics, and microbiome-informed nutrition can be tailored to specific genetic variants (e.g., FTO and MC4R), metabolic phenotypes (e.g., insulin resistance), and gut microbiota profiles. In real-world situations, mobile health apps, wearable devices, and AI-supported platforms improve self-monitoring, adherence, and dynamic feedback. To explain dietary disparities among individuals, modulation of the gut–brain axis, microbial fermentation, gene–diet interactions, and anti-inflammatory responses are investigated. Cost, accessibility, and patient motivation must be addressed to successfully deploy these integrated techniques in real-world settings. There is an importance of precision nutrition for tailored, scalable, and sustainable obesity therapies (Liu et al/, 2025).

The relationship between nutritional balance and recovery is essential for athletic performance, whereas AI-enhanced Smart HIIT programs improve cardiovascular fitness and physical performance via customization. These aspects collectively establish a contemporary, optimal training methodology in which nutrition enables the body to withstand the high-intensity demands dictated by AI, resulting in accelerated recovery, less injury risk, and enhanced performance.

2.3 AI-Based Athlete Stress Management and Nutrition

Stress can hinder athletes' performance and well-being. Poor stress management and lack of coping resources can impair physical output, decision-making, and well-being. Peak performance requires stress management. Sports psychology, stress management, and AI-powered integrative stress management. Cognitive-behavioral, mindfulness-based, relaxation, biofeedback, technology-based, social support, and team-based methods are used. The study classified AI-powered stress management strategies as wearable monitoring, virtual therapy and chatbot counseling, predictive analytics for stress forecasting, guided biofeedback training, enhanced injury and recovery support, cognitive behavior training, and AI integration with human support systems. AI-based athlete stress management offers the following benefits: improved performance and well-being, objective stress monitoring, all-around assistance for athletes, injury prevention, early identification and intervention, personalized training and recuperation, confidentiality, and stigma reduction. Advances in AI for stress management should include improved AI-powered injury-prevention models, biometric sensing, edge AI for real-time data processing, and wearable sweat analysis for feedback. Athletes should incorporate multimodal, targeted interventions into their training, warm-up, and recuperation to maximize performance and well-being. A hybrid approach by sport psychologists that uses AI to enhance athletes' stress management will yield faster and better results (Adebisi et al., 2025).

Endurance sports increasingly use AI to improve performance, recovery, nutrition, and supplement use. AI in endurance sports: metabolic health, nutritional methods, recuperation optimization, ethics, and future approaches. AI systems improve metabolic health monitoring, recovery prediction, and nutrition personalization by integrating multimodal physiological, environmental, and behavioral data. Continuous glucose monitoring and AI algorithms improve performance during extended events by managing carbs. AI-driven supplementing techniques based on genetic polymorphisms and metabolic responses have improved ergogenicity. However, measurement validity and reliability of sensor-derived signals, dataset quality (noise, missingness, labeling error), model performance and generalizability, algorithmic transparency, and equitable access remain issues. Homogeneous training datasets impede generalizability across varied sports populations. AI in endurance sports can improve performance, recovery, and nutrition through tailored techniques. Model performance, generalizability, ethical transparency, and fair accessibility must be addressed to realize this promise. Performance level (elite to leisure), sport discipline, climatic circumstances (heat, altitude), and device platforms (multi-vendor/multi-sensor) should be covered. To achieve scientifically robust, morally sound, and practically applicable AI solutions, thorough external and field validation, transparent and explainable deployment with proper governance, and fair access are essential (Grivas & Safari, 2025).

Precision exercise nutrition with AI is changing how athletes eat for performance, recovery, and well-being. Precision feeding techniques for athletes' physiological and metabolic needs using AI. AI-based mechanisms such as real-time diet monitoring, continuous glucose monitoring, and nutrient optimization systems offer insights into how AI can improve precision nutrition by analyzing complex datasets and integrating genetic, metabolic, and environmental factors to deliver adaptive dietary recommendations for athletes. AI challenges in this domain include ethical considerations, data confidentiality, and the need for homogeneity across diverse populations. Hiring AI helps athletes create more precise nutrition regimens, which improve workout performance and reduce fatigue and injury recovery time. AI might improve precision nutrition engagement for athletes and fitness aficionados (Nasb et al., 2025).

AI is increasingly impacting bodybuilding by providing data-driven insights for better training, nutrition, performance analytics, injury prevention, and supplement selection. AI affects five bodybuilding characteristics. AI-Based Training Optimization enhances progressive overload and movement precision through adaptive workout routines and real-time feedback. AI-Driven Nutrition & Diet Planning enhances macronutrient tracking, meal personalization, and genetics-based diet optimization. AI in Performance Monitoring & Biomechanics uses wearables and machine vision to correct exercise form and analyze body composition. AI addresses the fourth challenge of Injury Prevention and Recovery by utilizing advanced prediction models for muscle strain detection, individualized rehabilitation, and improved rest routines. AI in Supplementation & Pharmacology covers supplement initiatives, hormonal modulation, performance-enhancing substances, and detection.

Existing AI systems face challenges such as insufficient flexibility to individual physiology, biases in datasets, privacy concerns, and the lack of legal frameworks for AI-assisted supplements and doping detection. Future research trends include smart gym gear, AI-human instructors, AI-supported nutrigenomics, and regenerative medical methods (Al-Shareeda et al., 2025).

AI-driven stress management and nutrition solutions are revolutionizing athlete performance by leveraging real-time wearable data to deliver individualized, actionable insights that surpass traditional techniques. These systems employ machine learning (ML) and artificial intelligence (AI) to integrate physiological metrics—such as heart rate variability (HRV), sweat biomarkers, and continuous glucose monitoring (CGM)—to enhance training, recuperation, and nutrition.

2.4 Genetics & AI-Encourage Athletes' Nutrition Balance and Recovery

goFOOD™ is a specialized smartphone-based dietary assessment system designed to assist, monitor, and enhance the nutritional balance and recovery of athletes by overcoming the shortcomings of conventional, frequently unreliable, food diaries. It employs sophisticated deep learning techniques to examine food photos and deliver comprehensive, real-time analyses of nutrient intake. Accurate nutritional assessment may improve diets and clinical outcomes. goFOODTM, an AI-based dietary evaluation system. The technology uses smartphone photos of food to estimate meal calories and macronutrients. goFOODTM requires two meal photos or a short movie. Traditional single-camera smartphones must capture photographs from two viewing angles, whereas smartphones with two rear cameras need only one shutter button press. Deep neural networks detect, segment, and recognize food in both photos, while a 3D reconstruction method estimates the meal volume. Food type, volume, and nutrient database determine each meal's calories and macronutrients. goFOODTM supports 319 fine-grained food categories and has been validated on two multimedia datasets containing non-standardized and fast-food meals. The non-standardized meal database showed that goFOODTM outperformed expert dietitians, while the fast-food database yielded similar results. Dietary assessment is easy and fast with goFOODTM (Lu et al., 2020).

Genetics and nutrition science have advanced exponentially, changing our understanding of how genetics and diet affect metabolic responses and health. The convergence of genetics and nutrition science has led to the development of nutrigenomics and nutrigenetics, and to the rise of personalized nutrition in the media. Nutrigenomics examines how food affects human genetics. It helps us understand how diets affect gene expression, metabolic pathways, and physiological responses. Nutrigenomic studies reveal gene–nutrient interactions essential for nutrition sensing, metabolism, and homeostasis using high-throughput methods including microarray analysis and next-generation sequencing. The need for genetically targeted dietary therapies to promote metabolic health and prevent diet-related diseases. Nutrigenetics, on the other hand, studies genetic variants that alter an individual's response to dietary cues, underscoring the role of genetic variability in shaping nutritional needs and diet-related disorders. Single-nucleotide polymorphisms confer our uniqueness and enable genome-wide association studies and candidate-gene approaches to identify variants associated with nutrient metabolism pathways, thereby informing genotype-based dietary recommendations to reduce disease risk and improve nutritional adequacy. Nutrigenomic and nutrigenetic data combined with individualized nutrition could lead to genetically and metabolically adjusted diets. Incorporating omics data with clinical characteristics and lifestyle factors could enable detailed assessments of nutritional status and disease predisposition, as well as targeted preventive and management measures (Nongbet et al., 2026).

It appears that much of the extensively marketed food technology is still unready. Nutrition, food security, and sustainability are interwoven concerns in complex, adaptive food systems that need tackling biology, behavior, markets, policy, and environmental limits together. Nutrition science is crucial because it links human biology to the real-world variables that influence what people can access, afford, choose, and safely consume. As food systems become increasingly linked and sensitive to climate, conflict, and market volatility, reductionist problem-solving is giving way to context-aware techniques that can account for feedback, trade-offs, and equity. This scientific agenda and planetary health imperative require sustainable food systems to secure current and future nutrition while balancing environmental stewardship, health, and socio-economic stability across production, consumption, and waste. Overall, the agenda speaks to a new chapter in nutrition research that integrates the right level of complexity by combining deep disciplinary insight with better-integrated systems methods and mobilizing coordinated action (Berry et al., 2026).

Footballers have shown increased receptiveness to genetic testing for personalized nutrition, with many expressing greater willingness when it is linked to career prospects. Nutritionists exhibited overall support while exercising caution, demonstrating an understanding of the existing limits in evidence. Both groups exhibited diminished receptiveness to utilizing genetic information for selection eligibility and talent scouting. It underscores the need for enhanced education on genetic testing for both players and practitioners, and stresses the imperative to formulate ethical rules to prevent the misuse of genetic information in professional sports (Efstathiou et al., 2026).

Nutritional genomics is a burgeoning discipline that examines how foods affect gene expression and, in turn, their influence on skeletal muscle metabolism, athletic performance, and metabolic flexibility. Macronutrients act as essential regulators of metabolic programming by influencing cellular homeostasis and gene expression. An extensive examination of significant DNA polymorphisms associated with energy metabolism, specifically highlighting genes such as ACTN3, AMPD1 C34T (rs17602729), PPARA (rs4253778), PPARD (rs2016520), PPARG (rs1801282), PPARGC1A (rs8192678), and TFAM. The ramifications of these genetic polymorphisms are analyzed with respect to muscle fiber composition, athletic performance, and vulnerability to metabolic diseases. Personalized nutritional strategies are essential for maximizing individual genetic potential and enhancing metabolic health and physical performance (de Oliveira, 2025).

The integration of genetics and artificial intelligence (AI) is revolutionizing sports nutrition and recovery, shifting from a uniform approach to a highly individualized, data-centric framework. By integrating genomic data with real-time biometric monitoring, athletes may optimize their nutritional balance, expedite recuperation, and improve overall performance.

2.5 DAT Encourage Athletes' Nutrition Balance and Recovery

Artificial Intelligence is employed in nutrition to transition from generic dietary recommendations to tailored, data-driven, and real-time tactics. It advances nutritional science by automating dietary evaluations, providing customized meal plans, and managing chronic illnesses such as diabetes and obesity.

The intricate relationship among sports, nutrition, and sustainable foods highlights how a sustainability-based diet can enhance athletic performance, facilitate swift post-training recuperation, and aid in injury prevention. The enduring effects of these dietary selections on athletes' health and the environment are examined, providing a comprehensive perspective that links individual well-being to world health. The possible advantages of a sustainable diet for athletes by critically reviewing existing scientific literature and examining case studies and experimental research. It emphasizes that specific nutritional choices can enhance physical performance while fostering a more ethical and responsible lifestyle, amid the growing demand for global sustainability. The crucial role of dentists, especially those specializing in sports, in early diagnosis and in teaching and advising on optimal alternatives (Grosso & Turco, 2026).

Recovery is sometimes disregarded in athletic performance. Recuperation is not usually used immediately after training or during competition. Crisis increases psychological demands owing to uncertainty, which can affect the entire periodization cycle in team or individual sports. A crisis might be war, quarantine, or injury. Rehabilitation and recovery knowledge, along with sleep quality and psychological demands; nutritional techniques, including macronutrient timing, vitamin supplementation, and essential nutrients; sleep optimization; and recovery approaches such as cryotherapy and water, are addressed. The necessity of emotional management and understanding during such moments is significant. Finally, helping athletes focus on recovery can increase performance, self-reliance, and emotional stability. A paradigm that addresses physiological and psychological demands until the situational milieu normalizes can do this (Afshar Naseri, 2025).

Dietary adaptation was a gradual and interrelated process. In the beginning, participants reported decreased explosiveness, energy fluctuations, and mood instability. Some saw increased energy stability, physical awareness, and self-regulation with moderate exercise loads. Many athletes struggled with high-intensity efforts and late-session demands. Social dynamics, especially shared meals and carbohydrate-rich food culture, strongly influenced diet adherence and meaning-making. Understanding the perceived value of KD requires consideration of role expectations, team structures, and cultural eating habits. KD was a context-sensitive method that had varying ramifications for persons and situations, rather than delivering uniform performance outcomes. Sport nutrition that highlights athletes' lived experiences and contextualizes nutritional interventions within their socio-cultural and performance environments (Bo, 2026).

Research on measurement techniques for human energy intake and output has evolved considerably in recent decades. Wearables, sensors, software, and Web-based technologies are widespread in research and consumer settings. Self-report instruments have given way to advanced technologies that require coordination of optical and accelerometric data to estimate energy expenditure. Energy intake assessment still relies mainly on self-reporting. These tools have advanced from paper-based to online reporting, but they still need improvement, and novel, transformational techniques, such as spectroscopic and chemosensing, offer significant potential. The science and the pros and cons of present and emerging technologies from the perspectives of researchers, users, and developers. Researchers want validity, accuracy, data detail, and abundance, as well as ethical use; users want ease of use and privacy; and developers want high adherence and utilization, intellectual property, licensing rights, and monetization. Assessments depend on frequent updates and integration of food and nutrition databases, enhancing accessibility and reducing inequities in use, and providing reliable technical support. These contextual difficulties are addressed as possibilities and stages toward individualized health (Das et al., 2022).

AI-driven Dietary Assessment Tools (DAT) are advanced, technology-based solutions that automate the collection, analysis, and interpretation of dietary intake data, thereby replacing or augmenting conventional, subjective approaches such as paper diaries and 24-hour recalls. Utilizing artificial intelligence (AI)—particularly computer vision, deep learning (DL), and machine learning (ML)—these solutions mitigate reporting bias, conserve time for users and dietitians, and deliver objective, real-time nutritional data. DAT can be used to enhance nutritional balance, and recovery is essential for athletes to improve performance, mitigate injury risk, and sustain long-term health. Evidence-based techniques emphasize the "3 R's" of recovery—Refuel (carbohydrates), Repair (protein), and Rehydrate (fluids)—and the appropriate timing of meals (Panayotova, 2025).

3. METHODOLOGY

This chapter is integrated using the PRISMA method, with the related topic and keywords identified from scholarly papers indexed in Google Scholar, Scopus, and WOS from 2020 to 2025, as suggested by Siripipoatthanakul et al. (2025; a, b & c)

In PRISMA (Preferred Reporting Items for Systematic Reviews and Meta-Analyses), inclusion and exclusion criteria delineate the selection or rejection of studies based on PICOS (Population, Intervention, Comparator, Outcomes, Study design), providing a transparent and impartial assessment. These criteria are meticulously implemented during the screening step to refine outcomes from identification to final selection.

1. **Identification:** Scholarly journals are chosen via intentional sampling. The identifying procedure commences here. The identification of keywords and topics in the examined articles signifies the conclusion of the selection process. Data was gathered and analyzed from a collection of English-language articles that were initially published. A diverse array of sources yielded 589 scholarly articles on the topic and related themes throughout the identification process.
2. **Screening:** During the screening phase, papers are chosen for assessment. This systematic review involved the collection and analysis of secondary data through purposeful sampling. Thirty scholarly articles were selected from the preliminary compilation following this screening process. The key terms in this chapter include nutrition, AI-assisted fitness training, sports, athletic performance, and recovery.
3. **Eligibility:** To determine eligibility, the researchers excluded publications and copies lacking complete versions of the papers. Public presentations consist of the final 30 scholarly articles selected during the qualifying stage.
4. **Inclusion:** This phase involved the synthesis of thirty scholarly publications. The fourth phase entails completing the aggregation of research for inclusion in the systematic review. Ensure that all academic work adheres to the specified chapter sequence. Before the publication of the findings, the study's quality was evaluated by four independent reviewers. Grammarly was employed to detect occurrences of plagiarism and grammatical errors. Furthermore, Grammarly

detected occurrences of computer-generated content and plagiarism. Two English specialists assess and approve the article's content prior to the submission of the final edition.

4. RESULTS

Figure 1. Conceptual Framework

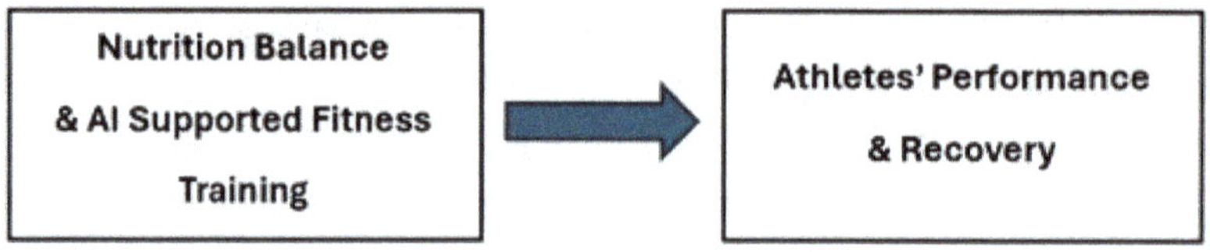

5. DISCUSSIONS

Hillen et al. (2025) discuss the use of AI for nutrition balance and recovery in healthcare, which could be applied to athletes. According to multimodal therapy, encompassing dietary assistance, physical exercise, and pain management, is crucial for addressing the intricate therapeutic problems associated with advanced pancreatic cancer. The global incidence of pancreatic cancer is rising, and the disease is frequently detected at an advanced stage, resulting in restricted treatment alternatives and a dismal prognosis. Advanced pancreatic cancer has numerous detrimental symptoms that impair patients' quality of life, necessitating early, comprehensive, and interdisciplinary patient care. The integration of digital health, especially through remote monitoring, is essential to overcoming therapeutic challenges and enhancing data-driven clinical decision-making. The European project RELEVIUM investigates the impact of a tailored, digitally facilitated, multimodal supportive care intervention on health-related quality of life in patients with pancreatic cancer, with the objective of enhancing early access to multidisciplinary, cost-effective palliative care. Thus, the AI data-driven approach is also effective for athletes.

Tertipi et al. (2025) conclude that skin quality depends on genetic, environmental, lifestyle, and exercise factors. Regular exercise boosts microcirculation, collagen synthesis, reduces oxidative stress, and modulates inflammatory pathways. Skin type, age, fitness level, and environmental exposures affect responses to physical exercise. AI enables personalized skin-health workout plans. Wearable sensors and smart fitness gadgets track physiological responses (heart rate, perspiration rate, oxidative stress) and environmental characteristics (UV exposure, pollution). Based on this data, AI algorithms develop dynamic, adaptive exercise routines to optimize skin benefits and minimize harm (e.g., exercise-induced oxidative stress in sensitive skin types). Exercise benefits the skin, and AI-driven, tailored physical activity is a new technique in cosmetic dermatology. AI in fitness planning may provide tailored, non-invasive skincare strategies to complement topical and procedural approaches, advancing precision dermatology. Thus, AI benefits athletes during recovery by helping them avoid sunburn.

Jud & Thalmann (2025) noted that the use of AI in sports coaching is increasingly promising, bringing both new potential and challenges for athletes and service providers. There is no thorough overview available, despite research on AI in sports coaching largely focusing on specific facets or technologies. AI in digital sports coaching is essential, given the coach's digital roles and the challenges of implementation. The need for additional empirical research on the application of digital coaches (DCs) in sports, and their use for the athletes' recovery and performance.

Moussa et al. (2026) concluded that there is a connection between women's psychological health and AI-assisted diet, with an emphasis on female college students. AI-assisted nutritional therapies have the potential to improve psychological well-being, encouraging the incorporation of AI technologies into women's dietary management and mental health. This study highlights the importance of tailored AI-driven food suggestions in fostering psychological and emotional stability. Thus, it could be applied for an AI-assisted diet for athletes' nutrition balance and recovery

Ghanem (2025) supports that in recent years, fitness and wellness training programs have gained popularity. One of the most popular is High-Intensity Interval Training (HIIT), which quickly improves cardiovascular efficiency and physical performance. With significant advances in artificial intelligence (AI), smart training systems that analyze biometric and physiological data to create personalized programs are possible. AI algorithms may assess users' biological and physical data and design physiologically-based training routines, enhancing exercise efficacy and reducing injury risk. AI-supported smart HIIT program affects cardiovascular fitness and physical performance in individuals aged 20–40. In a trial, 60 participants were randomly assigned to two groups: 30 who followed the smart HIIT program and an equal number who followed a traditional program. AI-driven HIIT program and standardized cardiovascular capacity and physical performance tests. The experimental group improved more than the control group on cardiovascular and performance measures. These data demonstrate the program's efficacy and the usefulness of technology-enhanced training for cardiovascular fitness. AI-supported technology in improving health and performance, accomplishing one of the UN's sustainable development objectives, Quality Education.

Rao & Rao (2026) state that Artificial intelligence uses interactive methods, like games and simulations, to enhance health education. Due to the rapid advancement of digital technology, AI is now recognized for helping individuals maintain optimal health through distinctive, interactive, and customizable instructional resources. AI-driven approaches may serve as a viable alternative to conventional methods, which often fail to engage learners or foster lasting behavioral change. Practical examples illustrate how AI facilitates mental health education, promotes nutritious diets, and encourages physical activity. Some issues arising from new technology include fairness, privacy concerns, and the risks of relying on algorithms in health education. AI assists educators, curriculum designers, and administrators in the effective and responsible utilization of AI tools.

Hillen et al. (2025) discussed that multimodal therapy, encompassing dietary assistance, physical exercise, and pain management, is crucial for addressing the intricate therapeutic problems associated with advanced pancreatic cancer. The global incidence of pancreatic cancer is rising, and the disease is frequently detected at an advanced stage, resulting in restricted treatment alternatives and a bleak prognosis. Patients with advanced pancreatic cancer endure numerous detrimental symptoms that impair their quality of life and necessitate early, thorough, interdisciplinary therapy. The integration of digital health, especially via remote monitoring, is essential for overcoming therapeutic obstacles and enhancing data-driven clinical decision-making. The European project RELEVIUM investigates the impact of a tailored, digitally facilitated multimodal supportive care intervention on health-related quality of life in pancreatic cancer patients, with the objective of enhancing early access to multidisciplinary, cost-effective palliative care.

Therefore, integrating nutritional equilibrium with AI-enhanced fitness training merges two vital components of athletic advancement—customized nutrition and intelligent, data-informed training—to optimize performance and expedite recovery. This collaboration uses artificial intelligence to tailor food and exercise to each athlete's physiological needs, objectives, and responses. The role of nutritional balance in athletic performance involves optimizing energy intake. Balanced nutrition ensures that athletes receive the appropriate combination of macronutrients (carbohydrates, proteins, fats) and micronutrients (vitamins, minerals) to support their training and competitive endeavors. Optimized recovery involves adequate nutrients that facilitate muscle regeneration, reduce inflammation, and restore energy reserves, thereby reducing recovery time between sessions. Injury prevention and immune support through sufficient nutrition fortify the immune system and diminish the risk of harm.

6. CONCLUSIONS

The integration of nutrition and AI-enhanced fitness training is transforming healthcare and physical endeavors, particularly in optimizing athletic performance and recovery. Using modern artificial intelligence technology, athletes and their coaches can now access training regimens dynamically modified based on real-time data, including physiological parameters, performance outcomes, and sleep habits. These AI-driven systems evaluate extensive data to propose individualized workout regimens tailored to each athlete's distinct strengths, weaknesses, and objectives. The integration of nutrition into this equation substantially amplifies the advantages. AI-assisted nutritional coaching can determine the precise balance of macronutrients, vitamins, and hydration required for optimal performance and effective recovery. AI can monitor nutritional consumption and correlate it with training results, recommending adjustments to enhance endurance, strength, or expedite muscle recovery. This comprehensive strategy mitigates injury risk by maintaining adequate nutrition and rest while also fostering sustained athletic excellence. The integration of nutritional science with AI-enhanced fitness training provides a comprehensive, evidence-based approach for athletes to achieve optimal health, set new performance benchmarks, and recover more efficiently from the physical strains of their sport.

The integration of nutritional equilibrium with AI-enhanced fitness training represents a transformative leap from conventional coaching to individualized, data-informed approaches to enhancing athletic performance and recovery. This method uses AI algorithms, wearables, and metabolic data to dynamically and in real time adjust training loads and food intake, resulting in accelerated recovery, improved metabolic efficiency, and reduced injury risk. A significant shift from generic, one-size-fits-all tactics to dynamic, data-driven, customized, “precision” approaches is evident in the combination of AI-supported physical training and personalized dietary balancing. This integration, which combines nutritional intake data with performance metrics from wearable technology, enables real-time, thorough monitoring to maximize training, accelerate recovery, and reduce injury risk. AI analyzes individual metabolic responses to suggest precise macronutrient and micronutrient intake, including optimizing carbohydrate timing for endurance events and improving recovery protein goals.

AI-driven precision nutrition and metabolic optimization leverage individual metabolic responses to prescribe specific macronutrient and micronutrient intake, including enhancing recovery protein goals and the strategic timing of carbohydrate consumption for endurance sports. Real-time nutrient monitoring can be achieved using AI-driven applications and wearables, exemplified by goFOODTM, which employs computer vision to identify food photos and tracks dietary intake while delivering immediate, context-sensitive feedback. AI-driven dynamic feeding utilizes

CGM data to tailor nutrition during exercise (e.g., gel timing, hydration) to mitigate the risk of "hitting the wall" and gastrointestinal issues. AI-Assisted Performance-Based Fitness Training uses adaptive training plans from AI algorithms (such as Athletica.ai) that analyze daily performance data to autonomously adjust training loads based on fatigue levels. This keeps athletes at an optimal training level, thereby avert burnout or overtraining. Biomechanical analysis using AI-driven motion-recognition technologies, including computer vision and 3DAT, can precisely detect injury risk, inefficient movement patterns, and gait asymmetries (approximately 85%), facilitating prompt technical modifications. Digital Twins are used to enhance performance while safeguarding athletes from risks such as overtraining. Sophisticated AI algorithms create virtual metabolic models of athletes to simulate their responses to various training and nutritional scenarios. Impact on Recovery and Injury Prevention. Predictive recovery metrics facilitate tailored rest and recovery protocols by employing AI to detect early signs of overtraining or illness and to anticipate next-day preparedness based on sleep, heart rate variability, and dietary logs. Customized Rehabilitation could be improved using AI by employing virtual reality and gamification to enhance compliance and accelerate recovery. AI-driven platforms evaluate surgical advancement to create individualized rehabilitation regimens. Nutritional assistance for recovery, provided by Evidence-based AI recommendations on protein and amino acid intake, can reduce post-exercise inflammation and expedite muscle recovery. Challenges and opportunities arise from its potential; this integration faces challenges, including the need for non-invasive, high-fidelity data and the risk of "hallucinations" in generative AI outputs. A "digital divide" exists: some individuals may lack access to advanced AI technologies, and models trained on homogeneous data may not generalize effectively to diverse groups. The future of advancements is in "Centaur coaching," where AI conducts complex data analysis and human coaches provide essential contextual, emotional, and strategic insights.

7. LIMITATIONS AND RECOMMENDATIONS

This chapter employs a systematic analysis without respondents. Thus, further studies recommend a survey, such as a questionnaire or a series of interviews. The recommendation for further research is that, when combined with nutritional insights—such as optimal macronutrient intake, hydration strategies, and recovery planning—these programs help maximize athletic performance, minimize injury risk, and accelerate recovery. This synergy enables a holistic, evidence-based approach that supports athletes in achieving peak performance while maintaining long-term health and well-being.

REFERENCES

Addolorato, S. (2025). Can Wearable and Digital Technologies Augment Business-to-Consumer Data Driven Outcomes in Health and Fitness Industry? *Sport i Turystyka, 8*(1), 161–175. https://www.ceeol.com/search/article-detail?id=1327735

Adebisi, E., Balogun, T. N., Oguntuase, S. B., & Olajide, F. O. (2025). Leveraging Artificial Intelligence (AI) for Stress Management in Peak Athletic Performance: An Integrative Review. *Scientific Journal of Engineering and Technology, 2*(2), 94–106. https://journals.stecab.com/sjet/article/view/999

Afshar Naseri, M. B. (2025). Beyond performance: A narrative review of prioritizing recovery and mental conditioning of athletes in times of crisis. *Journal of Sports and Rehabilitation Sciences, 3*(1), 26–38. https://www.jsportrs.com/article_229674 .html. DOI: 10.32598/JSRS.2505.1083

Al-Shareeda, M. A., Obaid, A. A., & Almajid, A. A. H. (2025). The role of artificial intelligence in bodybuilding: A systematic review of applications, challenges, and future prospects. *Jordanian Journal of Informatics and Computing, 2025*(1), 16–26. DOI: 10.63180/jjic.thestap.2025.1.3

Amawi, A., AlKasasbeh, W., Jaradat, M., Almasri, A., Alobaidi, S., Hammad, A. A., Bishtawi, T., Fataftah, B., Turk, N., Saoud, H. A., Jarrar, A., & Ghazzawi, H. (2024). Athletes' nutritional demands: A narrative review of nutritional requirements. *Frontiers in Nutrition, 10*, 1331854. DOI: 10.3389/fnut.2023.1331854 PMID: 38328685

Arslan, S. (2025). The Future of Nutrition in Esports: Integrating AI, Personalized Diets, and Holistic Approaches. In *Esports Nutrition: Enhancing Cognitive and Physical Performance in Competitive Gaming* (pp. 171–180). Cham: Springer Nature Switzerland. https://doi.org/DOI: 10.1007/978-3-031-99625-2_10

Berry, E. M., Cardoso, B. R., Cash, S. B., Cifuentes, A., Collado, M. C., le Coutre, J., German, J. B., Ibáñez, E., Lawrence, M., Nieman, D. C., Pravst, I., Raubenheimer, D., Rychlik, M., Scholey, A., Terranegra, A., & Zivkovic, A. M. (2026). Goals in Nutrition Science 2025–2030. *Frontiers in Nutrition, 13*, 1784021. https://pmc.ncbi.nlm.nih.gov/articles/PMC13006240/. DOI: 10.3389/fnut.2026.1784021 PMID: 41878571

Bo, Z. (2026). *Effect of Ketogenic Diet on Athletic Performance of Men's Basketball Players in Petaling Jaya.*, DOI: 10.6007/IJARPED/v15-i1/27578

Buceta, A. J. (2025). Nutritional Strategies in the Injury and Recovery Process in Athletes. In *Evaluating the Effectiveness of Functional Ingredients in Sports Nutrition* (pp. 75–90). IGI Global Scientific Publishing., DOI: 10.4018/979-8-3693-8699-6.ch003

Das, S. K., Miki, A. J., Blanchard, C. M., Sazonov, E., Gilhooly, C. H., Dey, S., Wolk, C. B., Khoo, C. S. H., Hill, J. O., & Shook, R. P. (2022). Perspective: opportunities and challenges of technology tools in dietary and activity assessment: bridging stakeholder viewpoints. *Advances in Nutrition*, *13*(1), 1–15. DOI: 10.1093/advances/nmab103 PMID: 34545392

de Oliveira, D. M., Silva, A. K. A. C., Macedo, A. G., Fernandes, M. B., & Fernandes, E. V. (2025). Global Research Trends in Sports Nutrition and Football over the Last 20 Years (2004–2024). *Sports (Basel, Switzerland)*, *13*(10), 365. DOI: 10.3390/sports13100365 PMID: 41150500

de Oliveira, T. V. P. (2025). Genetics and Sports Nutrition. In Genetics and Sports Performance (pp. 47-60). Cham: Springer Nature Switzerland. https://link.springer.com/chapter/10.1007/978-3-032-11647-5_4

Delany, L. V., Costello, N., Jones, B., & Backhouse, S. H. (2025). Dietary Recommendations for Body Mass and Composition Manipulation in Male and Female Athletes: a Scoping Review of Consensus Statements, Position Stands and Practice Guidelines from International Expert Groups: LV Delany et al. *Sports Medicine*, *55*(10), 2445–2487. https://link.springer.com/article/10.1007/s40279-025-02285-4

Efstathiou, E., Akam, L., & Mastana, S. (2026). Opinions and attitudes on genetic testing for personalised nutrition among professional footballers and sports nutritionists. *Performance Enhancement & Health*, *14*(1), 100385. DOI: 10.1016/j.peh.2025.100385

Fang, W., Fan, S., Zheng, H., Fang, Z., You, Y., Yin, B., Li, B., & Ye, X. (2025). How to improve mental health in the older adults through AI-enhanced physical activity: An emerging research topic. *Humanities & Social Sciences Communications*, *12*(1), 1–15. https://www.nature.com/articles/s41599-025-05155-6. DOI: 10.1057/s41599-025-05155-6

Ghanem, M. R. (2025). The Impact of an AI-Supported Smart HIIT Program on Cardiovascular Fitness and Physical Performance. *Modern Sport*, *24*(3), 370–384. DOI: 10.54702/2708-3454.2083

Grivas, G. V., & Safari, K. (2025). Artificial intelligence in endurance sports: Metabolic, recovery, and nutritional perspectives. *Nutrients*, *17*(20), 3209. https://www.mdpi.com/2072-6643/17/20/3209. DOI: 10.3390/nu17203209 PMID: 41156462

Grosso, F. D., & Turco, D. (2026). Nutrition in sport: An opportunity to balance performance, sustainability and Preventive Medicine. *Research in Sports Medicine, 34*(1), 61–70. https://www.tandfonline.com/doi/abs/10.1080/15438627.2025.2525854. DOI: 10.1080/15438627.2025.2525854 PMID: 40590526

Grosso, F. D., & Turco, D. (2026). Nutrition in sport: An opportunity to balance performance, sustainability and Preventive Medicine. *Research in Sports Medicine, 34*(1), 61–70. DOI: 10.1080/15438627.2025.2525854 PMID: 40590526

Heikura, I. A. (2020). *Dietary periodisation for health and performance in world-class endurance athletes* (Doctoral dissertation, Australian Catholic University). DOI: DOI: 10.26199/e8tq-dh06

Hillen, B., Oestreicher, G., Schwab, L., Enders, K., Simon, P., Elme, A., Ben-Aharon, I., Goshenlago, T., Neuzillet, C., Sclafani, F., Beltran, E. E. M., Schuster, M., Doncheva, H., Ruckes, C., Karlecik, M., Petrowski, K., Rosenbaum, D., Diou, C., Ballas, A., & Moehler, M. (2025). Digital and AI-assisted multimodal supportive care, combining physical activity, nutrition, and pain management during chemotherapy for advanced pancreatic cancer patients: Study protocol of the European multicenter randomized controlled trial of the RELEVIUM project. *BMC Cancer, 25*(1), 1610. DOI: 10.1186/s12885-025-14867-6 PMID: 41109944

Jud, M., & Thalmann, S. (2025). AI in digital sports coaching–a systematic review. *Managing Sport and Leisure, 30*(6), 1577–1593. DOI: 10.1080/23750472.2024.2449016

Kaufman, M., Nguyen, C., Shetty, M., Oppezzo, M., Barrack, M., & Fredericson, M. (2023). Popular dietary trends' impact on athletic performance: A critical analysis review. *Nutrients, 15*(16), 3511. https://www.mdpi.com/2072-6643/15/16/3511. DOI: 10.3390/nu15163511 PMID: 37630702

Liu, X., Xu, M., Wang, H., & Zhu, L. (2025). Integrating precision medicine and digital health in personalized weight management: The central role of nutrition. *Nutrients, 17*(16), 2695. https://www.mdpi.com/2072-6643/17/16/2695. DOI: 10.3390/nu17162695 PMID: 40871725

Lu, Y., Stathopoulou, T., Vasiloglou, M. F., Pinault, L. F., Kiley, C., Spanakis, E. K., & Mougiakakou, S. (2020). goFOODTM: An artificial intelligence system for dietary assessment. *Sensors (Basel), 20*(15), 4283. https://www.mdpi.com/1424-8220/20/15/4283. DOI: 10.3390/s20154283 PMID: 32752007

Mamta. (2025). The Role of Artificial Intelligence in Modern Healthcare: Transforming Diagnosis, Treatment and Rehabilitation. *AI-driven Innovations in Physiotherapy and Oncology 2*, 335–358. https://doi.org/DOI: 10.1002/9781394423552.ch17

Moussa, M. A., El-Safty, S. M., & Mahmoud, Y. A. H. (2026). Enhancing Psychological Well-being Through AI-Assisted Nutrition: A Study on Female University Students. *Port Said Journal of Educational Research, 5*(1), 30–58. https://journals.ekb.eg/article_477829.html

Nasb, M., Zhang, Y., & Chen, N. (2025). The role of artificial intelligence in precision exercise nutrition: A shift from data to diets. *Food Science and Human Wellness*. https://www.sciopen.com/local/article_pdf/10.26599/FSHW.2025.9250623.pdf

Nongbet, A., Chettry, U., Upadhaya, S., & Mohapatra, S. (2026). The future of personalized nutrition: AI, genomics, and precision medicine. In *Nanomedicine and Nutrigenomics* (pp. 269–285). Academic Press., DOI: 10.1016/B978-0-443-26761-1.00005-3

Okon, J. J. (2025). Leveraging Artificial Intelligence in Sports and Business Management for Enhanced Health and Performance Outcomes. *Applied Sciences, Computing, and Energy, 3*(2), 252-266. https://cemrj.com/index.php/volumes/article/view/58

Panayotova, G. G. (2025, October). Artificial Intelligence in Nutrition and Dietetics: A Comprehensive Review of Current Research. In *Healthcare* (Vol. 13, No. 20, p. 2579). MDPI. https://www.mdpi.com/2227-9032/13/20/2579

Pandya, N. N., Limbani, D. P., Ajmera, T., Prajapati, A., Kodwani, M., & Dadhania, A. J. (2026). AI-Driven Personalization of Sports Nutrition Supplements for Performance Optimization. *Advances in Consumer Research. Association for Consumer Research (U. S.), 3*(2).

Papadopoulou, S. K. (2020). Rehabilitation nutrition for injury recovery of athletes: The role of macronutrient intake. *Nutrients, 12*(8), 2449. DOI: 10.3390/nu12082449 PMID: 32824034

Raleigh, C. (2025). *An exploration of low carbohydrate dietary intake in endurance athletes: prevalence, knowledge and the potential effect on bone health and remodelling* (Doctoral dissertation). https://hdl.handle.net/10344/14017

Rao, S., & Rao, F. (2026). Transforming Health Education: AI-Driven Games and Simulations for Mental Health, Nutrition, and Physical Well-Being. In *AI-Powered Educational Games and Simulations* (pp. 273–306). IGI Global Scientific Publishing. DOI: DOI: 10.4018/979-8-3373-0035-1.ch008

Shlykov, S. N., Sycheva, O. V., Omarov, R. S., Trubina, I. A., & Skorbina, E. A. (2025). Sports Nutrition and Recovery: Key Nutrients and Supplements for Effective Regeneration. *Human Physiology, 51*(2), 201–216. DOI: 10.1134/S036211972570032X

Tertipi, N., Sfyri, E., Grech, V. S., Kefala, V., & Rallis, E. (2025). Optimizing Skin Quality via AI-Enhanced Physical Activity. *Cosmetics*, *12*(3), 104. DOI: 10.3390/cosmetics12030104

Wang, L., Koh, D., Li, F., Yaakop, N., & Wang, Y. (2026). The Construction of Personalized Sports Health Management System under Generative AI System. *Journal of Mechanics in Medicine and Biology*, *2640043*, 2640043. https://www.worldscientific.com/doi/abs/10.1142/S0219519426400439. DOI: 10.1142/S0219519426400439

KEY TERMS AND DEFINITIONS

AI & Nutrition Balance: AI improves nutrition balance by using machine learning to analyze data from genetics, microbiomes, and wearables, enabling highly personalized dietary plans and, in some cases, real-time calorie tracking. These AI-powered tools enhance accuracy in, for example, image-based food recognition and, in some cases, provide faster, more efficient dietary tracking. Key challenges include ensuring data quality, reducing algorithmic bias against certain demographics, protecting user privacy, and vetting AI-generated advice by professionals.

AI-Supported Fitness Training: AI-enhanced fitness training is rapidly transforming the industry by leveraging artificial intelligence, computer vision, and machine learning to deliver highly personalized, data-driven, and adaptable workout experiences, often serving as round-the-clock virtual trainers. This technology enables users to achieve expedited outcomes by evaluating performance data to enhance routines, rectify form in real time, and customize nutrition plans.

AI & Healthcare Well-Being: The incorporation of Artificial Intelligence (AI) into healthcare and wellness is revolutionizing the sector from a reactive, treatment-oriented paradigm to a proactive, individualized, and preventive framework. AI functions as a "co-pilot" for healthcare practitioners, improving diagnostic precision, optimizing administrative processes to alleviate burnout, and providing ongoing, individualized health surveillance.

AI & Physical Activities: Artificial intelligence enhances physical activity by providing individualized, data-driven insights and employing wearables and applications to monitor, analyze, and optimize exercise regimens. The principal uses motion tracking to support form correction, customized training regimens, injury avoidance, and enhanced participation through gamification. Artificial intelligence is utilized for both general fitness monitoring and the study of professional athletic performance.

AI & Athletes' Performance: Artificial intelligence enhances athletic performance by analyzing extensive, real-time data from wearables and video to refine training, prevent injuries, and improve tactical judgment. Through machine learning and computer vision, coaches can assess players' fatigue, refine approaches, and tailor workouts, moving beyond conventional methods toward data-driven insights.

AI & Athletes' Recovery: Artificial Intelligence (AI) is transforming athlete rehabilitation from a general, reactive approach to a tailored, proactive, and data-driven discipline. By analyzing extensive datasets from wearable devices, cameras, and, in certain instances, biological samples such as blood or saliva, AI systems can continuously monitor an athlete's physiological condition, facilitating customized rest, nutrition, and rehabilitation strategies that enhance recovery, avert overtraining, and reduce injury risk.

Chapter 2
Health Applications and E-Commerce Strategies for Promoting Nutritional Balance and Athletic Performance:
A Social Return on Investment Perspective in Thailand

Narisa Kamkaen
Pathumthani University, Thailand

Tanatorn Tanantong
http://orcid.org/0000-0002-8927-2365
Thammasat University, Thailand

Prapasri Siri
Chulabhorn Graduate Institute, Thailand

Tanpat Kraiwanit
http://orcid.org/0000-0002-5130-6427
Pathumthani University, Thailand

ABSTRACT

This chapter explores how health applications integrated with electronic commerce (e-commerce) strategies support nutritional balance and athletic performance in Thailand and examines their perceived social return on investment (SROI). Using

DOI: 10.4018/979-8-3373-9544-9.ch002

a qualitative approach, in-depth interviews were conducted with key stakeholders, including healthcare professionals, digital health developers, administrators, and end-users. The findings indicate that such applications enhance nutritional awareness, facilitate behavioural change, and translate dietary guidance into practical action through convenient access to health-related products and services, thereby supporting improved athletic performance. Beyond individual health benefits, stakeholders perceive broader social value in terms of improved quality of life, reduced caregiver burden, and potential long-term efficiency gains for the healthcare system.

1. INTRODUCTION

In the digital economy, the modern healthcare landscape is being reshaped by the "Fourth Industrial Revolution," a period defined by the fusion of biological sciences and digital innovation that is fundamentally altering patient care. In Thailand, this transition has progressed at a striking pace over the last decade. What began as a series of isolated attempts to digitize medical records for office efficiency has matured into a robust national mandate known as "Health 4.0" (Big Data Institute, 2021; Coelho et al., 2025; Marinescu et al., 2025). This shift is not merely a technological trend; it is a desperate systemic response to Thailand's unique demographic pressures. The nation is sprinting toward a "super-aged" society, one of the fastest transitions in the developing world, rendering the traditional, hospital-centric model of medical care increasingly fragile and unsustainable (Aekplakorn et al., 2011). The shadow of Non-Communicable Diseases (NCDs), including diabetes, hypertension, and obesity, now looms over 74% of all deaths in the country (UNDP & WHO, 2021). These conditions demand lifelong management rather than the "fix-it" approach of acute care, placing a crushing fiscal and operational weight on the Universal Coverage Scheme (UC) and the overstretched medical personnel who keep the system running (Tangcharoensathien et al., 2024).

The COVID-19 pandemic served as a definitive, albeit painful, catalyst for this digital evolution. It functioned as a nationwide "proof of concept" for mobile health (mHealth), with the *Mor Prom* platform leading the charge. This period fundamentally changed how the Thai public interacts with technology in relation to their own bodies (Chalardnarin et al., 2021). For the first time, millions of citizens, regardless of their economic background, began using smartphones as their primary interface for accessing medical data, tracking vaccines, and participating in remote consultations (Big Data Institute, 2021). This created a vital digital bedrock, proving that even "digitally hesitant" populations could adapt when the necessity was clear. As the crisis transitioned into an endemic phase, the focus of digital health has shifted from survival to the long-term promotion of wellness and disease prevention (Aekplakorn et al., 2011; Nguyen et al., 2019).

A central pillar of this preventive strategy is the pursuit of nutritional balance. While almost everyone agrees that nutrition is the cornerstone of metabolic health, there remains a stubborn "implementation gap" between a doctor's advice and a patient's actual dinner plate. In a typical clinical setting, a patient might leave with a list of dietary recommendations, only to find that follow-through is sabotaged by a lack of convenience, high costs, or limited access to healthy options. This is where the marriage of e-commerce and health applications becomes a game-changer. By moving beyond passive tracking, such as simple calorie counting, and toward an integrated "Online-to-Offline" (O2O) model, apps can finally trigger real-world action. Through embedded e-commerce strategies, a user can instantly book a tele-nutritionist appointment, order specialized supplements, or order healthy meal kits without ever leaving the app interface (Liu et al., 2025; Perez-Uribe et al., 2025; Rakshit, 2025). This synergy effectively turns a digital "nudge" into a tangible, healthy behavior.

However, the reality on the ground is complex. While policymakers at the Ministry of Public Health view digital tools as the only way to safeguard the national health budget, they also admit that the current ecosystem is dangerously fragmented. With various health applications currently on the market, the system has become a "spaghetti bowl" of competing platforms that often fail to communicate with one another, creating data silos that obscure the patient's holistic health journey. For hospital managers and frontline nurses, apps are seen as a vital "fiscal pressure valve" to reduce overcrowding and paperwork (Siri, 2025). Yet, there is deep concern regarding the "Digital Divide." If an application is too complex, it risks alienating the very people who need it most: the elderly and rural populations who may have low digital literacy but face the highest nutritional risks (Yuduang et al., 2022; van Dijk, 2006).

This shifting environment requires a new way to measure what "success" actually looks like in healthcare and digital health initiatives. Traditional financial metrics, such as Return on Investment (ROI), are too narrow; they account for the "baht saved" on medications or service delivery but fail to capture the broader human and societal dimensions of value creation. This study, therefore, employs the Social Return on Investment (SROI) framework as a more holistic evaluative approach. SROI is a principles-based method that quantifies value relative to the resources invested while explicitly incorporating "extra-financial" benefits (Nicholls et al., 2009; Siri, 2025). It enables the systematic measurement of social value, including invisible yet essential outcomes such as patient empowerment, improved quality of life, reduced burdens on family caregivers, enhanced preventive behaviors, and the narrowing of health disparities between Bangkok and provincial areas (Rauscher et al., 2012; Arunruangsirilert & Intanant, 2021; Siri, 2025).

By applying an SROI lens, an e-commerce-driven nutrition strategy can be understood as doing more than merely balancing a budget or improving short-term efficiency; it actively contributes to the development of a more resilient, inclusive, and socially responsive healthcare ecosystem. At present, a clear and significant gap exists in the academic literature concerning the Thai context. While prior studies have examined the technical functionality of health applications or documented the rapid expansion of e-commerce platforms in Southeast Asia, very few have systematically investigated how these two forces converge to address nutritional challenges through a social value– and impact-oriented perspective. In particular, limited attention has been given to how such integrations generate measurable social outcomes beyond conventional financial performance indicators. This research seeks to fill that critical gap by advancing an integrated analytical perspective grounded in SROI.

Accordingly, this chapter aims to explore how health applications integrated with e-commerce strategies support nutritional balance and athletic performance in Thailand and to examine the perceived social return on investment generated by their implementation. Drawing on in-depth qualitative interviews with key stakeholders, including digital health providers, healthcare professionals, and relevant ecosystem actors, the study focuses on understanding how these digital health initiatives influence health outcomes, encourage sustained behavioral change, and create broader social value across different population groups. The central research question guiding this chapter is therefore: How do health applications integrated with e-commerce strategies support nutrition balance and athletic performance in Thailand, and what social return on investment do stakeholders perceive from their use? By incorporating insights from multiple stakeholder perspectives, this chapter explores an emerging digital health paradigm for Thailand—one that is not only commercially viable and clinically effective, but also socially transformative, equitable, and sustainable in the long term. This chapter contributes to a deeper understanding of how digitally enabled nutrition strategies can generate sustained social value and inform more inclusive and impact-oriented health policy and practice in Thailand.

2. LITERATURE REVIEW

2.1 Health Applications in Nutrition Management

Telemedicine, also referred to as telehealth, involves the delivery of healthcare services and the exchange of medical information across physical distances through digital technologies. Although often viewed as innovative, telemedicine is not a novel medical practice. Telemedicine encounters can be categorized along two key dimensions: the mode of interaction between patients and healthcare professionals (synchronous or asynchronous) and the form of data communicated (text, audio, or video). While telemedicine has been most extensively implemented in developed countries, interest in its adoption is increasing in developing regions as populations become more familiar with and reliant on digital technologies in everyday life (Limna et al., 2022; Siripipatthanakul et al., 2023). In addition, the rapid growth of mobile health (mHealth) applications has reshaped how nutrition is understood, monitored, and managed. In the past, dietary management largely depended on occasional face-to-face consultations with healthcare professionals and self-recorded food diaries. These traditional approaches often suffered from inconsistent follow-up, recall bias, and limited patient engagement. In contrast, contemporary health applications enable a more continuous and interactive approach to nutrition management. Rather than functioning solely as digital record-keeping tools, many of these platforms now operate as behavior-oriented systems that offer real-time feedback, personalized recommendations, and ongoing metabolic monitoring (Nguyen et al., 2019; Limna, 2023; Sitthipon et al., 2022).

In Thailand, the importance of nutrition-focused health applications is particularly evident due to the country's growing burden of Non-Communicable Diseases (NCDs). Data from the UNDP and WHO (2021) indicate that NCDs such as diabetes, hypertension, and cardiovascular diseases are responsible for approximately 74% of all deaths nationwide. Poor dietary habits are widely recognized as a major contributing factor to these conditions. As a result, digital solutions that support personalized nutrition have gained increasing attention. By analyzing individual-level data, including age, physical activity, and health indicators such as blood glucose levels, these applications can deliver tailored dietary guidance designed to support sustainable behavioral change (Aekplakorn et al., 2011).

A notable development in this field is the shift from passive self-monitoring toward more active forms of intervention, particularly through the integration of e-commerce functionalities. Existing research highlights the persistent "implementation gap" in nutrition management, where individuals may understand what constitutes healthy eating but struggle to translate that knowledge into daily practice. To address this challenge, many health applications now incorporate e-commerce features that allow users to purchase recommended products directly, such as dietary supplements, healthy meal kits, or organic food items. By linking nutritional advice with immediate access to appropriate resources, these platforms reduce practical barriers and support healthier decision-making in everyday contexts.

The effectiveness of health applications in nutrition management is also closely associated with health literacy levels. Evidence from studies involving Thai healthcare stakeholders suggests that technological availability alone is insufficient to generate meaningful health outcomes. The social value of these applications emerges only when users can understand and apply nutritional information in their daily routines. From a SROI perspective, the benefits of nutrition-focused health applications extend beyond individual outcomes such as weight control. They also include broader societal gains, such as fewer hospital admissions related to NCD complications and reduced long-term healthcare expenditure for both individuals and the public health system (Chopvitayakun et al., 2025; Tangcharoensathien et al., 2024).

Overall, health applications in nutrition management function as a critical link between clinical dietary recommendations and everyday food practices within the home. By combining artificial intelligence for personalized dietary assessment with e-commerce platforms to improve access to healthy resources, these applications empower individuals in Thailand to take a more active role in managing their nutritional health. In doing so, they contribute to reducing the preventable disease burden and help ease pressure on the national healthcare infrastructure.

2.2 E-Commerce Strategies Embedded in Health Applications

In the contemporary digital landscape, e-commerce, defined as conducting commercial transactions through online platforms, has become a key engine of economic growth, particularly in emerging economies and digitally transforming societies. By enabling firms to transact beyond physical boundaries, e-commerce enhances operational efficiency, lowers transaction costs, and improves consumer accessibility, convenience, and market reach. In advanced economies, it has fundamentally reshaped industries such as retail, manufacturing, services, and healthcare through the integration of digital marketing, data-driven decision-making, and increasingly sophisticated supply chain systems. In developing contexts, e-commerce plays a critical role in supporting small and medium-sized enterprises by mitigating infrastructural limitations, facilitating entry into broader domestic and international markets, and generating employment opportunities in areas such as logistics, information technology, and digital services. The expansion of mobile commerce, social commerce, and electronic payment systems has further contributed to greater financial inclusion and consumer participation, particularly among previously underserved populations. Moreover, e-commerce has demonstrated its capacity to enhance economic resilience during periods of disruption, including the COVID-19 pandemic, by enabling business continuity, sustaining entrepreneurial activity, and supporting pathways toward inclusive and sustainable development (Amornkitvikai et al., 2022; Asanprakit & Limna, 2023; Hongsuchon et al., 2025; Limna et al., 2025; Liu et al., 2025; Perez-Uribe et al., 2025).

E-commerce strategies have become increasingly embedded in health applications as digital health platforms evolve from information-delivery tools into integrated commercial ecosystems. Contemporary health applications frequently incorporate transactional functionalities such as in-app purchases, subscription-based services, digital marketplaces for medical products, and integrated payment systems. These strategies enable health app developers to diversify revenue streams while enhancing service scalability and financial sustainability. By reducing intermediaries and enabling direct-to-consumer models, embedded e-commerce mechanisms allow healthcare providers and app developers to offer personalized health services and products more efficiently, thereby reshaping traditional healthcare delivery structures (Aggarwal & Travers, 2001; Yeung et al., 2023; Zacharia et al., 2024).

A central strand of the literature highlights personalization and data-driven marketing as core e-commerce strategies within health applications. Health apps leverage user-generated health data, behavioral analytics, and AI to recommend tailored products, premium features, or value-added services such as teleconsultations, wearable integrations, and personalized wellness plans. Such strategies enhance user engagement and perceived value, which in turn increase conversion rates and customer lifetime value. However, the literature also notes growing concerns regarding data privacy, algorithmic transparency, and ethical commercialization, particularly when sensitive health data are used to support commercial decision-making.

The integration of digital marketplaces within health applications has also received increasing scholarly attention (Hermes et al., 2020; Park et al., 2021; Wang et al., 2021). Health apps now function as platforms connecting users with third-party vendors offering pharmaceuticals, medical devices, nutritional supplements, and wellness products. Platform-based e-commerce strategies enable ecosystem expansion and network effects, positioning health applications as intermediaries rather than standalone service providers. The literature suggests that trust, regulatory compliance, and quality assurance mechanisms are pivotal in determining the success of such marketplaces, as users are particularly sensitive to risk in health-related transactions.

Ultimately, existing studies converge on the view that e-commerce strategies embedded in health applications play a crucial role in shaping digital health business models and user experiences. While these strategies contribute to financial sustainability, service innovation, and platform growth, the literature consistently underscores the need for careful governance to balance commercial objectives with ethical responsibility, user trust, and public health outcomes. This tension highlights a critical research gap concerning how e-commerce-driven health applications can achieve both economic viability and socially responsible healthcare delivery.

2.3 Nutrition Balance and Behavioral Change

The connection between nutritional balance and behavioral change is crucial to addressing the growing burden of non-communicable diseases (NCDs) in Thailand. Reports from the UNDP and WHO (2021) indicate that NCDs, most notably diabetes, hypertension, and cardiovascular diseases, account for approximately 74% of all deaths nationwide. Beyond their health impact, these conditions impose a substantial economic burden on the country, with estimated costs of 1.6 trillion THB annually, or nearly 10% of Thailand's GDP. Despite widespread access to health information and dietary guidelines, improved knowledge alone has proven insufficient to produce lasting changes in eating behavior.

As highlighted by Kotler (2017), consumer behavior is shaped by a combination of cultural norms, social relationships, and psychological influences. Food choices are deeply embedded in everyday life, family traditions, and social interactions. Nutritional balance is therefore not simply an individual decision, but a reflection of broader lifestyle patterns and social expectations. These factors help explain why conventional health education campaigns often struggle to achieve long-term behavioral change, even when awareness of healthy eating is relatively high.

Digital health applications attempt to address this challenge by incorporating principles from behavioral economics, particularly nudging and continuous feedback mechanisms. By monitoring physiological indicators such as blood glucose levels and heart rate, these applications provide users with immediate, tangible feedback on how their dietary choices affect their health (Okolo et al., 2024). This approach supports the *Theory of Reasoned Action*, which suggests that individuals are more likely to adopt a behavior when they perceive clear benefits. For many users, especially older adults, visualizing health data helps make the long-term consequences of poor nutrition more concrete and personally relevant.

Through these mechanisms, digital interventions help transform nutritional guidance from abstract medical advice into practical, everyday actions. By linking dietary behavior to real-time health outcomes, health applications strengthen the connection between health literacy and sustained adherence. In doing so, they play an increasingly important role in supporting balanced nutrition and encouraging healthier lifestyles.

2.4 Social Return on Investment in Digital Health

Conventional economic evaluations of healthcare interventions have typically relied on a narrow interpretation of Return on Investment (ROI), focusing primarily on direct financial outcomes such as reductions in medical expenditure. While these metrics are useful, they often overlook the broader social benefits generated by health interventions. As argued by Nicholls et al. (2009), many of the most meaningful outcomes in healthcare, such as improved quality of life, greater equity, and long-term social well-being, are not easily captured through standard financial accounting. The Social Return on Investment (SROI) framework was developed to address this limitation by offering a more holistic approach to measuring value.

Within Thailand's public health system, where financial and human resources are constrained, SROI provides a particularly relevant lens for evaluating digital health initiatives. Rather than asking only how much money is saved, SROI examines how each unit of investment translates into social value. For example, a single investment in a digital health application may generate benefits such as reduced patient anxiety, time savings for family caregivers, and the prevention of avoidable complications or long-term disability. By expressing these outcomes in comparable value terms, SROI helps decision-makers better understand the full impact of digital health beyond immediate budget considerations.

Recent studies have further expanded the application of SROI by incorporating environmental sustainability, often referred to as the "Green Health" dimension. Digital health solutions, especially telemedicine and remote monitoring, can substantially reduce the environmental footprint of healthcare delivery. Research by Serra et al. (2022) demonstrates that digital consultations can reduce carbon emissions by significantly reducing patient travel. In the Thai context, where access to healthcare often requires long-distance travel for rural populations, these environmental benefits also translate into social gains, including reduced travel time, lower transportation costs, and improved access to care.

When applied to digital health applications in Thailand, the SROI framework captures multiple layers of value: direct savings in medical costs, indirect benefits such as reduced travel and waiting times, and wider social impacts including decreased hospital congestion and improved system efficiency. Viewed through this lens, digital health should not be understood merely as a technological upgrade. Instead, it represents a strategic and sustainable investment in Thailand's human, social, and environmental capital, one that aligns healthcare innovation with long-term societal well-being.

2.5 Integrating Health Applications, E-Commerce, and SROI

The integration of health applications, e-commerce strategies, and the SROI framework represents a paradigm shift from fragmented digital interventions toward a cohesive "Techno-Social Ecosystem." In this conceptual model, each component plays a specialized yet interdependent role: health applications serve as the digital interface for data collection and user engagement; e-commerce acts as the functional engine that facilitates the procurement of health-related goods and services; and

SROI provides the evaluative lens through which the total value, both economic and social, is articulated. This triad is particularly critical in the Thai context, where the transition to "Health 4.0" necessitates a shift from hospital-centric care to community-based, self-managed wellness.

One of the most persistent challenges in nutritional management is the "implementation gap": the psychological and logistical distance between receiving medical advice and engaging in healthy behavior. In traditional Thai healthcare settings, a patient may receive dietary guidelines for managing NCDs, but the follow-through is often hindered by the "path of least resistance," which usually leads to convenient but unhealthy food options. By embedding e-commerce strategies within health applications, the platform moves beyond the role of a passive monitor. It becomes a facilitator of action. For instance, an AI-driven app that detects a user's high blood sugar can immediately "nudge" the user toward an e-commerce marketplace to purchase specialized nutritional supplements, low-glycemic meal kits, or a tele-consultation with a certified nutritionist. This "Online-to-Offline" (O2O) integration effectively lowers transaction costs for consumers, making nutritional balance as convenient as any other digital commercial transaction. This synergy transforms the app from a mere "information silo" into a lifestyle-integrated tool that supports practical, everyday adherence to nutritional goals (Amornkitvikai et al., 2022; Liu et al., 2025).

While the benefits of health apps are intuitive, their financial justification is often difficult to justify using traditional Return on Investment (ROI) metrics, which focus exclusively on direct cash flows or immediate cost savings. SROI, however, is a principles-based methodology that allows for the quantification of "extra-financial" value. In the context of Thai public health, where the Universal Coverage Scheme (UC) is under immense fiscal pressure, SROI is a vital tool for policymakers. The integration of SROI into digital health initiatives enables the valuation of intangible outcomes with long-term economic consequences. For example, a nutrition-focused application supported by e-commerce can be evaluated not just by the revenue it generates, but by the social value it creates: reduced patient anxiety, improved quality of life for family caregivers, and the prevention of NCD complications that would otherwise require expensive tertiary hospital care. Furthermore, as demonstrated by Serra et al. (2022), the SROI framework can incorporate the "Green Health" dimension, calculating the reduction in carbon emissions (Carbon Credits) achieved by replacing physical hospital visits with digital tele-nutrition consultations. By assigning a monetary value to these social and environmental benefits, SROI provides a compelling narrative for the sustained government and private sector investment required to maintain digital health infrastructure (Nicholls et al., 2009; Arunruangsirilert & Intanant, 2021).

A critical theme identified in stakeholder interviews with Thai healthcare executives is the role of digital integration in reducing health inequality. In Thailand, geographical disparities in healthcare access remain a significant concern, with rural populations often facing high travel costs and long wait times at provincial hospitals. The integration of health apps and e-commerce addresses this "last mile" problem by bringing specialized nutritional advice and health products directly to the user's doorstep. However, this integration is only socially valuable if it accounts for the "Digital Divide." To achieve a high social return, these integrated systems must be designed with high "Perceived Ease of Use" (TAM) to accommodate the elderly population, the group with the highest nutritional risk, and the lowest digital literacy. When applications are inclusive and culturally aligned, the SROI increases because the technology reaches the most vulnerable segments of society, thereby narrowing the health gap between urban and rural strata (Yuduang et al., 2022; Limna et al., 2025).

The sustainability of this integrated model is fundamentally dependent on trust, particularly concerning the handling of "Sensitive Personal Data" as defined by the Personal Data Protection Act (PDPA) B.E. 2562. Because nutrition management involves collecting metabolic data (glucose levels, BMI, heart rate) and e-commerce involves financial transactions, the ecosystem must operate within a high-security framework. Trust acts as the social currency that allows this triad to function. If users do not feel their data is secure, the "Word of Mouth" regarding the app will turn negative, leading to low adoption and a poor SROI. Therefore, rigorous compliance with PDPA is not merely a legal requirement but a strategic component of the e-commerce strategy. Ethical commercialization, ensuring that nutritional recommendations are based on clinical evidence rather than purely profit-driven algorithms, is essential to maintaining the "Social Value" that SROI seeks to measure (Office of the Personal Data Protection Commission, 2021; Tungtrakul et al., 2024).

At the macro level, the convergence of health apps, e-commerce, and SROI aligns Thailand with the United Nations' Sustainable Development Goals (SDGs), particularly Goal 3 (Good Health and Well-being) and Goal 10 (Reduced Inequalities). By shifting the NCD management burden from the state to an empowered, digitally enabled citizenry, Thailand can improve labor productivity and reduce the fiscal drain on GDP. The estimated economic loss of 1.6 trillion THB per year due to NCDs in Thailand provides a stark baseline for this study. If integrated digital interventions can reduce this burden by even a small percentage, the social and economic returns would be astronomical. In summary, integrating these three domains creates a resilient public health infrastructure. It empowers individuals to manage their nutritional balance autonomously, facilitates the commercial ease of doing so, and provides a rigorous evaluative framework to ensure that every baht invested in digital health delivers maximum returns to Thailand's digital economy (UNDP & WHO, 2021; Tangcharoensathien et al., 2024).

2.6 Nutrition Balance and Recovery for Athletic Performance

Nutritional balance plays a critical role in supporting recovery and optimizing athletic performance by ensuring athletes receive adequate energy and essential nutrients to meet the physiological demands of training and competition. A balanced intake of macronutrients—carbohydrates, proteins, and fats—supports glycogen replenishment, muscle protein synthesis, and hormonal regulation, while micronutrients such as vitamins and minerals contribute to immune function, oxidative stress reduction, and metabolic efficiency. Proper hydration further facilitates thermoregulation and nutrient transport, reducing fatigue and injury risk (Amawi et al., 2024; Ghazzawi et al., 2023; Heaton et al., 2017; Purcell, 2013).

Effective recovery nutrition has been shown to accelerate muscle repair, decrease inflammation, and restore neuromuscular function, thereby enhancing subsequent performance and training adaptation. Recent literature also emphasizes the timing and individualization of nutritional strategies, highlighting that nutrition plans tailored to sport type, training intensity, and individual metabolic needs can significantly improve recovery outcomes. Collectively, these findings underscore the importance of nutrition balance as a foundational component of recovery strategies that sustain athletic performance and long-term athlete health (Beck et al., 2015; Giraldo-Vallejo et al., 2023; Hwang & Yang, 2024; Martín-Rodríguez et al., 2024; Naderi et al., 2025).

3. METHODOLOGY

In qualitative research, the focus is on understanding meanings, experiences, and processes rather than measuring variables numerically. It seeks to explore how and why social phenomena occur by capturing participants' perspectives within their real-life contexts. Common qualitative approaches include in-depth interviews, focus group discussions, observations, and document analysis, which allow researchers to generate rich, nuanced data. Rather than aiming for statistical generalization, qualitative research emphasizes depth, contextual understanding, and analytical generalization through themes and patterns. Rigor is established through strategies such as credibility, dependability, reflexivity, and transparency in data collection and analysis. As such, qualitative research is particularly well suited to examining complex issues—such as stakeholder perceptions, behavioral change, and social value creation—where meanings and interactions are central to the research objectives.

This study employed a qualitative research methodology to examine how health applications integrated with e-commerce strategies support nutritional balance in Thailand and to explore stakeholders' perceptions of the SROI generated by these digital interventions. A qualitative approach was deemed appropriate because the study seeks to understand complex social processes, behavioral change, and perceived value creation that extend beyond measurable financial outcomes.

The study's data were collected between December 2025 and January 2026 through semi-structured, in-depth interviews, which enabled the researchers to obtain rich and nuanced insights while maintaining consistency across participants. The interview approach allowed respondents to articulate their experiences, perceptions, and judgments regarding the effectiveness of health applications, embedded e-commerce features, and their broader social implications. The interview guide and question development were developed based on the research objectives and relevant literature on digital health, nutrition management, behavioral change, and SROI. Key areas of inquiry included experiences with nutrition-focused health applications, the role of e-commerce functionalities in facilitating healthy dietary behavior, perceived health and social outcomes, barriers and facilitators to adoption, and views on social value creation, such as cost savings, quality-of-life improvements, and reduced burden on the healthcare system. The questions used in the interviews are listed in Table 1.

Table 1. Interview Questions

No.	Interview Question(s)
Q1	How do these health applications help users understand and maintain nutritional balance in their daily lives?
Q2	In your view, which features of nutrition-focused health applications are most effective in influencing dietary behavior?
Q3	How does real-time feedback or personalized dietary guidance provided by these applications affect users' food choices?
Q4	To what extent do health applications support physical recovery, energy management, or readiness for daily activities or exercise?
Q5	How do embedded e-commerce features (such as in-app purchasing or service booking) influence users' ability to follow nutritional recommendations?
Q6	Can you provide examples of how access to food products, supplements, or nutrition services through applications supports recovery or sustained physical performance?
Q7	What role does convenience play in encouraging users to adhere to nutrition and recovery-related guidance provided by health applications?
Q8	From your perspective, how do health applications help bridge the gap between nutritional knowledge and actual behavior?
Q9	What health or quality-of-life outcomes have you observed among users who consistently use nutrition-focused health applications?

continued on following page

Table 1. Continued

No.	Interview Question(s)
Q10	How do these applications affect users' confidence, self-management, or sense of control over their nutritional health?
Q11	In what ways do health applications contribute to reducing dependence on in-person healthcare services, such as hospital visits or consultations?
Q12	How do you perceive the social value generated by nutrition-focused health applications beyond direct health outcomes?
Q13	From a Social Return on Investment perspective, what types of benefits do these applications create for families, caregivers, or communities?
Q14	How do nutrition-focused health applications influence long-term healthcare costs or system efficiency in Thailand?
Q15	What challenges or barriers limit the effective use of health applications for maintaining nutritional balance or supporting recovery?
Q16	How does digital literacy affect users' ability to benefit from nutrition, athletic performance support, and recovery-related features of these applications?
Q17	What concerns, if any, do users have regarding data privacy or the commercial use of health information within e-commerce-enabled applications?
Q18	How can health applications be improved to better support nutritional balance, recovery, and physical performance across different population groups?
Q19	In your opinion, how can digital health applications be designed to maximize both financial sustainability and social return on investment in Thailand?

Within the survey design, not all questions were administered to every participant. Specific items were intentionally omitted to ensure their relevance to the characteristics and context of particular respondents.

Purposive sampling involves the deliberate selection of participants based on the researchers' judgment and subject-matter knowledge. This technique is widely used in qualitative research, as it enables the identification of information-rich cases. The primary objective of purposive sampling is to obtain an in-depth understanding of a specific phenomenon or population under investigation (Campbell et al., 2020; Kumar et al., 2023; Phuangsuwan et al., 2024; Siripipatthanakul et al., 2025; Jangjarat et al., 2026; Limna & Siripipattanakul, 2026). Thus, the study's participants were selected using purposive sampling to ensure the inclusion of information-rich cases directly relevant to the research objectives. The study involved key stakeholder groups, including healthcare professionals (such as physicians, pharmacists, and nutritionists), digital health application developers or managers, healthcare administrators or policy stakeholders, and end users managing nutrition-related conditions such as diabetes, hypertension, or obesity. A total of 12 participants were included in the study. The sample size was determined based on the principle of thematic saturation rather than statistical representativeness. All participants had direct experience with health applications that incorporate nutrition management and/

or e-commerce components. Interviews were conducted either face-to-face or via online communication platforms, depending on participant availability and location. Each interview lasted approximately 45–60 minutes, and data collection continued until thematic saturation was achieved, at which point no new substantive insights emerged. Ethical considerations were rigorously observed throughout the research process. Participation was voluntary, and informed consent was obtained from all participants prior to data collection. Participants were assured of confidentiality and anonymity, and all identifiable information was removed from transcripts and reporting.

All interviews were conducted in Thai and audio-recorded with participant consent. The recordings were transcribed verbatim to ensure data accuracy and analytical rigor. The qualitative data were analyzed using thematic analysis, following a systematic and iterative process. First, transcripts were repeatedly reviewed to achieve familiarity with the data. Initial coding was then undertaken to identify meaningful segments related to nutrition management, e-commerce integration, behavioral change, and perceived social outcomes. These codes were subsequently organized into broader themes and sub-themes that reflected recurring patterns across stakeholder groups. Throughout the analysis, particular attention was given to outcomes relevant to the SROI framework, including patient empowerment, improved health literacy, enhanced self-management, reduced caregiver burden, improved access to nutrition-related services, and perceived reductions in long-term healthcare costs. To ensure methodological rigor and trustworthiness, several strategies were employed. Credibility was enhanced through the inclusion of multiple stakeholder perspectives and iterative engagement with the data. Dependability was supported by maintaining a clear audit trail of interview procedures and analytical decisions. Confirmability was addressed through reflexive analysis and careful grounding of interpretations in participant narratives, while transferability was facilitated by providing contextual detail regarding Thailand's digital health and nutrition landscape.

4. RESULTS

The study comprised 12 respondents representing key stakeholder groups within Thailand's digital health and nutrition ecosystem. Participants were purposefully selected to capture diverse perspectives relevant to nutrition-focused health applications integrated with e-commerce strategies. The sample included healthcare professionals (e.g., physicians, pharmacists, and nutritionists), digital health application developers or managers, healthcare administrators or policy-related stakeholders, and end-users managing nutrition-related conditions such as diabetes, hypertension, or obesity. Respondents ranged in age from approximately 27 to 51 years, reflecting variation in professional experience, digital health exposure, and life-stage–related health needs. Healthcare professionals, developers, and administrators generally had several years of experience in their respective fields, while end-users were adult individuals actively managing nutrition-related health conditions through digital applications. All respondents had direct experience with health applications that support nutrition management and/or incorporate e-commerce functionalities. The inclusion of multiple stakeholder groups enabled the triangulation of perspectives across clinical, technological, administrative, and user domains, thereby enhancing the credibility and depth of the qualitative analysis.

The qualitative analysis revealed a set of interrelated themes that explain how health applications integrated with e-commerce strategies support nutritional balance and athletic performance support in Thailand and generate perceived SROI. The findings are organized into five main themes: (1) enhanced nutritional awareness and self-management, (2) translation of dietary advice into actionable behavior through e-commerce integration, (3) perceived health and quality-of-life outcomes, (4) system-level and economic value creation, (5) barriers affecting social value realization, and (6) nutrition balance and athletic performance support. Figure 1 presents the word cloud of key themes emerging from the qualitative results.

Figure 1. Word Cloud of Key Themes Emerging from the Qualitative Results

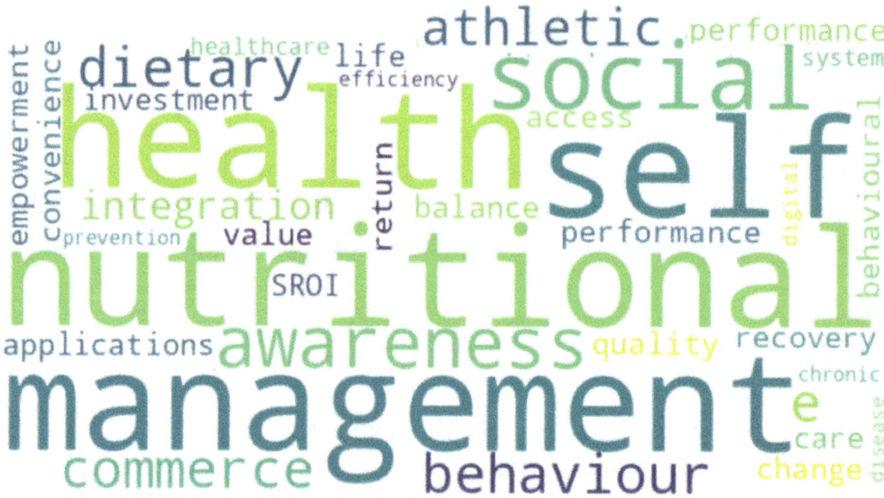

The word cloud in Figure 1 visualizes the relative prominence of key concepts identified in the qualitative analysis of stakeholder interviews. Terms such as nutrition, health, management, athletic performance, and awareness appear most frequently, highlighting the central role of nutrition balance and self-management in participants' accounts. The prominence of words related to e-commerce, integration, access, and convenience reflects the perceived importance of embedded commercial functionalities in translating nutritional advice into actionable behavior. Concepts such as behavior, change, recovery, and performance illustrate how digital health applications support sustained dietary practices, physical recovery, and functional readiness for daily activities and exercise. In addition, the visibility of terms such as social, value, quality of life, and SROI underscores stakeholders' recognition of broader social returns that extend beyond individual health outcomes to include system-level efficiency and long-term societal benefits. Overall, the word cloud reinforces the thematic findings by visually summarizing how nutrition-focused digital health applications generate interconnected health, behavioral, and social value within the Thai context.

4.1 Enhanced Nutritional Awareness and Self-Management

Across stakeholder groups, participants consistently reported that health applications significantly improved users' awareness of nutritional balance and health-related behaviors. Healthcare professionals emphasized that digital tracking features—such as calorie monitoring, blood glucose logging, and personalized dietary feedback—enabled users to better understand the relationship between food consumption and health outcomes. End-users described these features as making nutrition more concrete and manageable, thereby increasing their sense of control over daily dietary choices.

"The application helps patients clearly see how what they eat affects their health indicators, which was difficult to explain during short clinic visits." (R2, healthcare professional, personal communication)

Participants further highlighted that the continuous and real-time nature of app-based feedback was more effective than traditional, episodic clinical consultations. Immediate reflection after meals supported self-monitoring and encouraged greater personal responsibility for nutrition management, particularly among individuals with chronic non-communicable diseases.

"When I can see the data every day, I feel more responsible for what I eat." (R7, end-user, personal communication)

"Digital monitoring encourages patients to manage themselves instead of depending entirely on hospital visits." (R4, healthcare administrator, personal communication)

Overall, this theme demonstrates that nutrition-focused health applications strengthen self-management by transforming abstract dietary advice into continuous, personalized feedback. From an SROI perspective, enhanced nutritional awareness contributes to long-term behavior change, reduced reliance on clinical services, and improved individual capacity for preventive health management.

4.2 From Advice to Action: The Role of E-Commerce Integration

A central theme emerging from the interviews was the role of embedded e-commerce features in bridging the gap between nutritional knowledge and actual behavior. Participants viewed this integration as transforming health applications from passive monitoring tools into active facilitators of healthy lifestyles by enabling immediate access to recommended products and services.

"When advice is linked directly to products or services, users are more likely to act on it." (R5, digital health developer, personal communication)

Convenience was repeatedly identified as a decisive factor influencing adherence to nutritional guidance. Seamless in-app purchasing and consultation booking reduced time, effort, and uncertainty associated with making healthy choices.

"If I can order healthy food or supplements in the same app, I won't delay or forget." (R9, end-user, personal communication)

This theme highlights e-commerce integration as a key behavioral mechanism that converts nutritional intention into action. By reducing practical barriers, such integration enhances adherence and amplifies social value through improved dietary consistency and sustained engagement with nutrition management practices.

4.3 Perceived Health and Quality-of-Life Outcomes

Participants across all stakeholder groups reported positive health-related outcomes associated with using nutrition-focused health applications, including improved weight control, blood sugar regulation, and dietary discipline. Consistent use was perceived to reduce anxiety related to chronic disease management.

"Since using the app regularly, my blood sugar is more stable, and I feel less worried." (R8, end-user, personal communication)

Beyond physical health, participants emphasized improvements in quality of life, including increased confidence and reduced dependence on frequent hospital visits. These benefits were also perceived to extend to family members and caregivers.

"Patients feel more confident managing their own health, which reduces stress for both patients and families." (R3, healthcare professional, personal communication)

The findings indicate that nutrition-focused applications generate multidimensional benefits that extend beyond clinical indicators. From an SROI perspective, improvements in quality of life, emotional well-being, and reduced caregiver burden represent important forms of social value that complement measurable health outcomes.

4.4 System-Level and Economic Value Creation

Healthcare administrators and policy-related stakeholders highlighted broader system-level benefits arising from the adoption of digital nutrition applications. Improved self-management and preventive nutrition practices were perceived to contribute to reduced outpatient visits and lower long-term healthcare costs.

> *"If patients can manage nutrition better, hospitals can reduce repeated visits for preventable complications." (R1, healthcare administrator, personal communication)*

Participants also emphasized time and cost savings for both patients and healthcare providers, particularly through reduced travel and fewer in-person consultations.

> *"Digital consultations save time for both sides and reduce unnecessary hospital congestion." (R6, healthcare administrator, personal communication)*

This theme underscores the system-level social and economic returns associated with digital nutrition applications. Efficiency gains, cost savings, and reduced service demand collectively strengthen the SROI case by demonstrating value creation beyond individual users.

4.5 Barriers to Maximizing Social Return on Investment

Despite the perceived benefits, participants identified challenges that may limit the realization of full social return on investment. Digital literacy was frequently cited as a barrier, particularly among older adults and individuals with limited experience using mobile applications.

> *"Some elderly users struggle with complex features, which affects long-term use." (R10, healthcare professional, personal communication)*

Concerns regarding data privacy and trust were also prominent, particularly regarding the commercial use of health data on e-commerce-enabled platforms.

> *"I want to know clearly how my health data is protected before using paid features." (R11, end-user, personal communication)*

These barriers highlight critical governance and design considerations that influence the sustainability of social value creation. Addressing digital inclusion and data transparency is essential to ensuring that financial viability does not undermine equity or trust.

4.6 Nutrition Balance and Athletic Performance Support

An additional theme concerned the role of nutrition-focused health applications in supporting physical recovery and athletic performance. Participants perceived that balanced nutrition was essential for energy management, recovery, and physical readiness, particularly among physically active users.

"Balanced nutrition is important for recovery after exercise, and the app helps users adjust intake properly." (R12, healthcare professional, personal communication)

End-users engaged in regular physical activity reported that tailored guidance and monitoring supported recovery and reduced fatigue.

"The app helps me plan meals after workouts, so I recover faster and feel more energetic." (R7, end-user, personal communication)

This theme extends the application of digital nutrition tools to performance-oriented outcomes. From an SROI perspective, improved recovery and physical capacity contribute not only to sustained physical activity and productivity but also to long-term health maintenance, thereby reinforcing the broader social value of nutrition-focused digital health applications within the digital economy.

5. DISCUSSIONS

This study provides qualitative evidence that health applications integrated with e-commerce strategies contribute to nutritional balance and the development of athletic performance in Thailand, and generate social value beyond conventional financial returns. The findings demonstrate that integrating digital health tools and e-commerce mechanisms plays a critical role in bridging the long-standing gap between nutritional knowledge and sustained behavioral change, as well as in athletic performance. Consistent with prior research on digital health and behavior-oriented systems, the results show that real-time feedback, personalization, and continuous monitoring enhance users' awareness, self-efficacy, and accountability in nutrition management (Al Naabi et al., 2024; Chaudhry et al., 2024).

The findings further extend existing literature by highlighting the transformative role of e-commerce integration. While previous studies have emphasized self-monitoring and information provision as key benefits of health applications, this research shows that embedded e-commerce functionalities convert abstract dietary advice into actionable behavior. By reducing transaction costs, effort, and barriers to access, e-commerce-enabled health applications facilitate practical adherence to nutritional recommendations. This supports behavioral economics perspectives suggesting that convenience and immediacy are critical drivers of health-related decision-making (Chauhan & Sagar, 2023; Dogra et al., 2023).

Furthermore, from an SROI perspective, the study reveals multiple layers of value creation. At the individual level, users experience improved health outcomes, greater confidence in self-management, and reduced anxiety related to chronic disease control. At the family and community levels, improved self-care reduces caregiver burden and enhances overall quality of life. At the system level, stakeholders perceive potential long-term benefits in the form of reduced healthcare utilization, improved system efficiency, and eased fiscal pressure on Thailand's universal health coverage scheme. These findings reinforce arguments that traditional ROI metrics underestimate the true value of digital health interventions by failing to account for social, psychological, and preventive outcomes (Siri, 2025; Siri et al., 2025).

However, the discussion also underscores persistent challenges that may constrain the realization of social value. Issues related to digital literacy, trust, and ethical commercialization align with prior concerns in the digital health literature. Without inclusive design, transparent data governance, and appropriate regulatory oversight, the social return generated by these technologies may remain unevenly distributed. Thus, the findings suggest that technological innovation alone is insufficient; social, institutional, and governance factors play a decisive role in shaping impact.

6. CONCLUSION

This study examined how health applications integrated with e-commerce strategies support nutritional balance and athletic performance in Thailand and explored the perceived SROI generated by their use. The findings demonstrate that these digital platforms function as behavior-enabling systems that translate nutritional guidance into practical, sustained action. Through continuous monitoring, personalized dietary feedback, and convenient access to nutrition-related products and services, health applications support users in achieving balanced nutrient intake and developing athletic performance, which are essential not only for disease prevention but also for physical recovery and performance optimization.

From a nutrition balance perspective, the results highlight the role of digital health applications in aligning dietary intake with individual physiological needs. Participants perceived that real-time feedback and tailored recommendations helped users regulate macronutrient and micronutrient consumption, improve meal timing, and maintain dietary consistency. Such mechanisms are particularly relevant for individuals engaged in regular physical activity, where appropriate nutritional balance directly influences energy availability, muscle recovery, and overall physical performance. By facilitating timely access to functional foods, supplements, and professional nutrition consultations through embedded e-commerce features, these applications help reduce gaps between nutritional knowledge and effective recovery practices.

In terms of recovery and performance, stakeholders perceived that improved nutrition self-management contributed to faster physical recovery, reduced fatigue, and enhanced readiness for daily activities and exercise. Although the primary focus of the applications was health maintenance and chronic disease management, the same digital nutrition principles were viewed as transferable to athletic and physically active populations. From an SROI perspective, these outcomes represent important forms of social value, as improved recovery and physical performance can enhance productivity, reduce injury risk, and support long-term physical well-being.

Overall, the study concludes that health applications integrated with e-commerce strategies offer significant potential to support nutrition balance and recovery-oriented practices that underpin both general health and athletic performance. When designed and governed responsibly, these platforms extend beyond individual health benefits to generate broader social value by promoting sustained physical capability, reducing long-term healthcare burdens, and contributing to a more preventive and performance-supportive health ecosystem in Thailand.

7. IMPLICATIONS

The findings of this study offer several important implications for policy, practice, and the future development of digital health ecosystems. For policymakers, the results suggest that health applications integrated with e-commerce strategies should be viewed not merely as commercial innovations or standalone technological solutions, but as strategic social investments capable of generating measurable public value. Incorporating SROI principles into the evaluation of digital health policies and programs may support more informed decision-making, improved prioritization of public resources, and more effective long-term planning, particularly within publicly funded healthcare systems. Such an approach may also assist policymakers in aligning digital health initiatives with national objectives related to preventive healthcare, health equity, and sustainable development.

For healthcare practitioners and administrators, the findings highlight the value of integrating digital nutrition tools into routine care pathways and broader health promotion strategies. Encouraging patient engagement with user-friendly, evidence-based applications can enhance self-management capabilities, support healthier dietary behaviors, reduce unnecessary clinical visits, and alleviate pressure on overstretched healthcare services. Moreover, the provision of structured training and ongoing digital literacy support for both patients and healthcare professionals is a critical enabler of successful adoption. Strengthening digital competencies within healthcare organizations may help ensure that these technologies are used effectively, ethically, and consistently across different care settings.

For developers and platform providers, the study underscores the importance of balancing commercialization objectives with social responsibility and public health considerations. Ethical e-commerce design, transparent data governance, and responsible monetization practices are essential to building user trust and safeguarding long-term engagement. In addition, the development of inclusive and accessible interfaces—particularly for older adults, individuals with limited digital literacy, and other vulnerable populations—is critical to maximizing social impact. Applications that prioritize usability, cultural relevance, and affordability are more likely to generate higher social returns and contribute meaningfully to improved nutritional outcomes and social well-being.

8. LIMITATIONS AND FUTURE RESEARCH

Despite its contributions, this study has several limitations that should be acknowledged. First, the qualitative design and purposive sampling approach limit the generalizability of the findings. While the study provides rich and contextualized insights, the results may not fully represent all user groups or digital health platforms in Thailand. Second, the findings are based on perceived outcomes rather than objective clinical or economic measurements. Although this aligns with the principles of SROI and qualitative inquiry, future studies could strengthen the evidence base by triangulating qualitative insights with quantitative health indicators or cost data. Third, the study focused primarily on stakeholders with existing experience in digital health applications. As a result, the perspectives of non-users or individuals who have disengaged from such platforms may be underrepresented.

Future research could extend this study in several directions. Quantitative, such as questionnaire surveys, or mixed-methods research could be conducted to measure specific health outcomes, cost savings, and environmental benefits associated with nutrition-focused digital health applications. Such studies would complement qualitative insights and support more comprehensive SROI calculations. Longitudinal research is also recommended to examine sustained behavioral change and long-term social value creation. Understanding how user engagement evolves and which features most strongly influence adherence would provide valuable guidance for platform design and policy development. Finally, comparative studies across regions, population groups, or healthcare systems could offer deeper insights into the contextual factors that shape digital health effectiveness. Exploring equity, accessibility, and digital inclusion in greater depth would further strengthen future research's contribution to socially sustainable digital health innovation.

ACKNOWLEDGEMENT

The authors gratefully acknowledge the support and academic contributions of the Faculty of Pharmacy, the International College, and the Research and Innovation Center of Pathumthani University, Thailand; the Thammasat University Research Unit in Data Innovation and Artificial Intelligence and the Department of Computer Science, Faculty of Science and Technology, Thammasat University, Thailand; and the Chulabhorn Graduate Institute, Thailand.

REFERENCES

Aekplakorn, W., Chariyalertsak, S., Kessomboon, P., Sangthong, R., Inthawong, R., Putwatana, P., & Taneepanichskul, S. (2011). Prevalence and management of diabetes and metabolic risk factors in Thai adults: The Thai national health examination survey IV, 2009. *Diabetes Care*, *34*(9), 1980–1985. DOI: 10.2337/dc11-0099 PMID: 21816976

Aggarwal, A. K., & Travers, S. (2001). E-commerce in healthcare: Changing the traditional landscape. *Journal of Healthcare Information Management*, *15*(1), 25–36. https://pubmed.ncbi.nlm.nih.gov/11338906/ PMID: 11338906

Al Naabi, Y., Ibrahim, N., & Dhillon, J. S. (2024). Designing sustainable mobile weight management applications: Information technology (IT) experts perspectives. *mHealth*, *10*, 25. DOI: 10.21037/mhealth-24-4 PMID: 39114463

Amawi, A., AlKasasbeh, W., Jaradat, M., Almasri, A., Alobaidi, S., Hammad, A. A., Bishtawi, T., Fataftah, B., Turk, N., Saoud, H. A., Jarrar, A., & Ghazzawi, H. (2024). Athletes' nutritional demands: A narrative review of nutritional requirements. *Frontiers in Nutrition*, *10*, 1331854. DOI: 10.3389/fnut.2023.1331854 PMID: 38328685

Amornkitvikai, Y., Tham, S. Y., Harvie, C., & Buachoom, W. W. (2022). Barriers and factors affecting the e-commerce sustainability of Thai micro-, small-and medium-sized enterprises (MSMEs). *Sustainability (Basel)*, *14*(14), 8476. DOI: 10.3390/su14148476

Arunruangsirilert, T., & Intanant, S. (2021). Measuring social return on investment: A case study of a social project of a company in Thailand. *Journal of Federation of Accounting Professions*, *3*(7), 34–47. https://so02.tci-thaijo.org/index.php/JFAC/article/view/248043

Asanprakit, S., & Limna, P. (2023). Understanding the role of social influence in consumers' intention to use social commerce. *Rom Yoong Thong Journal, 1*(2), 103-121. https://so08.tci-thaijo.org/index.php/romyoongthong/article/view/2188

Beck, K. L., Thomson, J. S., Swift, R. J., & von Hurst, P. R. (2015). Role of nutrition in performance enhancement and postexercise recovery. *Open Access Journal Of Sports Medicine, 6*, 259-267. DOI: 10.2147/OAJSM.S33605

Big Data Institute. (2021). *Digital transformation of healthcare services*. Ministry of Digital Economy and Society.

Campbell, S., Greenwood, M., Prior, S., Shearer, T., Walkem, K., Young, S., Bywaters, D., & Walker, K. (2020). Purposive sampling: Complex or simple? Research case examples. *Journal of Research in Nursing : JRN, 25*(8), 652–661. DOI: 10.1177/1744987120927206 PMID: 34394687

Chaudhry, B. M., Siek, K. A., & Connelly, K. (2024). The usability and feasibility of a dietary intake self-monitoring application in a population with varying literacy levels. *Journal of Personalized Medicine, 14*(9), 1001. DOI: 10.3390/jpm14091001 PMID: 39338255

Chauhan, V., & Sagar, M. (2023). Healthcare decision making and choice: An empirical model of patient confusion. *Management Decision, 61*(11), 3454–3474. DOI: 10.1108/MD-11-2022-1488

Chopvitayakun, S., Rattanasiriwongwut, M., & Ketcham, M. (2025). Factors influencing mobile platform adoption for nutritional tracking among Thai elderly: A unified UTAUT and STAM approach. *Journal of Open Innovation, 11*(3), 100606. DOI: 10.1016/j.joitmc.2025.100606

Coelho, R. R., Bonato, S. V., Pacheco, D. A. D. J., & Brito, P. D. S. (2025). Moving Health 4.0 forward: A systematic literature review, challenges and future research agenda. *The TQM Journal*. Advance online publication. DOI: 10.1108/TQM-07-2024-0269

Dogra, N., Bakshi, S., & Gupta, A. (2023). Exploring the switching intention of patients to e-health consultations platforms: Blending inertia with push–pull–mooring framework. *Journal of Asia Business Studies, 17*(1), 15–37. DOI: 10.1108/JABS-02-2021-0066

Ghazzawi, H. A., Hussain, M. A., Raziq, K. M., Alsendi, K. K., Alaamer, R. O., Jaradat, M., Alobaidi, S., Al Aqili, R., Trabelsi, K., & Jahrami, H. (2023). Exploring the relationship between micronutrients and athletic performance: A comprehensive scientific systematic review of the literature in sports medicine. *Sports (Basel, Switzerland), 11*(6), 109. DOI: 10.3390/sports11060109 PMID: 37368559

Giraldo-Vallejo, J. E., Cardona-Guzmán, M. Á., Rodríguez-Alcivar, E. J., Kočí, J., Petro, J. L., Kreider, R. B., Cannataro, R., & Bonilla, D. A. (2023). Nutritional strategies in the rehabilitation of musculoskeletal injuries in athletes: A systematic integrative review. *Nutrients, 15*(4), 819. DOI: 10.3390/nu15040819 PMID: 36839176

Heaton, L. E., Davis, J. K., Rawson, E. S., Nuccio, R. P., Witard, O. C., Stein, K. W., Baar, K., Carter, J. M., & Baker, L. B. (2017). Selected in-season nutritional strategies to enhance recovery for team sport athletes: A practical overview. *Sports Medicine, 47*(11), 2201–2218. DOI: 10.1007/s40279-017-0759-2 PMID: 28702900

Hermes, S., Riasanow, T., Clemons, E. K., Böhm, M., & Krcmar, H. (2020). The digital transformation of the healthcare industry: Exploring the rise of emerging platform ecosystems and their influence on the role of patients. *Business Research, 13*(3), 1033–1069. DOI: 10.1007/s40685-020-00125-x

Hongsuchon, T., Chen, S. C., & Khan, A. (2025). Applying the S-O-R model to explore impulsive buying behavior driven by influencers on social commerce websites. *PeerJ. Computer Science, 11*, e3113. DOI: 10.7717/peerj-cs.3113 PMID: 40989320

Hwang, D. J., & Yang, H. J. (2024). Nutritional strategies for enhancing performance and training adaptation in weightlifters. *International Journal of Molecular Sciences, 26*(1), 240. DOI: 10.3390/ijms26010240 PMID: 39796095

Jangjarat, K., Shaengchart, Y., Limna, P., Suradinkura, S., & Bhumpenpein, N. (2026). The role of the 4Es in driving business performance and competitive advantage for cosmetic industry SMEs in emerging economies. *Business Performance Review, 4*(1), 33–44. DOI: 10.22495/bprv4i1p3

Kotler, P. (2017). Philip Kotler: Some of my adventures in marketing. *Journal of Historical Research in Marketing, 9*(2), 203–208. DOI: 10.1108/JHRM-11-2016-0027

Kumar, S. S., Muthukumaran, V., Devi, A., Geetha, V., & Yadav, P. N. (2023). A quantitative approach of purposive sampling techniques for security and privacy issues in IoT healthcare applications. In Zhao, J., Kumar, V., Natarajan, R., & Mahesh, T. (Eds.), *Handbook of Research on Advancements in AI and IoT Convergence Technologies* (pp. 281–299). IGI Global Scientific Publishing., DOI: 10.4018/978-1-6684-6971-2.ch016

Limna, P. (2023). The digital transformation of healthcare in the digital economy: A systematic review. *International Journal of Advanced Health Science and Technology*, *3*(2), 127–132. DOI: 10.35882/ijahst.v3i2.244

Limna, P., Shaengchart, Y., Kraiwanit, T., Asanprakit, S., & Nivornusit, R. (2025). Muketing: The fusion of *Mutelu* and marketing in e-commerce—Trends in Thailand's faith economy. *Frontiers in Communication*, *10*, 1662524. DOI: 10.3389/fcomm.2025.1662524

Limna, P., & Siripipattanakul, S. (2026). Sustainable clinic management based on practices and human resource management (HRM). In Siripipatthanakul, S. (Ed.), *Sustainable Development for Hospitals and Clinics* (pp. 65–96). IGI Global Scientific Publishing., DOI: 10.4018/979-8-3693-9800-5.ch003

Limna, P., Siripipattanakul, S., Sitthipon, T., Jaipong, P., & Auttawechasakoon, P. (2022). Telemedicine consultations among healthcare providers and patients during the COVID-19 pandemic: A review article. *Review of Advanced Multidisciplinary Sciences, Engineering & Innovation, 1*(1), 1-8. https://ssrn.com/abstract=4080873

Liu, J., Mao, S., Lu, L., Jing, Y., Yang, X., Xu, H., & Ren, Y. (2025). The impact of digital economy on the supply chain resilience of cross-border healthcare e-commerce. *Frontiers in Public Health*, *13*, 1570338. DOI: 10.3389/fpubh.2025.1570338 PMID: 40487520

Marinescu, M. R., Ionescu, O. N., Pachiu, C. I., Dinescu, M. A., Muller, R., & uchea, M. P. (2025). Next-gen healthcare devices: Evolution of MEMS and BioMEMS in the era of the Internet of bodies for personalized medicine. *Micromachines*, *16*(10), 1182. DOI: 10.3390/mi16101182 PMID: 41156428

Martín-Rodríguez, A., Belinchón-deMiguel, P., Rubio-Zarapuz, A., Tornero-Aguilera, J. F., Martínez-Guardado, I., Villanueva-Tobaldo, C. V., & Clemente-Suárez, V. J. (2024). Advances in understanding the interplay between dietary practices, body composition, and sports performance in athletes. *Nutrients*, *16*(4), 571. DOI: 10.3390/nu16040571 PMID: 38398895

Naderi, A., Rothschild, J. A., Santos, H. O., Hamidvand, A., Koozehchian, M. S., Ghazzagh, A., Berjisian, E., & Podlogar, T. (2025). Nutritional strategies to improve post-exercise recovery and subsequent exercise performance: A narrative review. *Sports Medicine*, *55*(7), 1559–1577. DOI: 10.1007/s40279-025-02213-6 PMID: 40221559

Nicholls, J., Lawlor, E., Neitzert, E., & Goodspeed, T. (2009). *A guide to social return on investment*. Cabinet Office.

Office of the Personal Data Protection Commission. (2021). *Guideline on personal data protection*. PDPA.

Okolo, C. A., Babawarun, O., Arowoogun, J. O., Adeniyi, A. O., & Chidi, R. (2024). The role of mobile health applications in improving patient engagement and health outcomes: A critical review. *International Journal of Science and Research Archive*, *11*(1), 2566–2574. DOI: 10.30574/ijsra.2024.11.1.0334

Park, J. I., Lee, H. Y., Kim, H., Lee, J., Shinn, J., & Kim, H. S. (2021). Lack of acceptance of digital healthcare in the medical market: Addressing old problems raised by various clinical professionals and developing possible solutions. *Journal of Korean Medical Science*, *36*(37), e253. DOI: 10.3346/jkms.2021.36.e253 PMID: 34581521

Perez-Uribe, R., Ocampo-Guzman, D., & Lozano-Correa, L. J. (Eds.). (2025). *Models, strategies, and tools for competitive SMEs*. IGI Global Scientific Publishing., DOI: 10.4018/979-8-3693-4046-2

Phuangsuwan, P., Siripipatthanakul, S., Limna, P., & Pariwongkhuntorn, N. (2024). The impact of Google Maps application on the digital economy. *Phuangsuwan, P., Siripipatthanakul, S., Limna, P., & Pariwongkhuntorn*, (2024), 192-203. https://virtusinterpress.org/IMG/pdf/cbsrv5i1art18.pdf

Purcell, L. K. (2013). Sport nutrition for young athletes. *Paediatrics & Child Health*, *18*(4), 200–205. DOI: 10.1093/pch/18.4.200 PMID: 24421690

Rakshit, D. (2025). Mobile applications in e-commerce and healthcare prescription management: Integrating AI-driven personalization, accessibility, and multi-domain services. *Journal of Computer Science and Technology Studies*, *7*(12), 46–54. https://al-kindipublishers.org/index.php/jcsts/article/view/11485

Rauscher, O., Grünhaus, C., & Millner, R. (2012). *Social impact measurement and social return on investment (SROI)-analysis*. Vienna University of Economics and Business. https://www.researchgate.net/publication/357335567

Serra, C. M., Aroca Tanarro, A., Cummings, C. M., Jimenez Fuertes, A., & Tomás Martínez, J. F. (2022). Impact on the reduction of CO2 emissions due to the use of telemedicine. *Scientific Reports*, *12*(1), 12507. DOI: 10.1038/s41598-022-16864-2 PMID: 35869274

Siri, P. (2025). *Evaluating the economic and social benefits of health application use in Thailand* (Doctoral dissertation). Rangsit University. DOI: 10.13140/RG.2.2.19760.67848

Siri, P., Kraiwanit, T., Keawngam, T., & Ponsri, R. (2025). The social impact of health applications: Transforming self-care and patient support. [Humanities and Social Sciences]. *Journal of Suvarnabhumi Institute of Technology, 11*(2), 213–225. https://so04.tci-thaijo.org/index.php/svittj/article/view/277401

Siripipatthanakul, S., Chaiprakarn, S., Rungsiyanont, S., & Phuangsuwan, P. (2025). A case study of sustainable development in hospitals in Thailand using ChatGPT. In *Sustainable development for hospitals and clinics* (pp. 1–32). IGI Global Scientific Publishing., DOI: 10.4018/979-8-3693-9800-5.ch001

Siripipatthanakul, S., Limna, P., Sriboonruang, P., & Kaewpuang, P. (2023). Applying the TPB and the UTAUT models predicting intentions to use telemedicine among Thai people during the COVID-19 pandemic. *International Journal of Computing Sciences Research, 7*(1), 1362–1384. https://stepacademic.net/ijcsr/article/view/350. DOI: 10.25147/ijcsr.2017.001.1.107

Sitthipon, T., Siripipatthanakul, S., Phayaphrom, B., Siripipattanakul, S., & Limna, P. (2022). Determinants of customers' intention to use healthcare chatbots and apps in Bangkok, Thailand. *International Journal of Behavioral Analytics, 2*(2), 1–15. https://ssrn.com/abstract=4045661

Tangcharoensathien, V., Adulyanon, S., Supaka, N., Munkong, R., Viriyathorn, S., Sirithienthong, S., Kanhachon, S., & Marten, R. (2024). The Thai health promotion foundation: Two decades of joint contributions to addressing noncommunicable diseases and creating healthy populations. *Global Health, Science and Practice, 12*(2), e2300311. DOI: 10.9745/GHSP-D-23-00311 PMID: 38448166

Tungtrakul, C., Thawornsujaritkul, T., & Silpcharu, T. (2024). The guide for information technology management regarding personal data protection of the industrial business sector in Thailand. *International Journal of Instructional Cases, 8*(2), 196–210. https://ijicases.com/menuscript/index.php/ijicases/article/view/159

UNDP & WHO. (2021, November 23). *Prevention and control of noncommunicable diseases in Thailand: The case for investment.* https://www.undp.org/thailand/publications/prevention-and-control-noncommunicable-diseases-thailand-case-investment

van Dijk, J. A. (2006). Digital divide research: Achievements and shortcomings. *Poetics, 34*(4-5), 221–235. DOI: 10.1016/j.poetic.2006.05.004

Wang, Q., Su, M., Zhang, M., & Li, R. (2021). Integrating digital technologies and public health to fight COVID-19 pandemic: Key technologies, applications, challenges and outlook of digital healthcare. *International Journal of Environmental Research and Public Health, 18*(11), 6053. DOI: 10.3390/ijerph18116053 PMID: 34199831

Yeung, A. W. K., Torkamani, A., Butte, A. J., Glicksberg, B. S., Schuller, B., Rodriguez, B., Ting, D. S. W., Bates, D., Schaden, E., Peng, H., Willschke, H., van der Laak, J., Car, J., Rahimi, K., Celi, L. A., Banach, M., Kletecka-Pulker, M., Kimberger, O., Eils, R., & Atanasov, A. G. (2023). The promise of digital healthcare technologies. *Frontiers in Public Health, 11*, 1196596. DOI: 10.3389/fpubh.2023.1196596 PMID: 37822534

Yuduang, N., Ong, A. K. S., Prasetyo, Y. T., Chuenyindee, T., Kusonwattana, P., Limpasart, W., Sittiwatethanasiri, T., Gumasing, M. J. J., German, J. D., & Nadlifatin, R. (2022). Factors influencing the perceived effectiveness of COVID-19 risk assessment mobile application "MorChana" in Thailand: UTAUT2 approach. *International Journal of Environmental Research and Public Health, 19*(9), 5643. DOI: 10.3390/ijerph19095643 PMID: 35565040

Zacharia, A., Thomas, A. C., Mathew, P. C., Cleetus, R. S., John, S. E., & Joseph, J. (2024). Exploring the intersection of e-commerce and healthcare: A visual analysis of research trends. *Cureus, 16*(9), e69865. DOI: 10.7759/cureus.69865 PMID: 39435212

KEY TERMS AND DEFINITIONS

Athletic performance: Athletic performance refers to an individual's capacity to effectively execute physical activities or sports-related tasks through the integrated application of physical, physiological, technical, tactical, and psychological attributes. It encompasses measurable components such as strength, endurance, speed, agility, coordination, and flexibility, as well as underlying physiological processes including energy metabolism, cardiovascular efficiency, neuromuscular function, and recovery capacity.

Behavioral Change: Behavioral change refers to the modification of individuals' habits, actions, and decision-making processes related to health and lifestyle. In nutrition-focused digital health interventions, behavioral change involves adopting healthier dietary practices, maintaining adherence to nutritional guidance, and sustaining long-term self-management behaviors. This study conceptualizes behavioral change as a gradual and socially influenced process facilitated by continuous feedback, convenience, and supportive digital environments.

Digital Health: Digital health refers to the use of digital technologies to enhance healthcare delivery, health promotion, and disease prevention. This encompasses mobile health (mHealth), telemedicine, health information systems, wearable devices, and data-driven decision-support tools. In the Thai context, digital health is increasingly positioned as a strategic response to rising non-communicable diseases, population ageing, and healthcare system constraints, enabling a shift toward preventive and patient-centered care models.

E-Commerce Integration: E-commerce integration refers to embedding commercial transaction capabilities within digital health applications. This includes features such as in-app purchasing, subscription services, digital marketplaces, and integrated payment systems, enabling users to directly access health-related products and services. In this study, e-commerce integration is understood as a mechanism that connects nutritional advice with practical action by enabling users to procure healthy food options, supplements, meal kits, or professional consultations, thereby reducing access barriers and supporting sustained behavioral change.

Health Applications: Health applications refer to digital software platforms, primarily mobile- or web-based, designed to support health-related activities such as monitoring, prevention, diagnosis, treatment, and self-management. In this study, health applications focus specifically on nutrition management, chronic disease monitoring, and health behavior support. These applications often incorporate features such as personalized dietary recommendations, health data tracking, real-time feedback, and remote consultations, enabling users to actively manage their health beyond traditional clinical settings.

Nutritional Balance: Nutritional balance refers to the appropriate intake and proportions of essential nutrients required to maintain optimal health and prevent disease. It involves aligning dietary consumption with individual physiological needs, lifestyle factors, and health conditions. Within this research, nutritional balance is viewed not only as a biological outcome but also as a behavioral and social process influenced by knowledge, accessibility, convenience, and digital support systems provided through health applications.

Preventive Healthcare: Preventive healthcare encompasses strategies and interventions aimed at preventing disease onset, delaying progression, and reducing health risks before clinical treatment becomes necessary. Within this research, preventive healthcare is closely linked to nutrition management supported by digital health applications. By encouraging early intervention, self-monitoring, and healthier lifestyle choices, such applications help reduce the burden of non-communicable diseases and improve population health outcomes.

Social Return on Investment (SROI): Social Return on Investment (SROI) is a principles-based framework used to measure and evaluate the social, health, and environmental value generated by an intervention relative to the resources invested. Unlike traditional financial ROI, SROI captures both tangible and intangible outcomes, such as improved quality of life, reduced caregiver burden, enhanced health equity, and system-level efficiency gains. In this study, SROI provides an analytical lens for understanding the broader societal impact of health applications integrated with e-commerce strategies in Thailand.

Chapter 3
The Role of User Experiences and Technology Adoption in Digital Business-Driven Nutrition Platforms for Athletic Performance

Pongsakorn Limna
http://orcid.org/0000-0002-7448-5261
Pathumthani University, Thailand

Yarnaphat Shaengchart
http://orcid.org/0000-0002-0157-3682
Pathumthani University, Thailand

Supakorn Suradinkura
http://orcid.org/0009-0008-4514-3546
Pathumthani University, Thailand

Saranchana Asanprakit
Pathumthani University, Thailand

Rattawut Nivornusit
Rangsit University, Thailand

Nalinpat Bhumpenpein
King Mongkut's University of Technology, North Bangkok, Thailand

ABSTRACT

The integration of artificial intelligence (AI) and digital business models is transforming sports nutrition from a product-oriented industry into a platform-based, intelligence-driven ecosystem. This chapter explores user experiences and examines how AI-enabled, digital business–driven nutrition platforms are adopted and valued in sport contexts. Drawing on qualitative interviews with athletes, performance nutritionists, coaches, and sports administrators, the study demonstrates that these

DOI: 10.4018/979-8-3373-9544-9.ch003

platforms function as socio-technical systems rather than simple technological tools. Their effectiveness depends on the alignment of technological capabilities with user experience design and organizational context. The findings reveal a clear shift from traditional product-based sports nutrition toward intelligence-driven, platform-based value creation, while also identifying institutional barriers—including digital literacy gaps, professional trust, and data governance concerns—that influence adoption and long-term use.

1. INTRODUCTION

The digital transformation of the global sports economy has precipitated a paradigm shift in how elite and amateur athletes approach nutritional periodization and performance optimization. Historically characterized by analog spreadsheets, static meal plans, and subjective coaching intuition, the sector is currently undergoing a radical restructuring driven by artificial intelligence (AI), machine learning (ML), and integrated digital platform ecosystems. The intersection of nutritional science and digital technology has birthed a rapidly expanding, data-intensive market segment that operates distinct from, yet parallel to, the traditional commodities market of supplements and sports drinks. This emerging "intelligence layer"—comprising software platforms, predictive algorithms, and interconnected wearable and monitoring devices—is redefining the economic value, scalability, and personalization of athletic performance (Chen, 2025; Choudhury et al., 2025; Du & Bi, 2025; Karnika et al., 2025; Santomier, 2026).

As reported by Research and Markets (2026), the global sports nutrition market is witnessing a robust expansion, with valuations projected to surge from approximately USD 52.32 billion in 2025 to USD 107.95 billion by 2035, representing a Compound Annual Growth Rate (CAGR) of 7.51%. Within this broader aggregate, the B2B sports nutrition sector—encompassing the software and enterprise solutions sold to professional teams, collegiate programs, and fitness institutions—demonstrates an even more aggressive trajectory, with forecasted CAGRs exceeding 10-11% (Precedence Research, 2025; Zion Market Research, 2025). This accelerated growth in the B2B sector is driven by a fundamental shift in the economics of elite sport. As player contracts and franchise valuations escalate, the financial penalty of injury or underperformance increases. Consequently, organizations are treating nutrition not as a consumable expense, but as a risk management asset. Platforms that can demonstrate a reduction in injury days or an extension of athlete career longevity command significant pricing power (Amawi et al., 2024; Can & Can, 2025; Jacobsson et al., 2023; Turnagöl et al., 2022).

Traditionally, sports nutrition businesses operated on a largely transactional model, focusing on the sale of discrete products such as protein supplements or hydration formulas. In contrast, the emerging digital model increasingly operates on an "Intelligence-as-a-Service" paradigm. Platforms such as Hexis and ZoneIn do not primarily sell food products; rather, they provide a data-driven decision-making framework that guides users on what to eat, when to eat, and in what quantities, thereby translating complex nutritional science into actionable, context-specific recommendations (Arenas-Jal et al., 2020; Hexis, 2023; Lemire, 2023; Teamworks, 2024). This shift is driven by the commercial necessity of extending the career lifespan of elite athletes. In a multi-billion dollar sports economy, the marginal gains derived from optimized recovery and metabolic flexibility are quantifiable financial assets. Consequently, nutrition platforms are migrating from simple "calorie counters" (like the early versions of MyFitnessPal) to complex metabolic predictive engines. The valuation of companies like Teamworks, which raised $235 million at a valuation exceeding $1 billion in 2025, validates the immense enterprise value placed on these "Operating Systems for Sports" (Teamworks, 2025).

According to Gabrišová et al. (2025) and PwC (2025), the global landscape is not monolithic; regional nuances dictate the pace and nature of technology adoption. The North America region remains the dominant market leader. This dominance is fueled by the unique structure of the NCAA (Collegiate Athletics) and the major professional leagues (NFL, NBA). The sheer volume of student-athletes in the U.S. creates a massive addressable market for "bulk personalization" tools like ZoneIn and Teamworks. The cultural emphasis on "bigger, faster, stronger" drives high adoption of performance-enhancing technologies. In Europe, the market is characterized by a high degree of fragmentation and a strong focus on privacy and data protection (GDPR). Innovation is often driven by the specific demands of football (soccer) and cycling, leading to highly specialized, science-first platforms like Hexis which are heavily utilized by UCI World Tour riders and Premier League teams. The European focus tends to be more on "efficiency" and "recovery" rather than just mass gain. Furthermore, Asia-Pacific is identified as the fastest-growing region with a CAGR of 10.8%. This growth is fueled by rising health awareness, urbanization, and the rapid proliferation of mobile technology. However, "digital divides" in connectivity and a lack of localized software interfaces remain significant barriers in developing sub-regions, potentially impeding the uniform adoption of cloud-based nutrition platforms (Hexis, 2023; Persistence Market Research, 2025; Stellar Market Research, 2025).

Despite the rapid growth of AI-enabled nutrition platforms within the global sports economy, existing scholarship remains fragmented and predominantly technology-centric. Prior studies have largely focused on algorithmic capabilities, performance analytics, or physiological outcomes of digital nutrition interventions, often adopting quantitative or experimental designs. While these approaches provide valuable insights into what these systems can achieve, they offer limited understanding of how and why such platforms are adopted, utilized, and sustained within real-world athletic and organizational contexts. Moreover, the literature tends to treat athletes and teams as homogeneous end users, overlooking the heterogeneity of user experiences across elite, semi-professional, and institutional settings. Some critical socio-technical dimensions remain underexplored. In particular, there is a paucity of qualitative research exploring the lived experiences of key stakeholders, including athletes, performance nutritionists, coaches, and sports administrators, who collectively shape technology adoption decisions. In addition, while the concept of "Intelligence-as-a-Service" has been discussed conceptually, empirical evidence explaining how this intelligence layer generates business value beyond traditional nutrition commodities is limited. Existing market reports emphasize market developments and valuations but do not sufficiently interrogate the micro-level mechanisms through which user experience and perceived value influence adoption, retention, and platform scalability. This gap is especially pronounced in non-Western and emerging markets, where cultural context, digital literacy, and institutional constraints may significantly alter adoption dynamics. Consequently, there is a clear need for an in-depth qualitative inquiry that captures stakeholder perspectives and contextual nuances to complement the predominantly quantitative and technology-driven literature.

To address the identified gaps, this chapter provides a comprehensive analysis of the role of user experience and technology adoption within digital business–driven nutrition platforms designed to enhance athletic performance. Specifically, the chapter pursues three research objectives: (1) to examine user experiences with digital business–driven nutrition platforms among athletes and sport-related professionals; (2) to investigate how digital nutrition platforms generate economic and performance value beyond traditional sports nutrition products; and (3) to identify the contextual and institutional challenges influencing the implementation and sustained use of AI-enabled nutrition platforms across diverse sporting environments. This study adopts a qualitative interview methodology to generate rich, contextualized insights that cannot be captured through survey-based or experimental designs alone. Semi-structured interviews allow participants to articulate their perceptions, motivations, and concerns in their own words, thereby revealing underlying cognitive, cultural, and organizational factors shaping technology adoption. From a theoretical perspective, the qualitative approach contributes to digital business and sports management literature by advancing a socio-technical understanding of AI-driven nutrition platforms. It moves beyond deterministic views of technology to highlight the role of human agency, user experience, and institutional context in shaping digital transformation outcomes. Practically, the findings offer actionable insights for platform developers, sports organizations, and policymakers by identifying design features, adoption barriers, and value propositions that matter most to users. By foregrounding stakeholder voices, this research supports the development of more user-centric, scalable, and context-sensitive digital nutrition solutions. Finally, methodologically, the insights from qualitative interviews are critical for advancing a more holistic understanding of digital business–driven nutrition platforms as socio-technical systems rather than purely technological tools. By adopting a qualitative interview-based approach, this study provides a nuanced, empirically grounded understanding of user experience and technology adoption in digital sports nutrition platforms, addressing a significant gap in both academic research and industry practice in the digital economy.

2. LITERATURE REVIEW

The rapid integration of AI, data analytics, and platform-based business models into sports nutrition has generated a growing yet fragmented body of scholarly work. Existing research spans multiple disciplines—including sports science, digital health, information systems, and digital business—resulting in conceptual and methodological silos that limit a holistic understanding of digital business–driven nutrition platforms. While prior studies have provided valuable insights into algorithmic design, physiological outcomes, and technological performance, they often underemphasize the experiential, organizational, and adoption-related dimensions that ultimately determine whether such platforms deliver sustained value in real-world sport contexts. This literature review synthesizes research across five interrelated domains: (1) the technological architectures underpinning performance nutrition platforms, (2) user experience design in digital nutrition systems, (3) technology adoption and acceptance in sports and health-related platforms, (4) digital business value creation in performance management systems, and (5) the emergence of digital business–driven nutrition platforms for athletic performance. By integrating insights from these streams, the review establishes a socio-technical foundation for examining how user experience and technology adoption jointly shape the performance and business outcomes of AI-enabled nutrition platforms.

2.1 Technological Architectures of Performance Nutrition

The effectiveness of contemporary digital nutrition platforms is largely contingent upon their technological architecture, defined as the integrated system of algorithms, databases, sensor interfaces, and interoperable applications that transform raw physiological, behavioral, and contextual data into actionable nutritional insights. Over the past decade, this architecture has evolved substantially, shifting from static, self-reported digital food logs toward dynamic, AI–driven ecosystems capable of real-time analysis, prediction, and adaptive decision-making. This transformation reflects a broader paradigm shift in sports science and health informatics toward data-intensive personalization, continuous feedback loops, and performance optimization supported by computational intelligence (Charfare et al., 2025; Kassem et al., 2025; Phalle & Gokhale, 2025; Prasad et al., 2025; Suarez & Adibi, 2025).

At the foundational level, modern performance nutrition platforms rely on multilayered data architectures that integrate diverse data streams, including dietary intake records, training load metrics, wearable sensor outputs (e.g., heart rate variability, energy expenditure, sleep quality), and contextual variables such as competition schedules and environmental conditions. Moreover, cloud-based databases and application programming interfaces (APIs) enable seamless data aggregation and interoperability across devices and services, facilitating longitudinal athlete monitoring and cross-platform functionality. Such infrastructures are essential for scaling digital nutrition services within digital business ecosystems while maintaining accuracy, responsiveness, and user accessibility (Ajibesin & Thangavel, 2025; Lee et al., 2025; Nikitjuk et al., 2025; Quan et al., 2026; Rao & Neethirajan, 2025; Sun et al., 2025; Tasmurzayev et al., 2025;).

Building upon this data infrastructure, machine learning and AI algorithms constitute the analytical core of advanced nutrition platforms. These systems employ predictive modeling, pattern recognition, and recommendation engines to translate complex datasets into personalized dietary strategies. In contrast to rule-based systems, AI-enabled architectures continuously learn from user behavior and performance outcomes, allowing nutrition recommendations to evolve in response to training adaptations, injury status, or changing performance goals. This adaptive capacity is particularly critical in high-performance sport contexts, where marginal nutritional mismatches can have disproportionate effects on recovery and competitive outcomes (Armand et al., 2024; Agrawal et al., 2025; Grivas & Safari, 2025; Quan et al., 2026).

One of the most influential applications of such technological architectures in sports nutrition is the operationalization of nutritional periodization within digitally enabled performance systems. Nutritional periodization involves the strategic modulation of nutrient intake—particularly carbohydrates and overall energy availability—in alignment with the varying physiological demands of training cycles, competition phases, and recovery periods. Widely regarded as a gold standard in elite performance nutrition, this approach has been empirically validated for enhancing metabolic flexibility, training adaptation, and endurance performance across diverse athletic contexts. However, despite its strong theoretical and empirical foundations, manual implementation remains highly complex and resource-intensive, requiring continuous and precise monitoring of training intensity, timing, macronutrient distribution, and individual metabolic responses over time (Chhabra et al., 2023; Jeukendrup, 2017; Macedo et al., 2024; Martín-Rodríguez et al., 2024; Morton et al., 2025; Turner et al., 2025).

Digital nutrition platforms address this complexity by embedding nutritional periodization logic into algorithmic decision frameworks. Through real-time synchronization with training data and wearable technologies, these systems can automatically adjust dietary recommendations to reflect daily training loads, recovery needs, and competition demands. For example, carbohydrate intake can be dynamically scaled in response to high-intensity sessions, while protein and micronutrient recommendations are recalibrated to support recovery and injury prevention. Such automation not only enhances precision but also reduces cognitive and time burdens on athletes and practitioners, thereby improving adherence and consistency (Balaji et al., 2025; Can & Can, 2025; Esco et al., 2025; Mundt et al., 2025; Suarez & Adibi, 2025).

These technological architectures also enable scalable personalization, allowing platforms to deliver elite-level nutritional intelligence to broader athletic and fitness populations. Subscription-based models, freemium services, and enterprise partnerships with sports organizations are increasingly built upon modular and extensible architectures that support continuous innovation and user engagement. Consequently, technological architecture functions not merely as a technical backbone but as a strategic asset that underpins value creation, competitive differentiation, and sustained user adoption in digital performance nutrition markets (Agrawal et al., 2025; Arshad et al., 2025; Mundt et al., 2025; Westerbeek & Schaik, 2025).

2.2 User Experience in Digital Nutrition Platforms

User experience has emerged as a critical determinant of engagement, adherence, and sustained use in digital nutrition and performance platforms. Unlike traditional nutrition tools that primarily function as static tracking systems, contemporary platforms operate as interactive decision-support environments that require frequent user input, interpretation, and behavioral response. As such, user experience extends beyond interface aesthetics to encompass usability, personalization, cognitive load, and the perceived relevance of recommendations to athletic goals. Platforms with intuitive navigation, clear data visualization, and minimal manual input requirements are more likely to sustain long-term engagement, particularly among athletes managing high training and competition demands (Adu et al., 2020; Fanani et al., 2023; Figueiredo et al., 2025; Gabrišová et al., 2025; Jiang et al., 2025).

Personalization plays a central role in shaping positive user experiences within digital nutrition platforms. Athletes and practitioners are more likely to trust and adhere to recommendations when systems account for individual training loads, performance objectives, and physiological responses rather than applying generic nutritional guidelines. Real-time feedback mechanisms, adaptive recommendations, and longitudinal performance tracking enhance perceived usefulness by making nutrition feel dynamically integrated into training routines rather than an external or burdensome task. Moreover, visual analytics that translate complex nutritional data into accessible insights have been shown to reduce decision fatigue and improve comprehension among both athletes and support staff (Cossich et al., 2023; Luczak et al., 2020; Mănescu, 2025; Naabi et al., 2024; Piskorz-Ryń et al., 2025; Prasad et al., 2025; Sah et al., 2024).

Importantly, user experience in performance nutrition platforms is inherently role-dependent. Athletes tend to prioritize immediacy, clarity, and actionable guidance, while performance nutritionists and coaches emphasize data accuracy, customization, and analytical depth. Administrators and decision-makers, in contrast, often interact with aggregated dashboards and summary reports rather than granular data. This heterogeneity underscores the need for multi-layered user experience design that accommodates diverse user groups within a single platform ecosystem. The literature increasingly suggests that platforms failing to align user experience with role-specific needs risk underutilization, regardless of their technological sophistication (Chatterjee & Sarkar, 2025; Chhabra et al., 2023; Dunne et al., 2022; Patra et al., 2024; Putra et al., 2024; Shanita et al., 2017; Sonnen, 2024).

2.3 Technology Adoption and Acceptance in Digital Sports Platforms

Technology adoption in digital sports and health platforms has traditionally been examined through established theoretical frameworks such as the Technology Acceptance Model (TAM), Unified Theory of Acceptance and Use of Technology (UTAUT), and Information Systems (IS) Success Model. These frameworks emphasize perceived usefulness, perceived ease of use, and performance expectancy as primary drivers of adoption. In athletic and institutional sport contexts, however, adoption dynamics extend beyond individual attitudes to encompass organizational culture, professional norms, and governance structures. Studies indicate that even highly advanced platforms may face resistance if they conflict with entrenched coaching philosophies or challenge professional autonomy (Cho et al., 2020; Liu et al., 2022; Liu et al., 2025; Marinescu et al., 2025; Westerbeek & Schaik, 2025).

Within performance nutrition, perceived usefulness is closely tied to demonstrable performance outcomes, such as improved recovery, reduced injury risk, or enhanced training consistency. Athletes and practitioners are more likely to adopt digital nutrition platforms when recommendations are clearly linked to measurable performance indicators rather than abstract health benefits. Ease of use remains equally critical, particularly in high-performance environments where time constraints are significant. Platforms that require extensive manual data entry or technical expertise often experience declining engagement over time, despite initial adoption driven by organizational mandates (Abeltino et al., 2025; Ahmad et al., 2025; Ajiye et al., 2025; Chopvitayakun et al., 2025; Wahyudi & Yunus, 2025; Yuxin et al., 2025).

At the organizational level, adoption is influenced by leadership support, resource availability, and institutional readiness (Amanollahnejad et al., 2026; Casey et al., 2012). Coaches and administrators play a pivotal role as gatekeepers, shaping whether platforms are framed as supportive tools or intrusive monitoring systems. Social influence, professional credibility, and trust in algorithmic decision-making further affect acceptance, especially among experienced practitioners who may be skeptical of automated recommendations. Consequently, the literature increasingly frames technology adoption in digital sports platforms as a socio-technical process in which human agency, institutional context, and technological capability interact dynamically rather than linearly (Christodimitropoulou et al., 2025; Jaswal et al., 2022; Roppelt et al., 2024; Saadati & Torres, 2024; Westerbeek & Schaik, 2025).

2.4 Digital Business Value in Performance Nutrition Platforms

The rise of AI-enabled nutrition platforms has coincided with a fundamental transformation in digital business models within the sports nutrition industry. Traditional models centered on product sales—such as supplements or meal plans—are increasingly being supplemented or replaced by subscription-based, platform-driven models that deliver continuous intelligence rather than discrete goods. These platforms function as performance management infrastructures, offering value through data integration, predictive analytics, and decision support rather than nutritional products alone (Agrawal et al., 2025; Kassem et al., 2025; Panayotova, 2025).

Furthermore, value creation in digital performance nutrition platforms extends beyond immediate consumption to encompass longer-term organizational benefits, including injury prevention, workload optimization, and career longevity across competitive seasons. From a business perspective, such outcomes translate into risk mitigation and measurable return on investment, particularly in elite and professional sport environments where athlete availability, performance continuity, and recovery efficiency carry substantial financial implications. As a result, organizations increasingly evaluate nutrition platforms not merely as operational expenses, but as strategic, data-driven assets embedded within broader performance management ecosystems that support sustained competitive advantage (Bangsbo et al., 2025; Budhiraja, 2025; Jalonen et al., 2018; Kanwal et al., 2025; Kretschmer et al., 2022; Qi et al., 2024).

Moreover, scalable personalization represents a key source of competitive advantage in digital nutrition markets. Modular architectures, interoperable systems, and data-driven learning mechanisms allow platforms to deliver individualized recommendations at scale, supporting both elite teams and broader fitness populations. This scalability underpins platform-based revenue models, including enterprise licensing and ecosystem partnerships, while reinforcing user lock-in and long-term retention. The literature suggests that sustained business value ultimately depends on the alignment between technological capability, user experience, and adoption dynamics, positioning digital nutrition platforms as socio-technical systems rather than purely commercial products (Arshad et al., 2025; Aydın et al., 2025; Boland et al., 2019; Prasad et al., 2025; Sah et al., 2024; Selvi et al., 2022; Sun et al., 2025; Tsolakidis et al., 2024).

2.5 Digital Business–Driven Nutrition Platforms for Athletic Performance

Digital business–driven nutrition platforms represent a convergence of sports science, data analytics, and platform-based business models aimed at optimizing athletic performance through continuous, intelligence-enabled decision support. Unlike traditional sports nutrition approaches that emphasize the consumption of standardized products or static meal plans, these platforms operate as integrated digital ecosystems that deliver personalized nutritional guidance aligned with training demands, recovery cycles, and performance objectives. The defining characteristic of such platforms lies not only in their technological sophistication, but also in their ability to translate complex nutritional and physiological data into scalable, market-oriented services that generate both performance and economic value. These platforms function as multi-sided systems connecting athletes, performance practitioners, organizations, and technology providers within a shared data environment. By leveraging cloud infrastructure, subscription-based access, and interoperability with wearables and training management systems, digital nutrition platforms enable continuous engagement and long-term user relationships. This shift reflects a broader trend toward servitization and platformization in the sports industry. Consequently, nutrition becomes embedded within performance management workflows, reinforcing its strategic importance in high-performance sport contexts (Agrawal et al., 2025; Christodimitropoulou et al., 2025; Gabrišová et al., 2025; Paul et al., 2024; Puce et al., 2024; Ratten & Thompson, 2020; Sutehall & Pitsiladis, 2025; Wang et al., 2025; Westerbeek & Schaik, 2025).

Performance outcomes remain central to the value proposition of digital business–driven nutrition platforms. Empirical studies suggest that when nutrition data are synchronized with training load, recovery metrics, and competition schedules, platforms can support proactive interventions that enhance adaptation and reduce performance variability. This integration enables organizations to move from reactive nutrition support to anticipatory performance management, aligning nutritional strategies with broader athletic development objectives. Importantly, such capabilities are particularly attractive in elite and institutional sport environments, where marginal gains and risk mitigation have disproportionate competitive and financial implications (Bangsbo et al., 2025; Bonilla et al., 2025; Can & Can, 2025; Chatterjee & Sarkar, 2025; Grivas & Safari, 2025; Hwang & Yang, 2025; Luo & Song, 2025).

However, the literature also highlights challenges inherent to digital business–driven nutrition platforms, particularly regarding data governance, trust, and contextual adaptability. As platforms increasingly rely on algorithmic recommendations, concerns related to data ownership, privacy, and transparency become more salient, especially within highly regulated or culturally diverse environments. Moreover, while global platforms offer scalability and efficiency, their real-world effectiveness may be constrained by limited localization capabilities, uneven digital literacy levels among users, and varying degrees of institutional readiness across regions. Collectively, these challenges underscore the importance of aligning digital business strategies not only with user experience design and technology adoption dynamics, but also with broader organizational, regulatory, and socio-cultural contexts in the digital age (Abeltino et al., 2025; Arslan, 2025; Boland & Bronlund, 2019; Brewer et al., 2021; Christ et al., 2025; Madhumanchi, 2025; Prasad et al., 2025; Siddika et al., 2024; Wang et al., 2025).

3. METHODOLOGY

This study adopted a qualitative research design to explore user experiences and technology adoption dynamics within digital business–driven nutrition platforms for athletic performance. A qualitative approach is particularly appropriate given the exploratory nature of the research objectives and the need to capture rich, contextualized insights into how diverse stakeholders perceive, utilize, and derive value from AI-enabled nutrition platforms.

3.1 Research Design and Approach

The study employed a qualitative, interpretivist approach grounded in semi-structured interviews. This design allows for in-depth exploration of participants' lived experiences while maintaining sufficient flexibility to probe emerging themes related to user experience, value creation, and institutional constraints. Semi-structured interviews are particularly well suited to examining socio-technical systems, as they enable participants to articulate both technological and organizational dimensions of platform use in their own terms.

3.2 Participant Selection and Sampling Strategy

Several studies support the use of purposive sampling for qualitative interviews (Phuangsuwan et al., 2024). A purposive sampling strategy was used to recruit participants with direct experience in the adoption, implementation, or use of digital nutrition platforms. To ensure a comprehensive and balanced representation of perspectives, the sample consisted of 20 key stakeholders drawn from four core groups: athletes, performance nutritionists, coaches, and sports administrators. Each group was represented by five participants, enabling systematic comparison across operational, professional, and strategic roles within sport organizations. Participants varied in age, professional experience, and levels of engagement with digital nutrition platforms, ranging from daily end users to senior decision-makers and budget holders. This diversity enhanced the analytical depth of the study by capturing heterogeneous user experiences and adoption rationales across different institutional levels. Such variation is critical in qualitative research aimed at understanding complex adoption dynamics.

3.3 Data Collection Procedures

Data were collected through in-depth, semi-structured interviews conducted in December 2025. Interviews were scheduled at times convenient for participants and were conducted either face-to-face or via secure online communication platforms, depending on participant availability and preference. Each interview lasted approximately 45–60 minutes, allowing sufficient time for detailed discussion while minimizing participant fatigue. The interview protocol was designed around the study's three research objectives and included open-ended questions addressing: (1) user experiences with digital business–driven nutrition platforms, (2) perceptions of value creation beyond traditional sports nutrition products, and (3) contextual, organizational, and institutional factors influencing adoption and sustained use. Follow-up probes were used to clarify responses, explore examples, and elicit deeper reflection where appropriate. All interviews were conducted in a professional and confidential manner, and participants provided informed consent prior to participation. Demographic profile used age, gender, etc., based on the studies of Phuangsuwan et al. (2025).

3.4 Data Analysis

Interview data were analyzed using qualitative thematic analysis. Audio recordings were transcribed verbatim and reviewed multiple times to ensure accuracy and familiarity with the data. The analysis followed an iterative coding process, beginning with open coding to identify meaningful units of text related to user experience, adoption drivers, value perception, and implementation challenges. These initial codes were then grouped into higher-order categories through axial coding, enabling the identification of relationships and patterns across stakeholder groups. In addition, through selective coding, core themes were refined and aligned with the study's research objectives. The final analysis yielded three overarching thematic domains: stakeholder user experiences, mechanisms of digital business value creation, and contextual and institutional challenges affecting adoption and sustainability. Throughout the analysis, constant comparison was employed to examine similarities and differences across roles, thereby enhancing interpretive rigor and analytical coherence.

3.5 Trustworthiness and Rigor

To enhance the credibility and trustworthiness of the findings, several qualitative rigor strategies were employed. First, data triangulation was achieved by incorporating perspectives from multiple stakeholder groups with differing roles and responsibilities. Second, rich, verbatim quotations were used to ground interpretations in participants' own words, supporting transparency and analytical validity. Third, reflexive analysis was applied throughout the research process to minimize researcher bias and ensure that interpretations remained closely aligned with the data. While the study does not seek statistical generalization, the systematic sampling strategy, transparent analytic process, and role-based comparisons enhance the transferability of the findings to similar sport and digital business contexts.

4. RESULTS

The results reveal a multidimensional understanding of how key stakeholders perceive and engage with digital business–driven nutrition platforms within contemporary sport systems. Consistent with the qualitative research design, the findings draw on in-depth insights from participants representing athletes, performance nutritionists, coaches, and sports administrators, each occupying distinct yet interconnected roles in the adoption and use of these platforms. This diversity provides a strong foundation for examining how user experience, perceived value creation, and institutional considerations jointly shape technology adoption and sustained use. To contextualize the analysis, Table 1 presents the demographic and professional characteristics of the 20 participants. These profiles highlight variations in age, experience, role responsibilities, and levels of platform engagement, offering a nuanced backdrop for interpreting the perspectives, challenges, and strategic priorities that emerge across the interview data.

Table 1. Respondents' Demographic Information

No.	Age	Gender	Primary Role	Years of Experience	Level of Involvement with Digital Nutrition Platforms
R1	22	Male	Elite Athlete	6	Daily End User (Mobile App + Wearables)
R2	25	Female	Professional Athlete	8	Daily End User (Team-Mandated Platform)
R3	29	Male	Professional Athlete	11	Frequent User (Nutrition Tracking + Recovery)
R4	34	Female	Professional Athlete	12	Voluntary User (Subscription-Based Platform)
R5	27	Male	Collegiate Athlete	7	Institutional User (Team-Provided Platform)
R6	31	Female	Performance Nutritionist	9	System Administrator and Analyst
R7	38	Male	Performance Nutritionist	14	Power User (Data Interpretation and Reporting)
R8	35	Female	Sports Dietitian	10	Platform Configurator and Advisor
R9	42	Male	Head Performance Nutritionist	18	Strategic Decision-Maker
R10	28	Female	Assistant Nutritionist	5	Operational User
R11	45	Male	Head Coach	22	Decision Influencer (Non-Technical User)
R12	39	Female	Coach	15	Regular Dashboard User
R13	51	Male	Senior Coach	27	Occasional User (Summary Reports Only)
R14	36	Male	Performance Coach	13	Integrated User (Training + Nutrition Systems)
R15	41	Female	Assistant Coach	17	Supportive User
R16	48	Male	Sports Administrator	21	Procurement and Evaluation Role
R17	44	Female	High-Performance Director	19	Strategic Adopter and Budget Holder
R18	53	Male	Sports Policy Administrator	28	Oversight and Compliance Role
R19	37	Female	Operations Manager	12	Implementation Coordinator
R20	46	Male	Club General Manager	20	ROI-Focused Decision-Maker

Table 1 presents the demographic profile of the 20 key stakeholders interviewed in this study, reflecting a deliberately diverse and balanced qualitative sample aligned with the research objectives. The participants comprise four core stakeholder groups—athletes, performance nutritionists, coaches, and sports administrators—with each group represented by five respondents, ensuring an equitable distribution of perspectives across operational, professional, and strategic roles. The respondents range in age from 22 to 53 years, capturing both early-career and highly experienced individuals, while the gender distribution (11 males and 9 females) demonstrates a reasonable balance that enhances the inclusiveness and credibility of the findings. In terms of professional experience, participants report between 5 and 28 years of involvement in their respective roles, allowing the study to incorporate both contemporary, technology-forward viewpoints and seasoned institutional perspectives. Importantly, levels of engagement with digital nutrition platforms vary substantially across respondents, ranging from daily end users to strategic decision-makers and budget holders. This variation enables a nuanced examination of user experiences, perceived value creation, and institutional challenges associated with the adoption and sustained use of digital business–driven nutrition platforms, thereby strengthening the depth and interpretive richness of the qualitative analysis.

The analysis of the interview data revealed three interrelated thematic domains corresponding to the study's research objectives: (1) stakeholder user experiences with digital business–driven nutrition platforms, (2) mechanisms of value creation beyond traditional sports nutrition products, and (3) contextual and institutional challenges shaping implementation and sustained use. Across stakeholder groups, participants articulated nuanced and sometimes contrasting perspectives that reflect differences in role responsibilities, professional priorities, and levels of engagement with AI-enabled nutrition systems.

4.1 User Experiences with Digital Business–Driven Nutrition Platforms

Athletes consistently framed their user experience around usability, immediacy, and the extent to which digital platforms translated complex nutritional information into clear, actionable guidance. Several athletes emphasized that real-time feedback and personalized recommendations enhanced daily adherence, confidence, and motivation. One athlete explained that *"the system makes nutrition feel connected to my training, not like a separate task I have to remember on my own"* (R1, personal communication, interviewed in December 2025). Similarly, another participant noted that automated suggestions reduced uncertainty and decision fatigue, stating that *"I don't need to guess what or when to eat anymore; the app adjusts based on my workload"* (R2, personal communication, interviewed in December 2025).

Furthermore, more experienced athletes highlighted the role of data visualization in sustaining long-term engagement. As one respondent remarked, *"seeing trends over time helped me understand how nutrition affects recovery, not just performance on one day"* (R3, personal communication, interviewed in December 2025). Others emphasized flexibility, noting that platforms were most useful when they accommodated individual preferences rather than imposing rigid plans: *"it works best when it adapts to me, not when it forces a fixed routine"* (R4, personal communication, interviewed in December 2025). Collegiate athletes, in particular, valued integration with team systems, with one participant explaining that *"having the same platform as the coaching staff makes communication easier and expectations clearer"* (R5, personal communication, interviewed in December 2025).

Performance nutritionists and dietitians evaluated user experience through a more analytical lens, emphasizing data accuracy, customization, and workflow compatibility. One nutritionist explained that *"the real value is not the meal plan itself, but the ability to adjust it continuously based on performance and recovery data"* (R6, personal communication, interviewed in December 2025). Another highlighted efficiency gains, noting that *"what used to take hours of manual tracking can now be reviewed in minutes"* (R7, personal communication, interviewed in December 2025). However, participants also cautioned against excessive complexity, with one stating that *"if the dashboard is too technical, it slows down practical decision-making"* (R8, personal communication, interviewed in December 2025).

Senior nutrition professionals emphasized strategic oversight rather than daily interaction. As one respondent noted, *"I use the platform less for daily inputs and more to identify patterns and risks across athletes"* (R9, personal communication, interviewed in December 2025). Early-career professionals echoed this perspective while emphasizing learning benefits, explaining that *"the system helps standardize best practices, especially for less experienced staff"* (R10, personal communication, interviewed in December 2025).

Coaches described user experience primarily in terms of clarity and relevance to training decisions. One head coach explained that *"I don't need all the data, just clear insights that link nutrition to performance outcomes"* (R11, personal communication, interviewed in December 2025). Others valued platforms that aligned nutrition with conditioning goals, noting that *"when nutrition data matches training phases, it becomes easier to plan workloads"* (R12, personal communication, interviewed in December 2025). More senior coaches expressed selective engagement, with one stating that *"I rely on summaries rather than raw data, but those summaries still influence my decisions"* (R13, personal communication, interviewed in December 2025). Performance-focused coaches emphasized integration, observing that *"nutrition makes more sense when it's part of the same system as training and recovery"* (R14, personal communication, interviewed in December 2025). Assistant coaches highlighted coordination benefits, explaining that *"shared access improves consistency across the support team"* (R15, personal communication, interviewed in December 2025).

The findings demonstrate that user experience with digital business–driven nutrition platforms is fundamentally role-dependent and shaped by the extent of interaction with the system. Athletes prioritize usability, immediacy, and personalization that translates complex nutritional data into actionable guidance supporting daily routines and behavioral adherence. In contrast, sport-related professionals emphasize analytical depth, data reliability, and workflow integration, viewing user experience as a function of decision support rather than interface simplicity alone. Administrators evaluate user experience through clarity and strategic relevance of aggregated insights rather than direct system engagement. Collectively, these perspectives indicate that effective platforms must accommodate heterogeneous user needs across operational, professional, and strategic levels, reinforcing the importance of adaptive, multi-layered design in sustaining engagement and perceived usefulness.

4.2 Value Creation Beyond Traditional Sports Nutrition Products

Across stakeholder groups, digital nutrition platforms were perceived as generating value that extends well beyond traditional product-based approaches. Nutritionists and coaches emphasized the role of these platforms in enabling proactive performance management and informed decision-making, with one participant stating that *"the platform helps us anticipate problems rather than reacting after performance drops"* (R6, personal communication, interviewed in December 2025). Moreover, another respondent observed a broader strategic shift, noting that *"nutrition has shifted from a supporting role to a strategic performance variable"* (R12, personal communication, interviewed in December 2025).

Athletes framed value in terms of confidence and accountability. One of the respondents explained that *"having data-backed recommendations makes me trust the process more"* (R1, personal communication, interviewed in December 2025), while another emphasized consistency, stating that *"it keeps me disciplined even when motivation is low"* (R5, personal communication, interviewed in December 2025). Moreover, from an organizational perspective, administrators highlighted economic and managerial value. One senior administrator observed that *"we now see nutrition as an investment in performance sustainability, not just a cost"* (R16, personal communication, interviewed in December 2025).

Decision-makers further emphasized return on investment and risk reduction. As one high-performance director explained, *"if the platform helps reduce injuries or downtime, the financial value is obvious"* (R17, personal communication, interviewed in December 2025). Policy-oriented stakeholders framed value in terms of governance and standardization, with one respondent noting that *"digital platforms provide transparency and documentation that traditional approaches cannot"* (R18, personal communication, interviewed in December 2025). Operational managers echoed this sentiment, explaining that *"data integration improves coordination and reduces inefficiencies across departments"* (R19, personal communication, interviewed in December 2025). Club executives emphasized strategic alignment, stating that *"these systems support long-term planning rather than short-term fixes"* (R20, personal communication, interviewed in December 2025).

The results indicate that digital nutrition platforms generate multidimensional value that extends beyond traditional product-based sports nutrition models. Rather than functioning as consumption tools, these platforms operate as intelligence-driven decision-support systems that enable proactive performance management, risk mitigation, and organizational learning. In addition, athletes derive value through enhanced confidence, consistency, and accountability, while professionals leverage data integration to anticipate performance issues and optimize interventions. At the organizational level, administrators and executives frame value in terms of cost efficiency, injury reduction, and long-term performance sustainability. This shift reflects a broader transformation of sports nutrition from a transactional expense to a strategic asset embedded within performance management infrastructures.

4.3 Challenges Affecting Adoption and Sustainability

Despite widespread recognition of the potential benefits, participants identified significant barriers to both initial adoption and sustained use of digital solutions. Digital literacy emerged as a recurring concern across stakeholder groups, with one respondent noting that *"not everyone is comfortable interpreting data, especially at the beginning"* (R8, personal communication, interviewed in December 2025). In parallel, budgetary constraints were frequently cited by administrators, who emphasized financial sustainability, with one stating that *"cost justification becomes challenging when benefits are long-term rather than immediate"* (R16, personal communication, interviewed in December 2025).

Cultural resistance also shaped adoption dynamics. One senior coach explained that *"there is still skepticism toward algorithm-driven recommendations, especially among experienced staff"* (R13, personal communication, interviewed in December 2025). Data governance and privacy concerns were highlighted by policy and executive stakeholders, with one participant emphasizing that *"data security and ownership must be clearly defined before full adoption"* (R18, personal communication, interviewed in December 2025).

Athletes also noted contextual challenges, particularly in maintaining consistent use over time. As one participant explained, *"the system works best when everyone commits, but consistency can drop during busy periods"* (R3, personal communication, interviewed in December 2025). Others highlighted the importance of organizational support, stating that *"without clear guidance from staff, it's easy to disengage"* (R4, personal communication, interviewed in December 2025). Ultimately, the adoption and sustainability are shaped not only by technological capability, but also by institutional readiness, cultural acceptance, and resource availability. As one executive succinctly summarized, *"technology alone does not transform performance; the organization has to be ready to use it"* (R20, personal communication, interviewed in December 2025).

Despite strong perceived benefits, the adoption and sustained use of AI-enabled nutrition platforms are constrained by contextual and institutional factors. Digital literacy gaps, budgetary limitations, and cultural resistance to algorithmic decision-making emerged as persistent barriers across stakeholder groups. Concerns related to data governance, privacy, and organizational readiness shape the pace and depth of implementation. These challenges underscore that technology adoption is not a purely technical process, but a socio-institutional one requiring alignment between technological capabilities, human competencies, and organizational structures. Sustainable adoption therefore depends on supportive leadership, clear governance frameworks, and ongoing capacity-building rather than technological sophistication alone.

4.4 Conceptual Model Development from Qualitative Findings

This study presents the conceptual model derived from the qualitative analysis, illustrating the socio-technical mechanisms through which digital business–driven nutrition platforms create value in athletic performance contexts.

Figure 1. A Socio-Technical Conceptual Model of User Experience, Technology Adoption, and Value Creation in Digital Business–Driven Nutrition Platforms

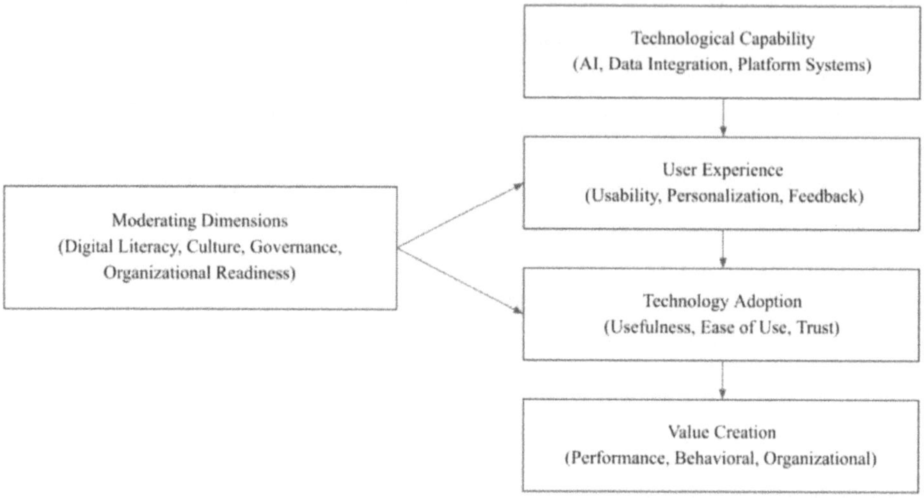

The model, presented in Figure 1, was developed through a thematic analysis of participant narratives, which revealed a sequential and interdependent relationship between technological capability, user experience, technology adoption, and value creation.

The findings indicate that technological capability—including artificial intelligence, data integration, and platform-based infrastructures—serves as the foundational enabler of digital nutrition systems. However, participants consistently emphasized that the mere presence of advanced technology does not guarantee effective outcomes. Instead, its impact is mediated through user experience, particularly in terms of usability, personalization, and real-time feedback. These elements shape how users interact with the platform and determine whether technological features are perceived as accessible and meaningful in practice. Furthermore, the analysis highlights that a positive user experience facilitates technology adoption, which is influenced by users' perceptions of usefulness, ease of use, and trust in algorithmic recommendations. Participants expressed that trust and interpretability are especially critical in contexts involving health and performance decisions, where reliance on digital systems must be justified through transparent and reliable outputs. The model also demonstrates that successful adoption leads to multidimensional value creation, encompassing enhanced athletic performance, improved behavioral adherence to nutritional plans, and organizational benefits such as efficiency gains and reduced risk of injury. Importantly, the qualitative findings revealed that these relationships are not linear but are shaped by a set of moderating socio-technical factors, including digital literacy, organizational readiness, cultural attitudes toward technology, and data governance concerns. These factors influence both user experience and adoption processes, either enabling or constraining the realization of value. Overall, the conceptual model underscores that value creation in digital nutrition platforms emerges from the dynamic interaction between technological systems and human actors within specific institutional contexts. It reinforces the importance of aligning technological innovation with user-centered design and organizational capabilities to achieve sustainable performance outcomes.

5. DISCUSSIONS

This study provides qualitative insight into how digital business–driven nutrition platforms are experienced, adopted, and valued within contemporary sport systems. By foregrounding stakeholder perspectives, the findings extend existing literature by demonstrating that AI-enabled nutrition platforms operate not merely as technological innovations, but as socio-technical systems whose effectiveness depends on the alignment between user experience, organizational context, and digital business strategy. While prior research has largely emphasized algorithmic capability or physiological outcomes, the present findings highlight the human and institutional mechanisms through which these platforms generate sustained performance and business value.

The findings reinforce existing evidence that user experience is a critical determinant of engagement and continued use in digital nutrition and health platforms (Adu et al., 2020; Fanani et al., 2023; Figueiredo et al., 2025). Athletes' emphasis on usability, immediacy, and actionable guidance aligns with prior studies showing that platforms which reduce cognitive load and integrate seamlessly into daily routines are more likely to support adherence in high-performance environments (Dunne et al., 2022; Jiang et al., 2025). Real-time feedback, adaptive recommendations, and longitudinal data visualization were perceived as particularly valuable, corroborating research suggesting that personalization and continuous feedback loops enhance perceived usefulness and trust in AI-driven systems (Cossich et al., 2023; Sah et al., 2024). Technological sophistication alone is insufficient; rather, value is realized when complex nutritional intelligence is translated into clear, context-sensitive guidance.

At the same time, the results extend the literature by illustrating that user experience is inherently role-dependent. Performance nutritionists and coaches evaluated platforms less in terms of interface simplicity and more in terms of data accuracy, customization, and workflow integration, echoing prior work on heterogeneous user needs within sport organizations (Luczak et al., 2020; Putra et al., 2024). Administrators and executives, by contrast, interacted primarily with aggregated dashboards and strategic summaries, reflecting research that highlights the importance of multi-layered platform design capable of supporting operational, professional, and strategic decision-making simultaneously (Chatterjee & Sarkar, 2025; Sonnen, 2024). These findings support a socio-technical view of user experience in which perceived value emerges from role-specific relevance rather than uniform usability standards.

The study also provides empirical support for the growing body of literature that frames digital nutrition platforms as intelligence-driven performance infrastructures rather than product-based nutrition tools. Participants consistently described value creation in terms of proactive decision-making, injury risk mitigation, and long-term performance sustainability, aligning with research on nutritional periodization and integrated performance management systems (Jeukendrup, 2017; Morton et al., 2025; Turner et al., 2025). By embedding nutritional logic within algorithmic architectures synchronized with training and recovery data, platforms reduce manual complexity while enhancing precision, supporting prior claims that automation and data fusion are central to scalable personalization in elite sport contexts (Grivas & Safari, 2025; Luo & Song, 2025; Quan et al., 2026; Wang et al., 2026).

From a digital business perspective, the findings reinforce the conceptual shift from transactional sports nutrition models toward "Intelligence-as-a-Service" paradigms. Administrators' emphasis on return on investment, cost efficiency, and performance sustainability mirrors prior research positioning digital platforms as strategic assets embedded within broader, data-intensive performance ecosystems (Boland & Bronlund, 2019; Jalonen et al., 2018; Qi et al., 2024). Furthermore, this transition reflects wider trends in platformization and servitization within the sports industry, where continuous, data-driven decision support and analytics-enabled learning loops, rather than discrete product consumption, underpin competitive advantage and long-term value creation (Kretschmer et al., 2022; Ratten & Thompson, 2020; Westerbeek & Schaik, 2025). The findings therefore move beyond conceptual discussion by providing grounded qualitative evidence of how this transformation is practically experienced, strategically rationalized, and organizationally justified by key stakeholders.

Despite strong perceived benefits, the findings also reveal persistent challenges that constrain adoption and long-term sustainability. Digital literacy gaps, cultural resistance to algorithmic recommendations, and financial constraints were repeatedly identified, aligning with prior research on technology adoption in sport and healthcare settings (Cho et al., 2020; Jaswal et al., 2022; Roppelt et al., 2024). In addition, skepticism among experienced practitioners reflects concerns about professional autonomy and trust in automated decision-making, supporting emerging literature on the social and ethical dimensions of AI adoption in elite sport (Saadati & Torres, 2024; Westerbeek & Schaik, 2025). Similarly, concerns related to data governance and privacy resonate with broader debates on digital responsibility and data ownership in platform-based systems (Brewer et al., 2021; Christ et al., 2025).

Crucially, the findings underscore that adoption is not a linear or purely individual-level process, as implied by traditional technology acceptance models, but a socio-institutional one shaped by leadership support, organizational readiness, and governance structures. This aligns with prior work emphasizing that sustainable digital transformation requires institutional alignment and capacity building rather than technological deployment alone (Alojail & Khan, 2023; Casey et al., 2012; Amanollahnejad et al., 2026). Athletes' reports of declining engagement during high-demand periods further highlight the need for structured support mechanisms and clear organizational expectations to sustain long-term use.

Overall, the study's discussion demonstrates that the effectiveness of digital business–driven nutrition platforms emerges from the dynamic interplay between technological capability, user experience, and institutional context. By integrating stakeholder perspectives across multiple organizational roles, this study advances existing literature by empirically framing these platforms as embedded socio-technical systems rather than standalone or purely technical digital tools. In doing so, it bridges important gaps between sports nutrition, digital business, and technology adoption research, offering a more holistic and practice-relevant understanding of how AI-enabled nutrition platforms generate both performance-related and economic value within contemporary, high-performance sport environments.

6. CONCLUSION

This chapter examined the role of digital business–driven nutrition platforms in supporting athletic performance, with a particular focus on user experience, technology adoption, and value creation. Drawing on qualitative insights from athletes, performance nutritionists, coaches, and sports administrators, the study demonstrated that AI-enabled nutrition platforms function as socio-technical systems embedded within organizational and institutional contexts, rather than as standalone technological solutions. The findings highlight that the effectiveness of these platforms depends not only on algorithmic sophistication, but also on their alignment with user needs, professional practices, and governance structures.

The study contributes to the literature by empirically substantiating the shift from traditional, product-centric sports nutrition models toward intelligence-based, platform-driven value creation. Digital nutrition platforms were shown to deliver value primarily through continuous decision support, personalized insights, and integrative performance management rather than through the provision of nutritional products alone. Importantly, the chapter underscores that sustained adoption and impact are contingent upon user trust, role-specific relevance, and organizational readiness. By integrating perspectives across multiple stakeholder groups, the study offers a holistic understanding of how digital nutrition platforms generate both performance and business value in contemporary sport ecosystems.

7. IMPLICATIONS

The findings of this study have several important implications for theory, practice, and digital business strategy. From a theoretical perspective, the results support socio-technical and platform ecosystem frameworks by demonstrating that technology adoption in sports nutrition cannot be adequately explained by individual-level acceptance models alone. Instead, adoption and value creation emerge through the interaction of technological capability, user experience design, and institutional context. This insight contributes to ongoing debates in digital business and sports management literature by positioning AI-enabled nutrition platforms as embedded performance infrastructures rather than discrete innovations. From a practical standpoint, the findings suggest that platform developers should prioritize role-specific user experience design, ensuring that interfaces, analytics, and decision-support tools are tailored to the distinct needs of athletes, practitioners, and administrators. Simplified, actionable outputs are critical for athletes, while advanced analytical capabilities and data integration are essential for nutritionists and coaches. For sport organizations, the results highlight the importance of leadership support, change management, and digital literacy development in facilitating sustainable adoption. Investment decisions should therefore account not only for technological features, but also for training, governance, and long-term integration into performance workflows. From a digital business perspective, the study underscores the strategic potential of "Intelligence-as-a-Service" models in sports nutrition markets. Platform-based revenue structures, scalable personalization, and ecosystem partnerships offer pathways for sustained competitive advantage. However, these benefits can only be realized if platforms successfully balance data-driven automation with transparency, trust, and ethical data governance.

8. LIMITATIONS

Despite its contributions, this study is subject to several limitations that warrant acknowledgement. First, the research adopted a qualitative design with a purposive sample of 20 participants, which constrains the generalizability of the findings beyond the specific organizational and sporting contexts examined. While this approach enabled rich, in-depth exploration of stakeholder experiences, the results may not fully capture variations across different sports, competitive levels, institutional settings, or geographical regions. Second, the study relied on self-reported perceptions and experiences, which may be influenced by recall bias or social desirability effects. As such, participants' accounts reflect subjective interpretations of platform use and perceived value, rather than objectively measured performance, health, or economic outcomes. Third, the cross-sectional nature of the data captures adoption and usage dynamics at a single point in time and does not account for how perceptions, practices, and value assessments may evolve as platforms mature, algorithms adapt, or organizational conditions change. Finally, although the study integrates multiple stakeholder perspectives, it does not incorporate direct analysis of platform usage logs or system-level performance metrics, which could provide more granular insight into actual behavioral patterns, decision-making processes, and measurable outcomes.

9. FUTURE RESEARCH

Future research should build on the study's findings by adopting mixed-methods or longitudinal research designs to examine how user experience, technology adoption, and value creation processes evolve over time. Quantitative studies incorporating platform usage analytics, performance indicators, and organizational outcomes would complement qualitative insights and enable stronger causal inferences regarding the effects of digital nutrition platforms on athletic, health, and economic performance. Further research could also pursue cross-sport and cross-cultural comparative analyses to investigate how institutional norms, regulatory environments, and resource availability shape platform adoption and utilization dynamics. Future studies should also examine ethical, governance, and data ownership considerations in greater depth, particularly as AI-driven nutrition platforms become increasingly embedded within elite, professional, and commercial sport ecosystems. Finally, there is substantial scope for theory development that integrates perspectives from sports nutrition, digital business, and platform ecosystem research. Conceptual frameworks that explicitly link user experience design, organizational readiness, and intelligence-based value creation would advance scholarly understanding while offering actionable guidance for practitioners seeking to leverage AI-enabled nutrition platforms in increasingly data-intensive sport environments.

REFERENCES

Abeltino, A., Riente, A., Bianchetti, G., Serantoni, C., Spirito, M. D., Capezzone, S., Esposito, R., & Maulucci, G. (2025). Digital applications for diet monitoring, planning, and precision nutrition for citizens and professionals: A state of the art. *Nutrition Reviews*, *83*(2), e574–e601. DOI: 10.1093/nutrit/nuae035 PMID: 38722240

Adu, M. D., Malabu, U. H., Malau-Aduli, A. E., Drovandi, A., & Malau-Aduli, B. S. (2020). User retention and engagement with a mobile app intervention to support self-management in Australians with type 1 or type 2 diabetes (My Care Hub): Mixed methods study. *JMIR mHealth and uHealth*, *8*(6), e17802. DOI: 10.2196/17802 PMID: 32525491

Agrawal, K., Goktas, P., Kumar, N., & Leung, M. F. (2025). Artificial intelligence in personalized nutrition and food manufacturing: A comprehensive review of methods, applications, and future directions. *Frontiers in Nutrition*, *12*, 1636980. DOI: 10.3389/fnut.2025.1636980 PMID: 40771216

Ahmad, M., Naqvi, R., & Ashfaq, Q. (2025). Developing a performance-based nutrition mobile application design and implementation. *Insights-Journal of Health and Rehabilitation*, *3*(2), 772–779. DOI: 10.71000/z873q831

Ajibesin, A. A. G., N., & Thangavel, S. K. (Eds.). (2025). *Synergizing data envelopment analysis and machine learning for performance optimization in healthcare.* IGI Global Scientific Publishing. DOI: 10.4018/979-8-3373-0081-8

Ajiye, O. T., Olajide, F. O., Ologunja, Y. S., Bamidele, S. O., Badmus, Y. K., & Appah, O. H. (2025). The impact of digital technologies, recreation, and nutrition on stress management and mental well-being in athletes. *Journal of Education, Learning, and Management*, *2*(2), 364–382. DOI: 10.69739/jelm.v2i2.1209

Alojail, M., & Khan, S. B. (2023). Impact of digital transformation toward sustainable development. *Sustainability (Basel)*, *15*(20), 14697. DOI: 10.3390/su152014697

Amanollahnejad, A., Fosso-Wamba, S., Shabbir, M. S., & Pakseresht, A. (2026). Aligning socio-technical systems: Rethinking AI adoption and digital transformation in SMEs. *Information Systems Management*, *43*(2), 1–15. DOI: 10.1080/10580530.2025.2612175

Amawi, A., AlKasasbeh, W., Jaradat, M., Almasri, A., Alobaidi, S., Hammad, A. A., Bishtawi, T., Fataftah, B., Turk, N., Saoud, H. A., Jarrar, A., & Ghazzawi, H. (2024). Athletes' nutritional demands: A narrative review of nutritional requirements. *Frontiers in Nutrition*, *10*, 1331854. DOI: 10.3389/fnut.2023.1331854 PMID: 38328685

Arenas-Jal, M., Suñé-Negre, J. M., Pérez-Lozano, P., & García-Montoya, E. (2020). Trends in the food and sports nutrition industry: A review. *Critical Reviews in Food Science and Nutrition*, *60*(14), 2405–2421. DOI: 10.1080/10408398.2019.1643287 PMID: 31352832

Armand, T. P. T., Nfor, K. A., Kim, J. I., & Kim, H. C. (2024). Applications of artificial intelligence, machine learning, and deep learning in nutrition: A systematic review. *Nutrients*, *16*(7), 1073. DOI: 10.3390/nu16071073 PMID: 38613106

Arshad, M. T., Ali, M. K. M., Maqsood, S., Ikram, A., Ahmed, F., Aljameel, A. I., Al-Farga, A., & Hossain, M. S. (2025). Personalized nutrition in the era of digital health: A new frontier for managing diabetes and obesity. *Food Science & Nutrition*, *13*(10), e71006. DOI: 10.1002/fsn3.71006 PMID: 41019177

Arslan, S. (2025). Artificial intelligence in food safety and nutrition practices: Opportunities and risks. *Academia Nutrition and Dietetics*, *2*(3), 1–11. DOI: 10.20935/AcadNutr7904

Aydın, S. K., Ali, R. H., Faiz, S., & Khan, T. A. (2025). An integrated AI framework for personalized nutrition using machine learning and natural language processing for dietary recommendations. *Applied Sciences (Basel, Switzerland)*, *15*(17), 9283. DOI: 10.3390/app15179283

Balaji, D. P., Kalayci, P. D., & Ramkumar, S. S. (Eds.). (2025). *Advances in sports science and technology* (1st ed.). CRC Press., DOI: 10.1201/9781003616283

Bangsbo, J., Hostrup, M., Hellsten, Y., Hansen, M. H., Melin, A., Kjær, M., Burr, J. F., Engebretsen, L., Egan, B., Hackney, A. C., Chambers, T. L., Jones, A. M., Pitsiladis, Y., Magnusson, S. P., Petersen, J., Deshmukh, A. S., Calbet, J. A. L., Elliott-Sale, K. J., Joyner, M. J., & Moesgaard, L. (2025). Consensus statements—Optimizing performance of the elite athlete. *Scandinavian Journal of Medicine & Science in Sports*, *35*(8), e70112. DOI: 10.1111/sms.70112 PMID: 40781883

Boland, M., Alam, F., & Bronlund, J. (2019). Modern technologies for personalized nutrition. In Galanakis, C. M. (Ed.), *Trends in Personalized Nutrition* (pp. 195–222). Academic Press., DOI: 10.1016/B978-0-12-816403-7.00006-4

Boland, M., & Bronlund, J. (2019). eNutrition-The next dimension for eHealth? *Trends in Food Science & Technology*, *91*, 634–639. DOI: 10.1016/j.tifs.2019.08.001

Bonilla, D. A., Stout, J. R., Gleeson, M., Campbell, B. I., Escalante, G., Rojas-Valverde, D., Petro, J. L., Kreider, R. B., & Odriozola-Martínez, A. (2025). The 4Rs framework of sports nutrition: An update with recommendations to evaluate allostatic load in athletes. *Life (Basel, Switzerland)*, *15*(6), 867. DOI: 10.3390/life15060867 PMID: 40566521

Brewer, S., Pearson, S., Maull, R., Godsiff, P., Frey, J. G., Zisman, A., Parr, G., McMillan, A., Cameron, S., Blackmore, H., Manning, L., & Bidaut, L. (2021). A trust framework for digital food systems. *Nature Food*, *2*(8), 543–545. DOI: 10.1038/s43016-021-00346-1 PMID: 37118166

Budhiraja, A. (2025). The winning edge: Leveraging data-driven decision making in modern sports management. *International Journal For Multidisciplinary Research*, *7*(4), 1–9. DOI: 10.36948/ijfmr.2025.v07i04.43883

Can, S., & Can, H. (Eds.). (2025). *Evaluating the effectiveness of functional ingredients in sports nutrition*. IGI Global Scientific Publishing., DOI: 10.4018/979-8-3693-8699-6

Casey, M. M., Payne, W. R., & Eime, R. M. (2012). Organisational readiness and capacity building strategies of sporting organisations to promote health. *Sport Management Review*, *15*(1), 109–124. DOI: 10.1016/j.smr.2011.01.001

Charfare, R., Desai, A., Keni, N., Nambiar, A., & Cherian, M. (2025). Smart healthcare framework: Real-time vital monitoring and personalized diet and fitness recommendations using IoT and machine learning. *International Journal of Robotics and Control Systems*, *5*(2), 1254–1277. DOI: 10.31763/ijrcs.v5i2.1839

Chatterjee, A., & Sarkar, T. (Eds.). (2025). *Examining physiology, nutrition, and body composition in sports science*. IGI Global Scientific Publishing., DOI: 10.4018/979-8-3693-6317-1

Chen, Z. (2025). Empowering sports in the digital economy: Change, opportunity and the future. *Highlights in Business. Economics and Management*, *59*, 34–39. DOI: 10.54097/ddqnsm75

Chhabra, G., Kumar, S., Gupta, S., & Nagpal, P. (2023). Technology for nutrition, fitness, and sports. In *Artificial Intelligence to Analyze Psychophysical and Human Lifestyle* (pp. 105–112). Springer Nature Singapore., DOI: 10.1007/978-981-99-3039-5_9

Cho, H., Chi, C., & Chiu, W. (2020). Understanding sustained usage of health and fitness apps: Incorporating the technology acceptance model with the investment model. *Technology in Society*, *63*, 101429. DOI: 10.1016/j.techsoc.2020.101429

Chopvitayakun, S., Rattanasiriwongwut, M., & Ketcham, M. (2025). Factors influencing mobile platform adoption for nutritional tracking among Thai elderly: A unified UTAUT and STAM approach. *Journal of Open Innovation, 11*(3), 100606. DOI: 10.1016/j.joitmc.2025.100606

Choudhury, T., Arya, P., Kotecha, K., Sharma, A., & Um, J. (Eds.). (2025). *AI and machine learning applications in sports analytics*. IGI Global Scientific Publishing., DOI: 10.4018/979-8-3693-5385-1

Christ, A. S., Carl, K. V., Kurtz, C., Lobschat, L., Mueller, B., & Zimmer, M. P. (2025). Taking digital responsibility for data: Toward a governance model for user-generated data. *Schmalenbachs Zeitschrift für Betriebswirtschaftliche Forschung = Schmalenbach Journal of Business Research, 77*(3), 527–556. DOI: 10.1007/s41471-025-00225-6

Christodimitropoulou, M., Choustoulakis, E., & Antonopoulou, P. (2025). Digital transformation in sports management: Technologies, trends, and strategic implications. *European Journal of Management and Marketing Studies, 10*(2), 135–152. DOI: 10.46827/ejmms.v10i2.2031

Cossich, V. R., Carlgren, D., Holash, R. J., & Katz, L. (2023). Technological breakthroughs in sport: Current practice and future potential of artificial intelligence, virtual reality, augmented reality, and modern data visualization in performance analysis. *Applied Sciences (Basel, Switzerland), 13*(23), 12965. DOI: 10.3390/app132312965

Du, T., & Bi, N. (2025). Application of artificial intelligence advances in athletics industry: A review. *Concurrency and Computation, 37*(3), e8372. DOI: 10.1002/cpe.8372

Dunne, D. M., Lefevre-Lewis, C., Cunniffe, B., Impey, S. G., Tod, D., Close, G. L., Morton, J. P., & Murphy, R. (2022). Athlete experiences of communication strategies in applied sports nutrition and future considerations for mobile app supportive solutions. *Frontiers in Sports and Active Living, 4*, 911412. DOI: 10.3389/fspor.2022.911412 PMID: 36172339

Esco, M. R., Fields, A. D., Mohammadnabi, M. A., & Kliszczewicz, B. M. (2025). Monitoring training adaptation and recovery status in athletes using heart rate variability via mobile devices: A narrative review. *Sensors (Basel), 26*(1), 3. DOI: 10.3390/s26010003 PMID: 41516438

Fanani, L., Az-Zahra, H. M., Akbar, M. A., & Sianturi, R. S. (2023). User experience design for nutrition information applications using design thinking. *MATICS: Jurnal Ilmu Komputer dan Teknologi Informasi, 15*(1), 43-50. DOI: 10.18860/mat.v15i1.23025

Figueiredo, T., Alcântara, L., Carrilho, J., Paúl, C., & Costa, E. (2025). Understanding adherence to digital health technologies: Systematic review of predictive factors. *Journal of Medical Internet Research*, *27*, e77362. DOI: 10.2196/77362 PMID: 41248309

Gabrišová, I., Koman, G., Soviar, J., & Holubčík, M. (2025). The adoption of modern sports technologies from professional settings to everyday life. *Administrative Sciences*, *15*(7), 249. DOI: 10.3390/admsci15070249

Grivas, G. V., & Safari, K. (2025). Artificial intelligence in endurance sports: Metabolic, recovery, and nutritional perspectives. *Nutrients*, *17*(20), 3209. DOI: 10.3390/nu17203209 PMID: 41156462

Hexis. (2023, December 7). *Technology unlocks the future of sports nutrition.* https://www.hexis.live/blog/technology-unlocks-the-future-of-sports-nutrition

Hwang, D.-J., & Yang, H.-J. (2025). Nutritional strategies for enhancing performance and training adaptation in weightlifters. *International Journal of Molecular Sciences*, *26*(1), 240. DOI: 10.3390/ijms26010240 PMID: 39796095

Jacobsson, J., Kowalski, J., Timpka, T., Hansson, P. O., Spreco, A., & Dahlstrom, O. (2023). Universal prevention through a digital health platform reduces injury incidence in youth athletics (track and field): A cluster randomised controlled trial. *British Journal of Sports Medicine*, *57*(6), 364–371. DOI: 10.1136/bjsports-2021-105332 PMID: 36564148

Jalonen, H., Tuominen, S., Ryömä, A., Haltia, J., Nenonen, J., & Kuikka, A. (2018). How does value creation manifest itself in the nexus of sport and business? A systematic literature review. *Open Journal of Business and Management*, *6*(1), 103–138. DOI: 10.4236/ojbm.2018.61008

Jaswal, R. S., Stergiou, P., & Katz, L. (2022). How Canadian high-performance coaches adopt and implement technology: Exploring the antecedents of intra- and interorganizational trust, technological proficiency, and subjective norms and social influence on technology adoption. *International Sport Coaching Journal*, *9*(2), 234–243. DOI: 10.1123/iscj.2020-0088

Jeukendrup, A. E. (2017). Periodized nutrition for athletes. *Sports Medicine*, *47*(S1, Suppl 1), 51–63. DOI: 10.1007/s40279-017-0694-2 PMID: 28332115

Jiang, X., Timmons, M., Boroda, E., & Onakomaiya, M. (2025). Impact of platform design and usability on adherence and retention: Randomized web- and mobile-based longitudinal study. *Journal of Participatory Medicine*, *17*, e50225. DOI: 10.2196/50225 PMID: 40152343

Kanwal, S., Ahsan, M. T, Khan, R. N., & Khan, A. (2025). Load management and injury prevention in elite athletes: A narrative review. *Premier Journal of Science*, 1-7. DOI: 10.70389/PJS.100088

Karnika, S., Sharma, S., Singh, A., Batth, S. S., & Sharma, A. (2025). From data to diet: The impact of artificial intelligence on nutritional science. *Journal of Scientific Research and Reports*, *31*(8), 449–458. DOI: 10.9734/jsrr/2025/v31i83388

Kassem, H., Beevi, A. A., Basheer, S., Lutfi, G., Cheikh Ismail, L., & Papandreou, D. (2025). Investigation and assessment of ai's role in nutrition—An updated narrative review of the evidence. *Nutrients*, *17*(1), 190. DOI: 10.3390/nu17010190 PMID: 39796624

Kretschmer, T., Leiponen, A., Schilling, M., & Vasudeva, G. (2022). Platform ecosystems as meta-organizations: Implications for platform strategies. *Strategic Management Journal*, *43*(3), 405–424. DOI: 10.1002/smj.3250

Lee, Y. K., Yoon, E. J., Kim, T. H., Kim, J. I., & Kim, J. H. (2025). Musculoskeletal digital therapeutics and digital health rehabilitation: A global paradigm shift in orthopedic care. *Journal of Clinical Medicine*, *14*(23), 8467. DOI: 10.3390/jcm14238467 PMID: 41375770

Lemire, J. (2023, April 12). *How Hexis is aiming to help athletes optimize performance with their AI-powered nutrition app.* Sports Business Journal. https://www.sportsbusinessjournal.com/Journal/Issues/2023/04/10/Technology/hexis/

Liu, J., Yu, H., Cheung, W. C., Bleakney, A., & Jan, Y. K. (2025). Societal attitudes and structural barriers in coaching para-athletes: A mixed-methods systematic review. *PLoS One*, *20*(6), e0326585. DOI: 10.1371/journal.pone.0326585 PMID: 40560855

Liu, Y., Lu, X., Zhao, G., Li, C., & Shi, J. (2022). Adoption of mobile health services using the unified theory of acceptance and use of technology model: Self-efficacy and privacy concerns. *Frontiers in Psychology*, *13*, 944976. DOI: 10.3389/fpsyg.2022.944976 PMID: 36033004

Luczak, T., Burch, R., Lewis, E., Chander, H., & Ball, J. (2020). State-of-the-art review of athletic wearable technology: What 113 strength and conditioning coaches and athletic trainers from the USA said about technology in sports. *International Journal of Sports Science & Coaching*, *15*(1), 26–40. DOI: 10.1177/1747954119885244

Luo, P., & Song, J. (2025). Beyond raw data: AI-driven biosensor fusion for enhancing athletic performance. *Array (New York, N.Y.)*, *26*, 100418. DOI: 10.1016/j.array.2025.100418

Macedo, A. G., Almeida, T. A. F., Massini, D. A., de Oliveira, D. M., Espada, M. C., Robalo, R. A. M., Hernández-Beltrán, V., Gamonales, J. M., Vilela Terra, A. M. S., & Pessôa Filho, D. M. (2024). Load monitoring methods for controlling training effectiveness on physical conditioning and planning involvement: A narrative review. *Applied Sciences (Basel, Switzerland)*, *14*(22), 10465. DOI: 10.3390/app142210465

Madhumanchi, C. (2025). AI-powered personalized nutrition: Transforming grocery retail into a public health partner. *International Journal of Computing and Engineering*, *7*(12), 11–23. DOI: 10.47941/ijce.2974

Mănescu, D. C. (2025). Big data analytics framework for decision-making in sports performance optimization. *Data*, *10*(7), 116. DOI: 10.3390/data10070116

Marinescu, . A., Oncioiu, I., & Ghibanu, A.-I. (2025). The digital transformation of healthcare through intelligent technologies: A path dependence-augmented–Unified theory of acceptance and use of technology model for clinical decision support systems. *Health Care*, *13*(11), 1222. DOI: 10.3390/healthcare13111222 PMID: 40508836

Martín-Rodríguez, A., Belinchón-deMiguel, P., Rubio-Zarapuz, A., Tornero-Aguilera, J. F., Martínez-Guardado, I., Villanueva-Tobaldo, C. V., & Clemente-Suárez, V. J. (2024). Advances in understanding the interplay between dietary practices, body composition, and sports performance in athletes. *Nutrients*, *16*(4), 571. DOI: 10.3390/nu16040571 PMID: 38398895

Morton, J. P., Hearris, M., Fell, M. J., Owens, D. J., Halson, S., & Trommelen, J. (2025). UCI sports nutrition project: Nutritional periodization: Strategies to enhance training adaptation and recovery. *International Journal of Sport Nutrition and Exercise Metabolism*, •••, 1–26. DOI: 10.1123/ijsnem.2025-0073 PMID: 41130458

Mundt, C., Yusufoğlu, B., Kudenko, D., Mertoğlu, K., & Esatbeyoglu, T. (2025). AI-driven personalized nutrition: Integrating omics, ethics, and digital health. *Molecular Nutrition & Food Research*, *69*(24), e70293. DOI: 10.1002/mnfr.70293 PMID: 41163310

Naabi, Y. A., Ibrahim, N., & Dhillon, J. S. (2024). Designing sustainable mobile weight management applications: Information technology (IT) experts perspectives. *mHealth*, *10*, 25. DOI: 10.21037/mhealth-24-4 PMID: 39114463

Nikitjuk, D. B., Korosteleva, M. M., & Tarmaeva, I. Y. (2025). Sports nutrition as an example of effective implementation of innovative trends in nutrition: Personalization and digitalization (Literature review). *Healthcare of the Russian Federation*, *69*(1), 65–69. DOI: 10.47470/0044-197X-2025-69-1-65-69

Panayotova, G. G. (2025). Artificial intelligence in nutrition and dietetics: A comprehensive review of current research. *Health Care, 13*(20), 2579. DOI: 10.3390/healthcare13202579 PMID: 41154258

Patra, E., Kokkinopoulou, A., Wilson-Barnes, S., Hart, K., Gymnopoulos, L. P., Tsatsou, D., Solachidis, V., Dimitropoulos, K., Rouskas, K., Argiriou, A., Lalama, E., Csanalosi, M., Pfeiffer, A. F. H., Cornelissen, V., Decorte, E., Dias, S. B., Oikonomidis, Y., María Botana, J., Leoni, R., & Pagkalos, I. (2024). Personal goals, user engagement, and meal adherence within a personalised AI-based mobile application for nutrition and physical activity. *Life (Basel, Switzerland), 14*(10), 1238. DOI: 10.3390/life14101238 PMID: 39459538

Paul, J., Ueno, A., Dennis, C., Alamanos, E., Curtis, L., Foroudi, P., Kacprzak, A., Kunz, W. H., Liu, J., Marvi, R., Nair, S. L. S., Ozdemir, O., Pantano, E., Papadopoulos, T., Petit, O., Tyagi, S., & Wirtz, J. (2024). Digital transformation: A multidisciplinary perspective and future research agenda. *International Journal of Consumer Studies, 48*(2), e13015. DOI: 10.1111/ijcs.13015

Persistence Market Research. (2025, October 29). *Sports nutrition market size, share, growth, and regional forecast, 2025–2032* (Report No. PMRREP2889). https://www.persistencemarketresearch.com/market-research/sports-nutrition-market.asp

Phalle, A., & Gokhale, D. (2025). Navigating next-gen nutrition care using artificial intelligence-assisted dietary assessment tools—A scoping review of potential applications. *Frontiers in Nutrition, 12*, 1518466. DOI: 10.3389/fnut.2025.1518466 PMID: 39917741

Phuangsuwan, P., Siripipatthanakul, S., Limna, P., & Pariwongkhuntorn, N. (2024). *The impact of google maps application on the digital economy. Corporate and Business Strategy Review, 5 (1), 192–203.* https://virtusinterpress.org/IMG/pdf/cbsrv5i1art18.pdf

Phuangsuwan, P., Siripipatthanakul, S., Siripipattanakul, S., & Jaipong, P. (2025). The impact of community participation in sustainable learning resource development: A case of Bangkok, Thailand. *Sustainability (Basel), 17*(10), 4620. https://www.mdpi.com/2071-1050/17/10/4620. DOI: 10.3390/su17104620

Piskorz-Ryń, O., Ballester-Ripoll, R., Gottschlich, D., Rostami, M., & Bulut, S. (2025). Understanding user perceptions of personalized feedback in digital health tools. *Health Nexus, 3*(4), 1–10. DOI: 10.61838/kman.hn.3.4.2

Prasad, G., Padhiary, M., Hoque, A., & Kumar, K. (2025). AI-driven personalized nutrition apps and platforms for enhanced diet and wellness. In Alhussaini Hamad, A., & Soni, R. (Eds.), *Food in the Metaverse and Web 3.0 Era: Intersecting Food, Technology, and Culture* (pp. 125–158). IGI Global Scientific Publishing., DOI: 10.4018/979-8-3693-9025-2.ch006

Precedence Research. (2025, December 18). *Sports nutrition market size, share and trends 2026 to 2035* (Report No. 1737). https://www.precedenceresearch.com/sports-nutrition-market

Puce, L., Ceylan, H., Trompetto, C., Cotellessa, F., Schenone, C., Marinelli, L., Zmijewski, P., Bragazzi, N., & Mori, L. (2024). Optimizing athletic performance through advanced nutrition strategies: Can AI and digital platforms have a role in ultraendurance sports? *Biology of Sport*, *41*(4), 305–313. DOI: 10.5114/biolsport.2024.141063 PMID: 39416500

Putra, I. P. O. D. J., Purnami, C. T., & Kartini, A. (2024). Overview of user experience in using nutrition information system: Scoping review. *Jurnal Multidisiplin Madani*, *4*(1), 45–56. DOI: 10.55927/mudima.v4i1.7670

PwC. (2025). *Sports industry outlook: Insights and opportunities for the Middle East.* https://www.pwc.com/m1/en/publications/2025/docs/sports-industry-outlook-2025-eng.pdf

Qi, Y., Sajadi, S. M., Baghaei, S., Rezaei, R., & Li, W. (2024). Digital technologies in sports: Opportunities, challenges, and strategies for safeguarding athlete wellbeing and competitive integrity in the digital era. *Technology in Society*, *77*, 102496. DOI: 10.1016/j.techsoc.2024.102496

Quan, W., Zhou, J., Wang, J., Huang, J., & Du, L. (2026). Machine learning-driven precision nutrition: A paradigm evolution in dietary assessment and intervention. *Nutrients*, *18*(1), 45. DOI: 10.3390/nu18010045 PMID: 41515163

Rao, S., & Neethirajan, S. (2025). Computational architectures for precision dairy nutrition digital twins: A technical review and implementation framework. *Sensors (Basel)*, *25*(16), 4899. DOI: 10.3390/s25164899 PMID: 40871763

Ratten, V., & Thompson, A. J. (2020). Digital sport entrepreneurial ecosystems. *Thunderbird International Business Review*, *62*(5), 565–578. DOI: 10.1002/tie.22160

Research and Markets. (2026, January). *B2B sports nutrition market - Global forecast 2026-2032.* https://www.researchandmarkets.com/report/b2b-sports-nutrition

Roppelt, J. S., Kanbach, D. K., & Kraus, S. (2024). Artificial intelligence in healthcare institutions: A systematic literature review on influencing factors. *Technology in Society*, *76*, 102443. DOI: 10.1016/j.techsoc.2023.102443

Saadati, N., & Torres, M. (2024). Dimensions of trust in AI coaching assistants among elite athletes: Interviews with users and non-users. *Game Nexus, 1*(2), 1-11. https://game-nexus.org/index.php/gamenexus/article/view/7

Sah, D., Kumar, A., Bhatia, R., Singh, K., Thakur, U., & Kesharwani, R. (2024). Unveiling the power of personalization in health and fitness apps. *International Journal for Research in Applied Science and Engineering Technology*, *12*(11), 755–761. DOI: 10.22214/ijraset.2024.64980

Santomier, J. P. (2026). Digital transformation: The global sport industry. *International Encyclopedia of Business Management, 2*, 414-419. DOI: 10.1016/B978-0-443-13701-3.00209-7

Selvi, M. K., Sowmya, B., Kannan, T., Latha, M., Jena, I., Kumar, V. A., & Vijayaraj, P. (2022). Advances in personalized food and nutrition. In Prakash, B. (Ed.), *Research and Technological Advances in Food Science* (pp. 31–60). Academic Press., DOI: 10.1016/B978-0-12-824369-5.00004-X

Shanita, S. N., Rahman, A. H. A., Azimah, A., Izham, M. M., Othman, N. E., Chan, Y. T., Pushpa, B. S., Poh, B. K., & Ruzita, A. T. (2017). DietScore™: Sports nutrition-based mobile application for athletes and active individuals. In Ibrahim, F., Cheong, J., Usman, J., Ahmad, M., Razman, R., & Selvanayagam, V. (Eds.), *3rd International Conference on Movement, Health and Exercise (MoHE 2016)* (IFMBE Proceedings, Vol. 58). Springer. DOI: 10.1007/978-981-10-3737-5_1

Siddika, M. A., Chakraborty, D., Noor, M. S., & Haque, M. N. (2024). Integrating business information systems in public health nutrition programs: Challenges and opportunities. *International Journal of Management Information Systems and Data Science*, *1*(04), 17–33. DOI: 10.62304/ijmisds.v1i04.178

Sonnen, J. (2024). *Framework for mobile applications aiding the visualization of performance data: A case study in swimming* (Master's thesis, KTH Royal Institute of Technology). DiVA. https://www.diva-portal.org/smash/get/diva2:1878986/FULLTEXT01.pdf

Stellar Market Research. (2025, February 12). *Sport nutrition market overview* (Report No. SMR_330). https://www.stellarmr.com/report/Sports-Nutrition-Market/330

Suarez, C., & Adibi, S. (2025). Integrating traditional nutritional wisdom into digital nutrition platforms: Toward culturally adaptive and inclusive health technologies. *Nutrients*, *17*(12), 1978. DOI: 10.3390/nu17121978 PMID: 40573089

Sun, S., Gu, B., & Tang, F. (2025). Cross-category innovation strategy and evolution of digital platform ecosystems: A technology-driven perspective. *Sustainability (Basel)*, *17*(11), 5113. DOI: 10.3390/su17115113

Sutehall, S., & Pitsiladis, Y. (2025). Personalized nutrition for the enhancement of elite athletic performance. *Scandinavian Journal of Medicine & Science in Sports*, *35*(4), e70044. DOI: 10.1111/sms.70044 PMID: 40164953

Tasmurzayev, N., Amangeldy, B., Imanbek, B., Baigarayeva, Z., Imankulov, T., Dikhanbayeva, G., Amangeldi, I., & Sharipova, S. (2025). Digital cardiovascular twins, AI agents, and sensor data: A narrative review from system architecture to proactive heart health. *Sensors (Basel)*, *25*(17), 5272. DOI: 10.3390/s25175272 PMID: 40942702

Teamworks. (2024, July 2). *Teamworks acquires ZoneIn performance nutrition.* https://teamworks.com/blog/teamworks-acquires-zonein/

Teamworks. (2025, June 17). *Teamworks raises $235M to accelerate AI-powered innovation.* https://teamworks.com/blog/teamworks-series-f/

Tsolakidis, D., Gymnopoulos, L. P., & Dimitropoulos, K. (2024). Artificial intelligence and machine learning technologies for personalized nutrition: A review. *Informatics (MDPI)*, *11*(3), 62. DOI: 10.3390/informatics11030062

Turnagöl, H. H., Koşar, Ş. N., Güzel, Y., Aktitiz, S., & Atakan, M. M. (2022). Nutritional considerations for injury prevention and recovery in combat sports. *Nutrients*, *14*(1), 53. DOI: 10.3390/nu14010053 PMID: 35010929

Turner, O., Chessor, R., & Mitchell, N. (2025). Fuelling gold medals: Developing a 'periodised nutrition system'for elite athletes and applying it in practice. *Performance Nutrition*, *1*(4), 1–23. DOI: 10.1186/s44410-025-00001-x

Wahyudi, N. T., & Yunus, M. (2025). Enhancing athlete performance with mobile health applications: Benefits and challenges. *Health Frontiers: Multidisciplinary Journal for Health Professionals*, *3*(1), 1–9. DOI: 10.62255/mjhp.v3i1.141

Wang, P., Wang, A., & Wang, S. (2026). Integrating multimodal AI technologies for sports injury prediction and rehabilitation: Systematic review. *Journal of Human Sport and Exercise*, *21*(1), 22–37. DOI: 10.55860/w6j5wc21

Wang, Y., Wen, Y., Wu, X., Wang, L., & Cai, H. (2025). Assessing the role of adaptive digital platforms in personalized nutrition and chronic disease management. *World Journal of Innovation and Modern Technology*, *8*(1), 24–31. DOI: 10.53469/wjimt.2025.08(01).05

Westerbeek, H., & Schaik, T. V. (2025). Platform power, athlete branding, generative AI, and the future of sport governance—A systematic review. *Frontiers in Sports and Active Living*, *7*, 1642180. DOI: 10.3389/fspor.2025.1642180 PMID: 41031328

Yuxin, L., Salih, S. A., & Shaari, N. (2025). Technical functions of digital wearable products (DWPs) in the consumer acceptance model: A systematic review and bibliometric analysis with a biomimetic perspective. *Biomimetics*, *10*(8), 483. DOI: 10.3390/biomimetics10080483 PMID: 40862856

Zion Market Research. (2025, May 15). *Global B2B sports nutrition market revenue estimated around USD 5.25 billion by 2034*. https://www.zionmarketresearch.com/news/global-b2b-sports-nutrition-market

KEY TERMS AND DEFINITIONS

Artificial Intelligence (AI): The application of computational algorithms and data-driven techniques that enable systems to simulate human cognitive functions—such as learning, prediction, and decision-making—to generate personalized insights and recommendations in sports nutrition contexts.

Digital Business–Driven Nutrition Platforms: Integrated digital systems that leverage AI, data analytics, and platform-based business models to deliver personalized, continuous nutrition decision support, shifting value creation from physical products to intelligence-based services.

Intelligence-Driven, Platform-Based Value Creation: A digital business model in which value is generated through continuous data collection, algorithmic analysis, and personalized decision support delivered via platforms, rather than through discrete, product-based transactions.

Socio-Technical Systems: Complex systems in which technological components interact with human actors, organizational structures, and institutional norms, emphasizing that technology outcomes are shaped by social, cultural, and organizational contexts.

Sports Nutrition: The scientific and practical application of nutritional strategies to support athletic performance, recovery, health, and long-term physical development across training and competitive environments.

User Experience: The overall perception and interaction of users with a digital platform, encompassing usability, clarity, responsiveness, and perceived usefulness, which collectively influence engagement, satisfaction, and sustained adoption.

Chapter 4

Building Trust in Sports' Nutrition and Supplementation for a Strategic Marketing Perspective in Athletic Performance and Recovery

Ira Mariyah Ulfah
http://orcid.org/0000-0003-3198-9061
Putra Indonesia University, Indonesia

Sutithep Siripipattanakul
http://orcid.org/0000-0002-5477-6723
Kasetsart University, Thailand

Sukumporn Sanguandeegul
http://orcid.org/0009-0004-7897-1496
Chiang Mai University, Thailand

ABSTRACT

The sports supplement market has been booming globally, and there has been a growing acceptance of a performance-based lifestyle. This chapter employs a systematic thematic content analysis. The findings show that building trust in the sports nutrition and supplementation market is essential to engaging athletes who

DOI: 10.4018/979-8-3373-9544-9.ch004

increasingly seek evidence-based products to improve performance and recovery, while navigating the risks of contamination and misinformation. Strategic marketing in this space requires moving beyond hype to demonstrate safety, efficacy, and individualization, particularly as the market matures beyond elite sports into general wellness and active lifestyles.

1. INTRODUCTION

The structure of the sports supplement industry impacts trust. Credibility, interconnected information imbalance, and digital amplification matter most. Supplement companies disclosed the origin of ingredients, manufacturing quality, and bioavailability. Package information, third-party certification, and marketing affect customers' behaviors. Nutritional science is technical. Trials must offer non-consumer data to verify amino acid absorption, micronutrient synergy, or anti-inflammatory benefits. Most specialized markets have information asymmetry, not disinformation. When combined with performance and regulatory harmonization, this discrepancy increases risk. Overusing celebrities, branding, and packaging design to indicate scientific excellence is possible. Sports supplements work. Frequent supplement use may not work. Training, sleep, diet, placebo, and nature boost performance. Since physiological responses are hard to measure, a product may not fail if nothing changes. This attribution enhances trust judgments.

An intrinsic assumption is that greater access to information enhances perceptions of brand transparency; yet customers still need clarity on pertinent issues. Customer–brand relationships by identifying the observable signals customers use to assess transparency and examining how consumer biases towards certain brands and product categories shape their perceptions of brand transparency. The obstacles in eliciting views of brand openness when information is prominent. The importance of open communication at all points of interaction to resolve consumer inquiries. consumer-oriented brand transparency by questioning certain assumptions in the accounting and governance (Sansome et al., 2024).

Numerous dimensions, including dietary, psychological, commercial, cultural, historical, and sociological concerns, were shown to have intricate interrelationships. Five factors are crucial for nutrition as follows: (a) Attitudes about Supplements and Doping due to the psychological factors affecting substance use; (b) Entryway to Doping. It draws attention to the development from the first usage of supplements to the adoption of illegal substances. (c) Networks and Key Players: This section charts the professional and social relationships that impact athletes' supplementing choices. (d) The Supplemental Grey Area addresses underrepresented groups and scientific ambiguities related to supplementation. (e) Ambiguity in Concepts: This theme addresses the field's persistent lack of accepted definitions and classifications, including a dual taxonomy that categorizes supplements into goods with several ingredients, ergogenic supplements, functional meals, and individual nutrients. Additionally, they create a hierarchy of scientific evidence, designating randomized controlled trials as the "gold standard." In addition to highlighting important dualities—health vs. energy metabolism, risk vs. benefit, and safety vs. effectiveness—this study also highlights how modern diets incorporate scientific discoveries, technological breakthroughs, and cultural traditions (Rojas & Cisterna, 2026).

Team sports athletes encounter nutritional issues during competition and rehabilitation. Nutrition for muscle regeneration, glycogen replenishment, fatigue, physical and immunological health, and training and competition preparation has been discussed. The competitive season limits athletes' recovery time between training bouts and games, so they must be deliberate. Recovery basics like protein, carbs, and hydration have been widely evaluated and recognized. Vitamin D, omega-3 polyunsaturated fatty acids, creatine, collagen/vitamin C, and antioxidants may aid recuperation. Curcumin and bromelain may help athletes recuperate during competition, but further research is needed before adding them to their diets. Air travel poses challenges for nutrient timing and quality. Seasonal athlete recovery requires effective micronutrient and ingredient consumption (Heaton et al., 2017).

The global public agenda includes the Sustainable Development Goals (SDGs) for Food and Nutrition, which help organize international science and research. The creation of suitable approaches is based on the acquisition and analysis of large datasets, and nutritional science has emerged as a crucial component in bolstering work on the SDGs. Research on the human microbiome is shedding new light on how immunity, diet, and illness are related. We are finally seeing a peek at the possibilities for brain health and nutrition, thanks to enhanced characterization of the gut-brain axis. Numerous significant milestones have been reached, and any assessment of the future must take into account the lessons learned from COVID-19, as well as the sobering realization of food systems' vulnerability to the challenge of ensuring global food security. The majority of future scientific research will focus on sustainability and health (Bassaganya-Riera et al., 2021).

Brand integrity and science are trusted when product efficacy is unknown. Supplemental digitalization offers pros and downsides. Social media virilizes performance claims, transformation stories, and success stories. Emotionally algorithm-friendly content may eclipse science. Influencer marketing builds trust. Fitness gurus can give women non-commercial advice and parasocial connections. Impact marketing sells items but replaces choice with science. Phantomization permits direct-to-consumer transactions without middle-verification, unlike retail. Influencer endorsements, fragmented regulation, and internet amplification promote transparency. Professional athletes must balance anti-doping measures because inadvertent drug use can ruin careers. Not all third-party testing certifications are validated. Financial issues arise from augmentation. High-quality, evidence-based formulations are popular. Intra-workout, pre-workout, and recovery blend memberships cost more. Evaluation preparation increases the financial risk in the credible goods market. Long-term supplementation is possible without efficacy. If performance doesn't improve, consumers must use, switch brands, or quit. Attribution ambiguity does not affect financial risk. Next, the level of investment in supplements depends on belief rather than causality. Sports may be the riskiest performance scenario. Competition athletes synchronize recovery, muscle adaptation, and energy-restoration workouts. Organizations foster mental independence using supplements. Two techniques measure performance. Supplements improve athletic performance. Athletes may fear failure without evidence. Such worries may lead to a cycle of competing standards from supplements.

2. LITERATURE REVIEW

2.1 Growth of the Global Nutritional Supplement Industry

The market for nutraceuticals and dietary supplements is one of the fastest-growing industries, driven by consumers' increasing emphasis on natural ingredients and preventive health management. Functional foods, probiotics, vitamins, and prebiotics that support health and help prevent lifestyle-related illnesses such as diabetes, heart disease, and obesity are referred to as nutraceuticals. Probiotics and functional foods account for the majority of growth in this market. The bioavailability of nutrients has increased due to technological advancements in product composition, such as nanotechnology and biofortification, and the industry has followed suit. As customers became more conscious of artificial additives, they began to gravitate toward items without them. Their product preferences contributed to the growth in demand for natural excipients and clean-label goods. A few disadvantages of this industry are a tight regulatory framework, significant development costs, and limited product accessibility in some areas. The market for dietary supplements and nutraceuticals has the potential to affect the world economy (Chhabra et al., 2025).

Food supplements are currently governed by various laws around the world, but they must be safe for final consumers in the global market. In light of a global market that frequently transcends national regulatory barriers, this search sought to compare the legislative frameworks currently in place in the European Union (EU) and the United States (USA), the two major markets in which dietary supplements are purchased, with an emphasis on the strengths, similarities, and potential shortcomings. Food supplements are subject to strict laws in both the USA and the

EU to guarantee their quality and safety. In several instances, though, the regulatory strategies diverge significantly. In Western markets, it is anticipated that an increasing number of operators will introduce new dietary supplements. To regulate and protect the dietary supplements market, it is imperative that responsible food safety authorities expand and develop new regulatory tools (Zovi et al., 2025).

Increasing health awareness has increased demand for traditional and complementary medicines (T&CM), including nutraceuticals, functional foods, and FAMS. Chronic illness loads and preventative healthcare trends boost this growth. Global trade and consumer trust are hindered by fragmented regulatory frameworks, conflicting definitions, and regional safety evaluation systems. T&CM governance in China, the US, the EU, Japan, South Korea, Australia, India, Russia, African nations, and faith-based Kosher/Halal certification systems is compared, along with legislative milestones and risk management strategies. Standardization, ingredient approvals, and evidence requirements differ. Asian and Western countries have strict safety laws, while African nations struggle to comply. T&CM safety and efficacy depend on emerging technologies like AI-powered quality control, multi-omics-based validation, and blockchain traceability. There is a necessity for a globally coordinated regulatory framework with strategic positive/negative ingredient lists and cross-border cooperation. Policy recommendations emphasize integrating traditional knowledge with scientific evidence to maximize market access and consumer safety. Cultural heritage and global public health provide policymakers with actionable insights to promote equitable trade and innovation in the wellness industry (Shan et al., 2025).

Concentrating on essential regulatory documents and directives from the Dietary Supplement Health and Education Act (DSHEA) in the United States, the Food Safety and Standards Authority of India (FSSAI), and the European Food Safety Authority (EFSA). Market entry procedures, safety regulations, toxicity assessments, and health-claim stipulations across various areas are significant factors. The United States of America (USA) prioritizes post-market surveillance and manufacturer accountability for product safety, whereas India follows a more straightforward registration process. Europe requires stringent pre-market authorization and scientific substantiation of health assertions. These inequalities hinder the smooth integration of nutraceutical products into global markets. The growing need for global harmonization of nutraceutical legislation. Standardized rules could enhance product safety, streamline foreign market access, and cultivate increased consumer confidence. Regulatory convergence will be crucial for the sustainable development of the nutraceutical sector (Bose & Sharma, 2025).

The plant-based food sector is a rapidly expanding industry with numerous opportunities for growth and innovation. In recent decades, consumer preferences have shifted significantly towards plant-based foods due to a convergence of factors, including concerns about animal welfare, environmental sustainability, ethical considerations, and culinary innovation. The recent years have seen heightened diversity, expansion, and innovation. The trends shaping the plant-based food sector's current trajectory. The plant-based food sector: its historical development, current market conditions, and future potential. It explores a range of plant-based goods, including meat and dairy substitutes, plant-derived protein sources, and novel plant-based additives. The catalysts driving the rapid expansion of this sector include evolving consumer preferences for sustainability, health, and ethical considerations. The chapter also emphasizes significant trends influencing the plant-based food sector, including technical innovations, strategic partnerships, and regulatory changes. The potential and challenges facing consumers in the plant-based food business, through a critical analysis of industry data and market statistics. The crucial importance of plant-based meals in promoting a more sustainable and inclusive food system for the future (Prasad et al., 2025).

Nutraceuticals are increasingly recognized worldwide as functional foods that provide health benefits beyond basic nutrition, often serving as preventive or therapeutic agents. Regulatory classifications differ by region, with items classified as dietary supplements in the USA, functional foods in Japan, and traditional herbal products in India. India and China have a rich heritage of using botanicals in traditional systems, establishing them as significant contributors to the nutraceutical industry. India possesses significant potential owing to its abundant herbal heritage; nevertheless, the absence of uniform rules and scientific validation constrains its global market accessibility. The increasing consumer demand for natural health solutions necessitates aligning global regulations and scientific breakthroughs to support the sustainable development of the nutraceutical industry (Silpi, 2025).

One of the biggest structural revolutions in the modern health and performance market is the growth of the international sports supplement market. What was once a niche market, with the main consumers being elite athletes and the bodybuilding community, has now become a universal ecosystem where the global recreational athlete and fitness enthusiast, lifestyle consumer, and older person who prefers to maintain their performance at the required level are the primary consumers. But not just a quantitative development, but a development of bigger change in social construction and commercialization of performance, recovery, and optimization of the body.

2.2 Expanding the Sport Nutrition Market and Commercialization

The sports industry exerts a beneficial impact on the advancement of the health sector. The diverse analysis indicates geographical disparities in the influence of the sports business on the advancement of the health sector. In the various regions, the sports industry exerts the most significant promotional influence on the development of the health industry in the western regions, followed by the eastern and central regions. In contrast, the effect in the northeastern regions is quite minimal. The sports sector can effectively advance the health industry by substantially increasing R&D intensity. Moreover, the examination of the threshold effect reveals that the influence of the sports business on the health sector demonstrates a dual threshold and non-linear declining marginal effects (Zhao & Huang, 2025).

The worldwide growth in chronic inflammatory disorders has heightened the demand for functional beverages that incorporate bioactive substances with anti-inflammatory effects. A thirteenfold surge in publications, with China, India, the USA, and Brazil in the forefront of research output. Principal themes encompass polyphenols, curcuminoids, fermentation, encapsulation, and non-thermal processing. The mechanisms relate to antioxidant processes, metabolic and cytokine modulation, plant-derived flavonoids, and phytochemical profiling. Analysis of consumer behavior indicates that flavor, clean-label appeal, and health claims affect market performance. Although technological advancements such as nanoencapsulation and high-pressure processing enhance bioavailability and sensory attributes, gaps remain in clinical validation and regulatory standardization. Consolidated insights for researchers, industry experts, and policymakers to inform innovation and evidence-based advancement of anti-inflammatory functional beverages (Munarso et al., 2026).

In the contemporary world, sport and technology are inextricably linked, influencing how sports are observed and understood. Technology in sports encompasses a diverse array of advances, ranging from fundamental tools like video analysis and heart rate monitors to sophisticated systems such as VAR (Video Assistant Referee). Each of these technologies has significantly transformed the way sports are played, viewed, and analyzed. The significant technical advancements that have revolutionized sports in recent years, along with an analysis of new technologies shaping the current sports landscape. Emphasis is placed on technologies such as Instant Replay, Hawk-Eye, and Goal-Line Technology, which have enhanced precision and equity in sports. Contemporary innovations such as artificial intelligence, virtual reality, and nanotechnology are examined for their roles in performance analysis and athlete training (Hoxha, 2025).

National Sports Industry Bases (NSIBs) function as a reliable metric for assessing the concentration of sports companies and sports-related initiatives, together referred to as sports brand resources, within a specific region. Four key aspects: distribution pattern, distribution density, spatial orientation, and affecting variables. The findings reveal several notable trends: Initially, in the early stage of sports brand resource development within Chinese urban agglomerations, the spatial distribution exhibited random dispersion, which later transformed into a statistically significant clustering pattern. Secondly, the resources of sports brands in Chinese urban agglomerations have shifted from a dispersed distribution to a more concentrated structure, while spatial distribution remains markedly uneven. Thirdly, the center of gravity of NSIBs has exhibited a dynamic migration pattern, transitioning from "northwest-northeast-southwest," while the developmental imbalance between the eastern and western regions, as well as between the southern and northern regions, is progressively diminishing. Fourthly, elements such as the economic foundation, prospective market, and policy environment substantially interact with other variables to propel the advancement of sports brand resources (Zhong et al., 2025).

The rapid advancement of Metaverse technology has led the sports sector to increasingly incorporate it to enhance event experiences and fan engagement. The influence of event characteristics in Metaverse sporting events on immersion, satisfaction, and team attitude. Relational transcendence in event features greatly enhanced relational immersion, whereas cognitive image had a substantial impact on spatial immersion. Spatial immersion considerably affected personal fulfillment, while relational immersion notably influenced relational satisfaction. Subsequent analysis revealed that both personal happiness and relational satisfaction positively influenced team attitude. Consumers with low engagement have heightened perceptions of relational transcendence and relational immersion. The immersive experiences in Metaverse sports events markedly improve consumer happiness and cultivate a more favorable disposition toward the team. Future sports marketing strategies must integrate virtual and physical events to deliver highly engaging, tailored experiences for consumers with diverse participation levels (Li & Jia, 2025).

The use of nutritional supplements in athletics presents both potential advantages and considerable regulatory and ethical dilemmas. The legal framework governing dietary supplements under international anti-doping laws, namely the World Anti-Doping Agency (WADA) Code, and evaluates the risks associated with supplement contamination. The discrepancies between international and national regulatory frameworks lead to varying degrees of safeguarding for athletes against inadvertent doping infractions. Case studies of athletes penalized for using tainted supplements underscore the pressing need for stronger regulatory controls and increased athlete education. Ethical issues pertaining to equitable competition, athlete accountability, and the marketing of supplements are also examined. The study indicates that a unified regulatory framework, mandatory third-party certification for supplements, and improved teaching programs are essential to mitigate the hazards associated with dietary supplement use in sports and maintain competitive integrity (Borecki, 2025).

In the long run, international market trends indicate high single-digit growth for protein powders, creatine, electrolyte drinks, vitamin complexes, and recovery supplements. Many factors contributed to this expansion. Performance optimization has become mainstream, diversifying the target market and including more professionals than athletes. Digital fitness clubs, performance-tracking tools, and analytics apps have popularized physiological monitoring. Consumers are paying more attention to heart rate, recovery, calories, and macronutrients. Data-driven training uses quantified supplementation to increase accuracy. Second, social media changed marketing. Product sales are rising due to influencer endorsements, user-generated testimonials, and algorithmically generated fitness content. To promote identity-based consumption, supplement brands utilize aspirational visuals, transformation stories, and performance metaphors. Performance measures self-discipline, hence supplementation and identity indicators are related. Third, e-commerce is easier to distribute. Direct-to-consumer sales allow brands to introduce products quickly and globally. More consumers use dietary supplements because subscription services make them a daily habit. Internet markets are increasing but overloaded with information.

2.3 Nutrition Affecting Athletes' Performance Enhancement Professionalization

E-sports nutrition, emphasizing new trends and future paths. The use of artificial intelligence (AI) to create customized nutritional plans, the growing significance of holistic approaches that incorporate physical activity, sleep hygiene, and mental health, and the expected evolution of nutrition's role in the competitive esports landscape are all highlighted. Dietary practices might change, guiding esports athletes, teams, and professionals toward sustainable performance and health outcomes, benefiting market forecasts (Arslan, 2025).

The use of advanced technology in professional sports training has transformed the methods by which athletes prepare for competition. The influence of advanced technology on improving performance, efficiency, and results in professional ST programs. The impact of new technologies on training efficacy in professional sports, with an emphasis on performance enhancement, injury prevention, and comprehensive athlete development. Athletes employing virtual reality (VR), augmented reality (AR), and wearable technology (WT) in their training demonstrate notable improvements in performance metrics (PM) and reduced injury risk compared with those using conventional training methods. Technology-assisted training enhances cognitive skills, decision-making, and psychological factors such as motivation and concentration. Moreover, advanced analytics and artificial intelligence (AI) enable more efficient, tailored coaching methods, improving overall training outcomes. Exhibiting that virtual and augmented reality, wearable technology, and advanced analytics boost sports training by improving performance, customer satisfaction, and resilience, while simultaneously minimizing injuries and accelerating recovery (Huang & Yongquan, 2025).

Elite athletes train and recover using new gear. This progress has smashed endurance records worldwide. Increased access to scientific knowledge, improved practical and scientific interchange among interdisciplinary support teams, and technological innovation have been key drivers of performance development. Professional and health-oriented lifestyles, better comprehension of sport-specific needs, improved competition execution, larger and more targeted training loads, and better training quality were observed from these expert observations. Technology, greater environmental and nutritional precision, improved athlete–equipment interactions, and a deeper focus on the prevention of injury, illness, and maladaptation will drive future growth. Athletes improve and perform better when coaches use their expertise and experience to practice. Their perspective complements and occasionally challenges scientific methods. Coaching opinions on best-practice training and performance improvement have been scarce over time, despite their relevance (Sandbakk et al., 2025).

Another thing is that the industry has become professional. Brands work together with scientists, advisory boards, and elite athletes. There are increased third-party certifications and anti-doping tests. Professionalization, however, is not even. Big companies allocate funds towards research and testing; smaller digital brands might not. This brings hierarchical quality levels and confuses consumers. The scientifically supported ingredients might not be at an accurate dosage or even have proper formulation integrity. Professionalization improves symbolic legitimacy and does not eradicate asymmetry. Consumers need to be able to assess both its existence and its relevance.

2.4. Organizational Specificities of Trust in Nutrition and Supplement Markets

Pharmaceuticals or health products used in illness prevention, treatment, management, rehabilitation, and palliative care may be relevant to nutrition-related diseases across the life course. The accessibility and availability of these nutrition-related health items are crucial. priority, given the persistent trends in undernutrition across many regions of the world. Malnourished children, especially those experiencing severe malnutrition (World Health Organization, 2019).

Precision Nutrition (PN) uses genetics, microbiome, metabolic profile, health status, physical activity, dietary pattern, food environment, socioeconomic status, and psychosocial factors to create personalized nutritional recommendations. PN can answer "What should I eat to be healthy?" Recognizing that what is healthy for one person may not be for another, and that diet and health change with time. The PN market has grown due to customer demand for personalized products and services and improvements in technology, analytics, and omics sciences. The quality of scientific evidence supporting current product and service claims is questionable. Diagnostic testing and wearable gadgets are expensive, limiting PN access. Despite these obstacles, PN has enormous potential to increase health span and save healthcare costs. Investing in multidisciplinary collaborations to develop user-friendly tools using technological advances in omics, sensors, artificial intelligence, big data management, and analytics; engaging healthcare professionals and payers to support equitable and broader adoption of PN as medicine shifts toward preventive and personalized approaches; and system-wide collaboration between stakeholders will accelerate PN advancement (Berciano et al., 2022).

The correlation between diet and human health has been consistently supported by robust scientific evidence, and advanced cultures seek food products that offer value beyond mere hunger satisfaction and nutrient provision. Functional foods, dietary supplements, and nutraceuticals occupy the intersection of nutrition and pharmaceuticals, facilitating the exploration of novel therapeutic options for the prevention of nutrition-related disorders. Functional foods, dietary supplements, and nutraceuticals could outline their regulatory frameworks in Europe, the United States, and Japan. A specific harmonized rule for these products is necessary. Functional foods, dietary supplements, and nutraceuticals offer health-enhancing benefits and may serve as viable options for managing chronic diseases alongside prescribed medications. Additional studies are necessary to determine the most appropriate and advantageous nutritional-pharmaceutical combinations for each chronic condition (Domínguez Díaz et al., 2020).

Agencies and industry are now more aware of adverse health outcomes resulting from dietary supplement fraud (DSF). Awareness that this issue is a major public health danger is growing. Supplement use is expanding, with both favorable and unfavorable effects on food science and safety. "Dietary supplements" are complete goods (such as vitamin D tablets) containing one or more nutritional constituents. "Dietary ingredients" are the components of finished products, such as vitamin D in breakfast cereal. Several variables allow dangerous dietary supplements to reach the market and stay there. The FDA classifies food fraud as Economically Motivated Adulteration (EMA) and DSF as product fraud. DSF may pose a greater public health risk than typical dietary supplement safety issues due to its unconventional adulterants (adulteration is simply one form of fraud). Criminology concepts such as situational crime prevention and the crime triangle help explain fraudsters' opportunities and barriers to fraud. This research aims to inform the public health community about the danger posed by DSF and to change current intervention- and response-based approaches to prevention (Wheatley & Spink, 2013).

The interplay between subjective and objective food knowledge influences consumer preferences for fad diets, whereas demographic considerations shape the types of information available. According to the Heuristic–Systematic Model (HSM), subjective knowledge denotes confidence that promotes heuristic processing, whereas objective knowledge denotes the factual ability to engage in systematic assessment.

Subjective knowledge positively influences the propensity for fad diets, whereas objective knowledge has no direct effect. Conversely, objective knowledge influences this relationship: confidence exerts a greater effect when factual knowledge is minimal, aligning with defensively driven reasoning. Demographic characteristics elucidate the diversity in both types of information, indicating that specific populations are more susceptible to confidence-driven dietary decisions. It underscores the unique yet interrelated functions of perceived and factual knowledge, highlighting the need to align confidence with precise nutritional understanding (Zhan, 2025).

Exercise and sports-related nutritional supplements can facilitate exogenous replenishment. Men comprised the majority of the study, and the female group focused primarily on postmenopausal women. Research is still dominated by cardiovascular and coronary heart disorders. With an annual increase, research on exercise- and sports-related nutritional supplements is expanding rapidly. The current study focuses on insulin resistance, female sex, gut microbiota, inflammation, limb strength performance, sports nutrition, and alpha-linolenic acid. Future studies should concentrate on enhancing the general public's quality of life and training, as well as the scientific training system for athletes (Fu et al., 2024).

The absence of regulation in the commercialization and digitalization of the sports supplement industry has created a vacuum that false information and pseudoscientific systems could fill. Although science has made the discipline of sports nutrition persuasive in its use of certain supplements, it can also be disproportionate, time-consuming, or even exaggerated in its use of scientific findings as marketing messages. These manipulations in a computerized, amplified space can be more viral, compromising consumer information and disrupting ideologies. Wrong information in the supplement business does not always constitute an overview. It is more frequently expressed through overgeneralized statements, the abuse of research findings, out-of-context information, or inaccurate wording that lead to unrealistic performance expectations. This dynamic, together with regulatory asymmetry and an influencer-based marketing system, also increases consumers' vulnerability due to the complexity of the information

3. METHODOLOGY

According to the studies of Andriani & Siripipatthanakul (2026), Siripipatthanakul et al. (2025; a & b) and Phuangsuwan et al (2024); A systematic review with thematic content analysis was typically employed for book chapter reviews. A systematic review with thematic content analysis synthesizes qualitative literature by identifying, analyzing, and reporting patterns (themes) across studies. It rigorously searches and selects studies, then uses thematic synthesis—coding findings, developing descriptive themes, and generating analytical themes—to answer complex research questions and provide in-depth insights into qualitative data

Based on related topics and keywords, purposive sampling was conducted as follows: Information asymmetry, Credence goods, Signaling theory, Scientific credibility, Adoption intention, Perceived recovery, Influencer, Regulatory asymmetry, Pseudoscience, Sports' Nutrition Supplementation, Strategic Marketing, Athletic Performance, and Recovery.

Scholarly papers from 2020 to 2026 are mainly selective in this review, and were published in English. Grammarly was used to detect plagiarism and for grammar checking.

4. RESULTS

In this chapter, a model of marketing strategy has been constructed that elaborates on the following: scientific transparency, perceived scientific credibility, brand trust, adoption intention, and perceived recovery optimization.

Figure 1. Transparency-Based Trust Sports Supplementation

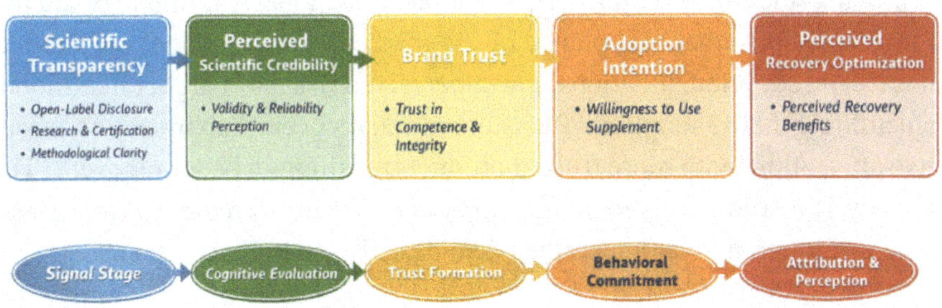

To suggest transparency as a strategy for competitive differentiation and a regulatory tool in the supplement market, this chapter combines signaling theory, trust

theory, and credibility economics. The framework supports an interdisciplinary perspective that incorporates marketing research methodology and sports nutrition science. It will remain relevant to ethical marketing, reducing digital disinformation, and sustainable ecosystems that promote performance. The dynamics of growth in the industry, the structural disinformation, the weaknesses in athletes' decision-making, and the use of transparency tactics are discussed in the next section. The chapter presents a strategic rationale for companies and lawmakers interested in enhancing long-term legitimacy in the market for evidence-based sports supplements, as well as the rationale for the framework and the recommended conceptualizations.

4.1 Conceptual Framework Development

The above segments have created three necessary conditions for structural expansion and commercialization of the sports supplement market: (2) misinformation and regulatory asymmetry, and (3) the multidimensional vulnerability of the decisions taken by athletes. All these reasons support the idea that there should be a systematic system of governance that will help stabilize trust in market performance in terms of credibility. The transparency-Based Trust Framework, which views scientific transparency mechanisms as strategic cues that reduce information asymmetry, boost scientific credibility, build brand trust, and influence adoption intentions and recovery optimization. The conceptual framework develops confidence in sports supplements in stages. Scientific transparency reduces information asymmetry by exposing substantial ingredients, dosage, research support, and third-party confirmation, improving scientific credibility. Competence and honesty promote brand trust, which increases consumer acceptance of the market's trustworthiness. Trust has a similar effect on adoption intentions: lower perceived risk and a higher likelihood of supplementing. Finally, adoption affects perceived recovery maximization through cognitive attribution, with more trusted products resulting in better recovery. Thus, transparency is a strategic governance approach that uses credibility and trust to impact behavior and perceptions rather than directly affecting conduct.

4.2 Model Overview

The initial assumption of this model is that the supplement market operates under information asymmetry and high credibility. Consumers are unable to assess product efficacy on their own and must rely on cues. Transparency is a strategic variable that influences subsequent cognitive and relational outcomes. There are three theoretical pillars of this framework: 1) Signaling Theory - uality is an invisible quality that is signaled, at cost, observably; 2) Trust Theory - Trust is a readiness to be vulnerable, depending on the opinions about competence and integrity; and 3) Trust Goods

Economy - There must be a governance of evaluation cessation on institutional and relational mechanisms. Rather than making direct causal assumptions about the relationship between transparency and behavioral adoption, this framework focuses on cognitive mediation mechanisms. Transparency does not always create trust, but in the first instance, it must demonstrate perceived scientific credibility, which in turn leads to the formation of relational trust.

4.3 Construct Elaboration

4.3.1 Scientific Transparency

Scientific transparency refers to the disclosure of sufficient, useful scientific data about a product and its ingredients, including dose, reference methodology, quality assurance operations, and the limits of evidence. This is a multidimensional construct that consists of 1) Transparency of ingredients and dosage levels; 2) Relevance of research mentioned and credibility; 3) Third-party certification disclosure; and 4) Methodological boundaries of communication. This should be economical and reliable so as to indicate dependability. Symbolic transparency (e.g., a vague label like "has been clinically tested") has no signaling power, since it can be easily lied to. Scientific transparency is the primary exogenous construct in this model.

4.3.2 Perceived Scientific Credibility

Perceived scientific credibility is a consumer's cognitive evaluation of a product based on solid, trustworthy, and verifiable evidence (Hendriks et al., 2020). Trust is not the same as credibility. It represents a judgment of epistemic validity, and not relational acceptance vulnerability. Transparency helps increase credibility by reducing ambiguity and maximizing clarity. Trust in a highly complex area like nutritional sciences requires credibility. A lack of credibility may lead people to form beliefs based purely on affective or identity-based cues, leaving them vulnerable to misinformation. Thus, scientific transparency relates to perceived scientific credibility.

4.3.3 Brand Trust

Brand trust is an indicator of a brand's readiness to take risks and is grounded in the brand's perceived ability, integrity, and reputation. Health, physiological, financial, and performance risks are associated with trust in the supplement market. Scientific credibility is perceived to have a positive effect on competence and integrity. Relational trust can be boosted when consumers believe the claims are evidence-based and well-explained. Trust and credibility are not the same; trust is the assurance that someone will act in undesirable circumstances. Credibility enlightens judgments; trust is the actor. Thus, perceived scientific credibility affects brand trust.

4.3.4 Adoption Intention

Adoption intention refers to consumers' desire to use a supplement product or to obtain more of it, regardless of the level of involvement. Trust minimizes the risk perceptions and maximizes willingness to exchange. Direct verification is also commonly substituted with confidence in the credibility of the product market. The intention to adopt can take the form of a purchase at first instance, a subscription, or the addition of a supplement to a formal training program. Thus, brand trust positively relates to adoption intention.

4.3.5 Recovery Optimization Subjectively

Perceived recovery optimization is a subjective impression that positively influences the efficacy of supplement recovery, readiness, and performance persistence. This construct is specifically differentiated in objective physiological recovery. Objective recovery can be quantified using biomarkers or performance testing, whereas perceived recovery is a cognitive process shaped by beliefs and expectations. Trust can be beneficial to positive attribution processes. As soon as sportspeople have a positive attitude toward a brand, they will be inclined to view the recovery process positively, which will further reinforce their perception of its effectiveness. Thus, Perceptions about recovery maximization are positively correlated with adoption intention.

5. DISCUSSIONS

Signal regulatory imbalance is another structural misleading source. Dietary supplements have separate pre-market approval, clinical trial, labeling accuracy, and post-market surveillance criteria. Others include producers' responsibility to ensure product safety without pre-market efficacy testing. These regulatory discretions allow performance claims that may be stronger than the proof. Despite ingredient studies, commercial products may not include the same dosage as controlled trials. It may have low elite and general consumer population-specific communication. This structural flaw occurs when customers believe a product's market availability means it is scientifically confirmed. Regulatory climates may ensure safety, but they cannot assure efficacy or dose. One reason for the discrepancy between evidence legitimacy and strength is this. Regulatory asymmetry complicates global digital trade. Products with a single guarantee can be marketed and exported, even to local control systems, without authorization. Bold platforms reduce geographic boundaries, involving law enforcement. Consumers must make sophisticated, non-institutional cross-border decisions in these instances. Structured gaps in regulation aid volunteer privacy and third-party verification. Brands' transparency practices vary because different parts of openness require different disclosure requirements.

The Internet has revolutionized how supplemental information is created, shared, and analyzed. Social media, short videos, and fitness forums spread product stories faster. Influencers use stories and technical terms to promote supplements as part of a training program. Likes, shares, and comments are algorithmically boosted. Change stories or dramatic before-and-after photos are more important than research limitations. Thus, visibility does not ensure quality. Online information also confuses causality. Performance can be affected by supplements without training, nutrition, or a placebo. Deterministic efficacy and experienced knowledge are encouraged by causal scripts. Persuasion increases with parasocial contacts. Therefore, buyers will view influencers as friends rather than entrepreneurs. It can be more powerful than traditional advertising, especially when buy recommendations are embedded in human stories. Trust in connections can replace scientific judgment for customers without scientific understanding. Remember that digital misinformation can be positive. Influencers probably think their things work. Overconfidence can originate from confirmation bias and performance-induced optimism. Viral stories can persist after corrections. Supplement marketing uses scientific vocabulary and methodological transparency to frame pseudoscience. Packaging and marketing materials say "research-proven or bio-optimized clinically" without mentioning study design, sample size, or statistical significance. Cherry-picking can taint believability. Unmatched or limited ingredient efficacy studies may be rejected by brands. Laboratory-tested supplements may work for all people, workout levels, and meal patterns. Recovery pills with exaggerated claims are perfect for pseudoscience. Sleep, hydration, exercise, nutrition, psychological stress, and genetics affect recovery. Supplements simplify complex body processes, not recovery. In competitive web marketing, basic messages work. Confusing ingredient-level proof with product-level efficacy is another aspect of pseudoscience presentation. Even with empirically established ingredients, interactions can alter absorption or efficacy in multi-ingredient combinations. Such claims cannot be assessed without dose and consumer testing. These tactics may not deceive audiences due to competition and marketing. However, they cause long-term epistemic perplexity. Consumers may doubt businesses and research when faced with contradicting or exaggerated claims.

Trust building, fake news, and pseudoscience are linked. Competence, integrity, and generosity build trust. Inconsistencies in statements, outcomes, or brand reports might weaken insights into integrity. Trust loss can take many forms. This may cause some consumers to distrust commercial supplements. Others can rely on informal groups or influencers, creating echo chambers that misunderstand evidence. Consumers can take health risks by using unapproved supplements. Consumer well-being goes beyond spending. In addition to drugs, exercise, and diseases, supplements can be taken. The wrong dosage or use pattern can cause unintended physiological effects. Despite no injury, excessive expectations about a faster recovery can lead to training miscalibration or performance dissatisfaction. Mass disinformation undermines the industry's market credibility. Major scandals, such as pollution or over-automation, can have industry-wide reputational implications. Even with valid research, compliance, and investment, reputable brands may face broad distrust. Misinformation still corrects it, reducing psychological and structural causes. When the initial communication matches identity or motivational goals, corrective messages are less salient.

Performance-oriented consumers can be convinced to believe in fast optimization treatments, which drives frequent confirmation. Digital amplification, pseudoscientific framing, and regulatory asymmetries complicate the supplement business. Supplements are essential in a digital economy, so athletes must consider time, performance, and limitations. The next section discusses athletic decision-making problems, specifically supplementing as a high-risk choice integrated into psychological, epistemological, and identity-based decision-making. Comprehending why transparency and credible signals are crucial governance tools in the evidence-based sports supplement market requires comprehending this issue. Industry development, regulatory imbalance, digital amplification, and pseudoscientific framing force athletes to buy supplements under unclear conditions. They are built in a high-performance environment with risk exposure, identity, and time pressure. Three factors make athletes vulnerable to decision-making errors: supplementation is a high-stakes decision, sports supplements are credibility goods, and psychological and epistemic dependency processes influence information processing and belief formation.

Despite their popularity and safety assurances, dietary supplements offer risks. Training pills can harm athletes, especially competitive ones. Health risks matter most. Although metabolism, underlying diseases, and combinations of supplements and medications can produce adverse effects, the drugs are safe at the specified dose. Compound compositions strain senses due to unknown synergy. Undeclared contaminants can still contaminate some sectors. Professional athletes must balance anti-doping rules, and even accidental drug use might hurt their careers. Third-party testing certification is available, but not all are validated. Financial difficulties accompany supplementing. High-quality, evidence-based formulations are popular. Supplement subscriptions (pre-workout, intra-workout, recovery blend) increase costs. Evaluation preparation increases the financial risk in the credible goods market.

Customers can commit to long-term supplementation without proof of efficacy. If performance doesn't improve, consumers must use it, switch brands, or stop. Attribution ambiguity does not affect financial risk. Without causative evidence, the next investment in supplements hinges on credibility. Sports may be the most perilous performance-reliance scenario. Contest athletes usually follow well-coordinated training schedules that promote recovery, muscle adaptation, and energy restoration. Organizations promote psychological independence with supplements. Two techniques depend on performance. Supplements boost athletic performance. Despite the lack of objective data, athletes may worry about performing poorly. Due to such concerns, supplementation may become a cycle of achieving competitive standards.

Sports supplements are reliable. Unlike product enjoyment, trustworthiness is immeasurable after consumption. Training factors and supplements are inseparable. Training intensity, sleep, hydration, macronutrient balance, status, psychological readiness, and heredity affect performance. Supplements' marginal effects are hard to identify, especially in performance-enhancing situations. Most large consumers cannot get laboratory, biomarker, and controlled trial tests. Evaluations are subjective. Brand name, scientific listing, and certification insignia become more essential without self-efficacy checks. Attribution issues hinder assessment. Sports supplements may reduce muscle pain. Enhancements, sleep, activity, placebos, and scale changes can help. Insufficient, delayed, or inadequate nutrients may hinder improvement. One reason to use the belief heuristic is non-attribution. When causality is unknown, customers trust credibility. Evaluation requires transparency and credibility. Institutional and relational trust depend on trustworthiness. Customers can use brand or influencer endorsements unpromoted. Psychological and structural variables influence supplement decision-making. The workplace is dynamic, and thinking and feeling affect information processing. Complex information processed rather than organized will make customers more heuristic in nutrition. Scientific terminology, influencer authority, brands, and packaging quality are heuristics. Heuristics help with information overload. Based on the reliance heuristic, persuasive framing is more credible. Clinically tested product labels can boost credibility without methodological specificity. Heuristics are also used due to time restrictions. Athletes speed up recovery before competition. Sometimes prescription evidence analysis can be delegated. Other factors include performance anxiety. Competition, comparison, and evaluation are typical sporting settings. Performance anxiety can boost optimization responsiveness.

Recovery aids that may offer faster recovery or greater endurance may seem especially attractive in high-pressure conditions. Cognitive narrowing can also be caused by performance-related anxiety, which raises the level of receptivity to persuasive socialization in the direction of motivational goals. Fear and intimidation can make an individual more prone to exaggerated narrative assertions. In cases where the stakes are high, the threshold of admissibility can be reduced. Athletic identity also influences supplementation. Most athletes construct self- concepts on the basis of meticulousness, scientific awareness, and exposure to maximalists. The involvement in supplementation may become a facade of professionalism and seriousness. Identity-based consumption habits should be self-reinforced to promote adherence to habits perceived as improving performance. It is possible to add supplements to identity scripts that define what it means to be an optimal athlete. Identity coherence in such cases may be in conflict with the adoption of supplementation. Identify investment results in increased emotional attachment to a brand perceived as scientifically acceptable. Trust will result in integration with the self-concept upon establishment, thereby enhancing adoption intentions.

Epistemic dependency means that unskilled people rely on external information. Some sports supplement buyers aren't nutritionists. They hire complex evidence analysts. The science advisory board can comprise doctors, nutritionists, coaches, trainers, and celebrities. Evaluation is easier and more credible with expert advice. Official membership and authority blur online. Without a true opponent, influential people with large followings or poor performance can appear informed. Popularity confuses consumers about expertise, increasing epistemic risk. When customers lack evidence, trust substitutes for membership. Cognitive shortcuts accelerate judgments. Without knowing the brand, people may admire its vulnerability. Trust substitution makes sense in the credibility market: one cannot learn everything. Doubts surround trust signals. Symbolic widgets lower trust. The dynamic should be clear. Transparency reduces knowledge asymmetry, improving well-being. Some openness builds trust. Credibility, psychological heuristics, high-stakes decision-making, and epistemic reliance expose athletes. supplements identification, affective-motivational sentiments, and trust, not performance. A reasonable risk. It prides itself on perfecting the structure and ideas of the supplement market. Marketing and governance require openness and integrity, yet they have drawbacks. The strategy and evidence signal, and how substantive openness affects credibility and trust-building in evidence-based sports supplements, are examined in the second part. Openness and Proof: Sports supplements' growth, deception, and athletes' choice indicate unequal market circumstances. Performance alone cannot differentiate consumer marketing here. Governance variation is noted. Disclosure and evidence signaling boost confidence in the supplement market. Transparency is expensive but reduces information asymmetry and promotes scientific confidence.

Credible signals can reduce distractions and improve trading in asymmetric-information markets. Sports supplements cannot demonstrate a scientific basis for product efficacy. Customers have no input on material, dosage, manufacture, or laboratory research quality. Therefore, corporations should organize tacit qualities into messaging. Transparency measures substantive information, not symbolic signals.

Substantial disclosure includes: 1) Complete ingredient and dosage withdrawal (open-label medicines); 2) Dosage and population-related peer-reviewed publications are mentioned; Purity and third-party laboratory testing of illegal substances; 3) Brief access to clinical trial technique; 4) Research funding and partnerships. Financial, operational, and image costs accompany transparency procedures. Clinical trials, third-party testing, and documentation need long-term commitment. Transparency is another clue because low-quality enterprises may not be able to pay. It's surprising that transparency must be readable to indicate. Technical disclosure can please customers since interpretation is improved. A good signal reduces methodological rigor but improves communication. Visibility, which is hard to understand, may not reduce transparency. Scientific transparency includes information, procedural, certification, and communicative transparency.

Openness includes disclosing substance combination, dosage, and expected effects. Open-label disclosure enables consumers and experts to assess dose levels within research parameters. Creatine supplements have daily loading and maintenance dosages in controlled research; consumers may not follow them. Product risk perception decreases with transparency. Showing context lacking is not enough. Consumers want proof and ingredient interpretation. Sharing production, sourcing, and quality management techniques is procedural openness. Compliance with GMP, batch testing, and contamination screening is needed. Health and regulatory hazards are reduced by procedure transparency. Procedure clarity builds trust between anti-doping athletes. They may reduce contamination when guided rather than responding to quality assurance. Third-party certification signifies an institution. Quality assurance certifications, anti-doping verification seals, and independent laboratory testing limit self-reporting. Extrinsic certificates improve accuracy. Certification transparency is crucial in online markets because products are not physically inspected. Institutional support touches instead of evaluating. Communicative transparency describes brand evidence and limits. Communication that identifies boundaries, population features, and performance requirements is ethical. Communicative transparency resists overstated universal or deterministic findings. Depth and perspective improve integrity, which builds trust. Ironically, honesty highlights flaws.

Trust transparency does not influence scientific credibility. Credibility requires cognitive talent and performance ratings. Consumers regard claims as scientific when methodological rigor and institutional support are transparent. Scientific credibility reduces epistemic clarity. This helps buyers discern evidence-based from rhetorically appealing products. Credibility mediates apparent and perceived credibility in the credibility market. Cognitive styles change views. Heuristic processing might use certification seals or research references. Systematic scheduling aids consumer research evaluation. Expert judgment and downloaded cues are transparent. Market governance requires competition and openness. Governance systems that legitimize markets and reduce opportunism set expectations. Institutional, trust-based, and market-oriented governance can be asymmetric. Transparency holds three. Voluntary disclosure boosts regulatory oversight, trust, and reputation. Governance opportunism is reduced by transparency. Marketing to certification and research publications. Disclosure risks reputation and encourages misconduct. Through transparency, groups earn credibility. Industry norms may alter if a major brand adopts transparency standards. Openness may differentiate and standardize markets. Online governance becomes harder. Complete platform algorithm proof wins. Opacity advises online communication. Governance system-consumer touchpoint connections allow peer-reviewed research and testing. Transparency increases in consumer choices, brand strategy, and industry governance.

6. CONCLUSIONS

The blistering growth of the global sports supplement market can be seen as a manifestation of a broader structural change in the modern culture of performance. Supplementation has become more than a peripheral support to a central part of athletic identity and lifestyle optimization. Although the current state of knowledge in sports nutrition has strengthened the empirical foundation of specific supplementation strategies, commercialization, digital amplification, and asymmetric regulatory processes have also increased informational complexity and market uncertainty. This chapter holds that sports supplements are a type of credence good, whose effectiveness consumers are uncertain about even after use. Trust is essential to governance in such markets. Nevertheless, trust is not a priori; it has to be built up through a systematic signaling procedure in which epistemic uncertainty is diminished, and the correlation between commercial and scientific claims is established. This chapter combines signaling theory, trust theory, and the economics of credence goods to establish a Transparency-Based Trust Framework between scientific transparency, perceived scientific credibility, brand trust, adoption intention, and perceived recovery optimization. In this model, transparency is not only informative but also strategic and expensive- it is a signal of credibility that distinguishes actors of high quality in asymmetric markets. However, commercialization without regulatory harmonization and consumer education has accelerated. The regulatory frameworks for dietary supplements vary widely, and these new structural differences are evident in quality control, labelling, and evidence requirements. In the meantime, health claims have become more prevalent due to influencer endorsements, social media tests, and visibility-driven designs resulting from algorithms in the digital marketing ecosystem. In this case, one must address the use of a diverse mix of scientifically proven facts, misinterpreted research findings, personal experience, and pseudoscience on consumers. These forces augment the state of asymmetry in which manufacturers have more information about how the product should be formulated, the quality of the information material, and the scientific content than consumers do. Conventional quality assessment systems are not applicable in markets with high information asymmetry. Sports supplements will become credibility goods, i.e., consumers cannot properly assess the product's effectiveness after taking it. Credibility goods do not require external validation, unlike search or experience goods, whose quality can be ascertained before or even at the point of purchase.

Trust is a crucial performance-market governance mechanism grounded in believability. Trust is consumers' propensity to be vulnerable to a brand or system's perceived competence, virtue, and benevolence. Supplements offer physiological, financial, and reputational hazards for athletes. Brand statements, certifications, professional advice, and scientific proof that can change performance and health behaviors are their preferred criteria. Trusting does not always require scientific evidence. Evidence should be admissible, communicated, evaluated, and perceived. The operation strategically places the supplement market. Marketing under unexpected conditions demands that enterprises demonstrate product quality without being able to see it. According to signaling theory, expensive, well-known signals that are hard to imitate can reveal organizational traits. Disclosure of supplement components, third-party certification, study summaries, clinical studies, and open-label dose form are sports-related signals. Not all transparency is meaningful. Imprecise references to ingredient clinical trials, lacking methodological depth, provide formal transparency and legitimacy without reducing knowledge asymmetry. The gap between transparency as marketing jargon and transparency as an expensive governance exercise is crucial. High operational openness can boost scientific credibility and brand trust.

The concepts of objective physiological and subjective recovery optimum differ greatly. Biomarkers and performance indicators measure physiological repair, but cognitive attribution processes based on trust and credibility determine perceived healing. This discrepancy shows how the supplement business combines marketing, psychology, and physiology. Transparency becomes multi-level governance. It clarifies individual decision-making, boosts competitive differentiation and reputational capital, and legitimizes the industry in a digitalized, misinformed world. Sustainable brands should connect their image and content with openness through open label disclosure, third-party certification, ethical influencer governance, and expectations-based management. Policymakers can reduce structural asymmetries by standardizing evidence-disclosure rules, encouraging digital platform collaboration, and improving consumer literacy. The long-term validity of the sports supplement market depends on epistemic compatibility, meaning that performance claims must be supported by science. Thus, in evidence-based performance markets, transparency is a strategic resource and a compliance need for competitive advantage and ethical legitimacy. Building trust in sports nutrition and supplementation is a marketing goal since brand trust and reputation drive purchasing behavior in a market with efficacy doubts. Beyond advertising, strategic marketing must emphasize openness, scientific validation, and true partnerships to convert customers. Sports nutrition and supplementation must move from flashy marketing to evidence-based, open, and tailored communication to build trust. Marketers must stress safety certifications, scientific validation, and sport-specific instruction to influence athletes focused on performance and recuperation.

7. IMPLICATIONS

The sports supplement market is no longer considered a niche market; several products are used by elite athletes, and it has become a multi-billion-dollar international market that is a normal part of health and fitness culture. It is now assuming a crucial role in contemporary lifestyle profiles rather than being an attribute of sporting institutions. The pursuit of viable physiological modifications has been customized by the spread of wearable devices, self-measuring health applications, a high-evidence training community, and a fitness culture moderated by the digital realm. Today, dietary supplements can be considered strategic for increasing endurance, boosting recovery rates, stimulating muscle growth, and reducing inflammation in this broader performance-based ecosystem, rather than add-ons. It has been found that the world is experiencing a supplementation. It is this scientific premise that has been used to justify supplementation in elite and then recreational sport. Transparency and trust have a linear relationship; this is not just that, cognitive evaluation processes mediate the relationship between them. Consumers perceive cues through heuristic and systematic processing. Specifically, among consumers of highly complex sciences, such as nutritional science, the majority do not consider methodological analysis and instead focus on credibility cues. Therefore, confidence in the knowledge, institutional support, and compliance with the regulations have proved to be key components in the construction of trust. Moreover, the psychological context influences the course of supplement decisions, i.e., the performance anxiety, competitive identity formation, and recovery urgency. Athletes are typically subject to performance cycles and time constraints, and recovery optimization is seen as an indispensable tool for providing a competitive advantage. Subjective perceptions can be as useful as objective physiological indicators in assessing recovery in such situations. This creates a large conceptual gap between physiological recovery, which is objective, and maximization of perceived recovery. In contrast to biomarkers and performance indicators of physiological recovery, the concept of perceived recovery is based on the cognitive attribution process, which relies on perceptions of trust and credibility. Endless demand for protein supplements, pre-workout and recovery solutions, electrolytes, and micronutrient-enriched functional compounds. Along with the evolution of the commercial sphere, scientific findings in sports nutrition have generated a body of evidence supporting various supplementation programs, including protein timing, carbohydrate periodization, creatine loading, and anti-inflammatory omega-3 supplementation. It can be attributed to the persistent issues of misinformation, exaggeration, and regulatory asymmetry, which perpetuate information asymmetry in the supplement market. As sports supplements gain more and more credibility as a commodity, consumers become less informed about ways to degrade the product's effectiveness, even after consumption. This chapter develops an evidence-based marketing strategy for developing trust in sports supplements. The chapter relies on the economics of credibility goods and trust signaling theory to develop a model of scientific transparency and credibility, brand trust, adoption intention, and perceived recovery optimization. The chapter presents strategic guidance on governance for brands and policymakers to reinforce positive marketing behavior and legitimacy in the industry by highlighting transparency as an expensive yet strategic indicator.

REFERENCES

Andriani, A. D., & Siripipatthanakul, S. (2026). Technology-Driven Organization Policies: E-Waste Governance Framework. In *Technology Policy and Its Impact on Green Governance and Sustainability* (pp. 31–62). IGI Global Scientific Publishing. DOI: DOI: 10.4018/979-8-3373-6821-4.ch002

Arslan, S. (2025). The Future of Nutrition in Esports: Integrating AI, Personalized Diets, and Holistic Approaches. In *Esports Nutrition: Enhancing Cognitive and Physical Performance in Competitive Gaming* (pp. 171-180). Cham: Springer Nature Switzerland. https://link.springer.com/chapter/10.1007/978-3-031-99625-2_10

Bassaganya-Riera, J., Berry, E. M., Blaak, E. E., Burlingame, B., Le Coutre, J., Van Eden, W., El-Sohemy, A., German, J. B., Knorr, D., Lacroix, C., Muscaritoli, M., Nieman, D. C., Rychlik, M., Scholey, A., & Serafini, M. (2021). Goals in nutrition science 2020-2025. *Frontiers in Nutrition*, *7*, 606378. DOI: 10.3389/fnut.2020.606378 PMID: 33665201

Berciano, S., Figueiredo, J., Brisbois, T. D., Alford, S., Koecher, K., Eckhouse, S., Ciati, R., Kussmann, M., Ordovas, J. M., Stebbins, K., & Blumberg, J. B. (2022). Precision nutrition: Maintaining scientific integrity while realizing market potential. *Frontiers in Nutrition*, *9*, 979665. DOI: 10.3389/fnut.2022.979665 PMID: 36118748

Borecki, M. (2025). Legal and ethical analysis of dietary supplement use in the light of anti-doping regulations. *Quality in Sport, 39*, 58988-58988. https://orcid.org/0009-0009-4678-5986

Bose, A., & Sharma, S. (2025). Global regulatory trends and comparative insights: Nutraceuticals in the USA, India, and Europe. *PharmaNutrition*, *31*, 100430. DOI: 10.1016/j.phanu.2025.100430

Chhabra, N., Shiriskar, J., & Srinivasan, G. (2025). Current and future market of the dietary supplements and nutraceuticals in the global Economy. In *Dietary Supplements and Nutraceuticals* (pp. 1–48). Springer Nature Singapore., https://link.springer.com/rwe/10.1007/978-981-97-9936-7_29-1

Domínguez Díaz, L., Fernández-Ruiz, V., & Cámara, M. (2020). The frontier between nutrition and pharma: The international regulatory framework of functional foods, food supplements and nutraceuticals. *Critical Reviews in Food Science and Nutrition*, *60*(10), 1738–1746. DOI: 10.1080/10408398.2019.1592107 PMID: 30924346

Fu, T., Liu, H., Shi, C., Zhao, H., Liu, F., & Xia, Y. (2024). Global hotspots and trends of nutritional supplements in sport and exercise from 2000 to 2024: A bibliometric analysis. *Journal of Health, Population and Nutrition*, *43*(1), 146. DOI: 10.1186/s41043-024-00638-9 PMID: 39267150

Heaton, L. E., Davis, J. K., Rawson, E. S., Nuccio, R. P., Witard, O. C., Stein, K. W., Baar, K., Carter, J. M., & Baker, L. B. (2017). Selected in-season nutritional strategies to enhance recovery for team sport athletes: A practical overview. *Sports Medicine*, *47*(11), 2201–2218. https://link.springer.com/article/10.1007/s40279-017-0759-2. DOI: 10.1007/s40279-017-0759-2 PMID: 28702900

Hoxha, S. (2025). Technological innovations in sports: Advancing performance, accuracy, and global impact. *The Journal of Bio based Marketing©*, 135.

Huang, M., & Yongquan, T. (2025). Tech-driven excellence: A quantitative analysis of cutting-edge technology impact on professional sports training. *Journal of Computer Assisted Learning*, *41*(1), e13082. https://onlinelibrary.wiley.com/doi/abs/10.1111/jcal.13082. DOI: 10.1111/jcal.13082

Li, Z., & Jia, L. (2025). Bridging the virtual and the real: The impact of metaverse sports event characteristics on event marketing communication effectiveness. *Communication & Sport*, *13*(6), 1090–1123. DOI: 10.1177/21674795251321754

Munarso, S. J., Elmatsani, H. M., Djafar, M. J., Kailaku, S. I., Lukas, A., Susetyo, E. B., Setianto, W. B., & Warsono, S. Y. (2026). Global Trends and Innovations in Anti-Inflammatory Functional Beverages: A Bibliometric and Consumer Insights Analysis (2006–2025). *Beverages*, *12*(1), 7. DOI: 10.3390/beverages12010007

Phuangsuwan, P., Siripipatthanakul, S., Chaiprakarn, S., & Rakpathum, W. Muthmainnha, Pariwongkhuntorn, N., & Wattanakul, P. (2024, June). Sustainable Development Adopting Artificial Intelligence (AI) in Marketing and Consumer Behaviour Analysis. In *International Conference on Data Analytics & Management* (pp. 569–587). Singapore: Springer Nature Singapore. https://link.springer.com/chapter/10.1007/978-981-96-3372-2_39

Prasad, S., Gupta, E., Yadav, S., Babulal, K. S., & Mishra, S. (2025). Plant-based food industry: overview and trends. *The future of plant protein: innovations, challenges, and opportunities*, 73-97. https://link.springer.com/chapter/10.1007/978-981-96-4190-1_4

Rojas, A. S., & Cisterna, M. Z. (2026). Dialogue and sports supplementation: reflections from the social sciences: a systematic review. *Frontiers in Sports and Active Living*, *7*, 1719247. https://pmc.ncbi.nlm.nih.gov/articles/PMC12867773/. DOI: 10.3389/fspor.2025.1719247 PMID: 41647279

Sandbakk, Ø., Herzog, S., McGawley, K., Pyne, D. B., Talsnes, R. K., Millet, G. P., & Sandbakk, S. B. (2025). Perspectives of World-Class Endurance Coaches on the Evolution of Athlete Training and Performance. *International Journal of Sports Physiology and Performance*, *21*(1), 98–105. https://journals.humankinetics.com/view/journals/ijspp/21/1/article-p98.xml. DOI: 10.1123/ijspp.2025-0317 PMID: 41248624

Sansome, K., Conduit, J., & Wilkie, D. C. H. (2024). Consumer-based conceptualisation of brand transparency: Scope, characteristics and contextual determinants. *European Journal of Marketing*, *58*(12), 2637–2669. DOI: 10.1108/EJM-12-2022-0885

Shan, F., Liu, L., Li, L., Wang, W., Bi, Y., & Li, M. (2025). Management, safety, and efficacy evaluation of nutraceutical and functional food: A global perspective. *Comprehensive Reviews in Food Science and Food Safety*, *24*(4), e70222. https://ift.onlinelibrary.wiley.com/doi/full/10.1111/1541-4337.70222. DOI: 10.1111/1541-4337.70222 PMID: 40613254

Silpi, C. (2025). Nutraceuticals traditional practices, regulatory guidelines, opportunities and challenges. *Discover Food*, *5*(1), 191. https://link.springer.com/article/10.1007/s44187-025-00437-z. DOI: 10.1007/s44187-025-00437-z

Siripipatthanakul, S., Rakpathum, W., Siripipattanakul, S., Kaewnaknaew, C., Phuangsuwan, P., & Jaipong, P. (2025, a). The Future Artificial Intelligence (AI) for the Hotel and Hospitality Industry: The Case of Hotels' Human Resource Management (HRM). In *Best Practices for Human Resources Management in Tourism and Hospitality* (pp. 395–422). IGI Global Scientific Publishing.

Siripipatthanakul, S., Rungsiyanont, S., & Siripipattanakul, S. (2025, b). Sustainable dentistry using artificial intelligence (AI) for digital education and business among university dental hospitals. In *Sustainable development for hospitals and clinics* (pp. 33–64). IGI Global Scientific Publishing. DOI: DOI: 10.4018/979-8-3693-9800-5.ch002

Wheatley, V. M., & Spink, J. (2013). Defining the public health threat of dietary supplement fraud. *Comprehensive Reviews in Food Science and Food Safety*, *12*(6), 599–613. https://ift.onlinelibrary.wiley.com/doi/abs/10.1111/1541-4337.12033. DOI: 10.1111/1541-4337.12033 PMID: 33412717

World Health Organization. (2019). *Meeting report: WHO technical consultation: nutrition-related health products and the World Health Organization model list of essential medicines–practical considerations and feasibility: Geneva, Switzerland, 20–21 September 2018* (No. WHO/NMH/NHD/19.1). World health organization. https://iris.who.int/bitstream/handle/10665/311677/WHO-NMH-NHD-19.1-eng.pdf

Zhan, Z. (2025). *The Distinct Roles of Subjective and Objective Food Knowledge in Fad Diet Preference: A Heuristic-Systematic Perspective* (Doctoral dissertation, University of Guelph). https://atrium.lib.uoguelph.ca/items/aceaac13-ea09-4432-9b98-0acf5b96ca49

Zhao, S., & Huang, H. (2025). The impact of the sports industry on the development of the health industry: An exploration of mediating and threshold effects. *Frontiers in Public Health, 13*, 1691241. DOI: 10.3389/fpubh.2025.1691241 PMID: 41341443

Zhong, X., Wang, J., & Zhong, Z. (2025). Spatial evolution characteristics and influencing factors of sports brand resources in Chinese urban agglomerations. *Scientific Reports, 15*(1), 22138. https://www.nature.com/articles/s41598-025-09706-4. DOI: 10.1038/s41598-025-09706-4 PMID: 40594806

Zovi, A., Vitiello, A., Sabbatucci, M., Musazzi, U. M., Sagratini, G., Cifani, C., & Vittori, S. (2025). Food supplements marketed worldwide: A comparative analysis between the European and the US regulatory frameworks. *Journal of Dietary Supplements, 22*(1), 25–40. https://www.tandfonline.com/doi/full/10.1080/19390211.2024.2389397. DOI: 10.1080/19390211.2024.2389397 PMID: 39221704

KEY TERMS AND DEFINITIONS

Adoption Intention: The behavioral willingness of consumers to start or continue using a product based on perceptions of trust and scientific merit, rather than direct performance verification.

Athletic Performance and Recovery: An organized strategy that incorporates healthy eating, restful sleep, and focused methods like massage, foam rolling, and active recovery (low-intensity movement) is essential for both athletic performance and recuperation. Making rest a priority promotes muscle recovery, which lowers the chance of injury and improves performance. Specialized equipment, such as compression clothing and cold plunges, can also help reduce tiredness.

Brand Trust: A consumer's willingness to rely on a brand's competence and integrity, which serves to minimize perceived physical, financial, and performance risks.

Credibility Goods: Products whose quality or effectiveness remains difficult for consumers to assess independently even after consumption, necessitating reliance on external evidence.

Epistemic Dependence: A condition where individuals rely on external knowledge sources (such as experts or certifications) due to a lack of specialized expertise in interpreting complex information.

Evidence Signaling: A communication strategy used to convey unobservable product qualities through credible, high- cost signals that are difficult for competitors to imitate.

Information Asymmetry: A market situation where manufacturers possess significantly more information regarding product quality and formulation than consumers.

Recovery Optimization as Perceived: A subjective attribution or cognitive belief that supplementation has improved recovery efficiency and readiness, as distinct from objective physiological measurements.

Scientific Transparency: The factual disclosure of ingredients, dosages, research methodology, and quality control as strategic tools to reduce information imbalances.

Sport Nutrition Strategic Marketing: Building trust through open, fact-based content, influencer collaborations, and individualized experiences is a key component of successful sport nutrition marketing campaigns. Social media storytelling, using athletes and gym trainers for credibility, and employing event-based sampling to directly interact with active customers are important strategies. A customized message for varying skill levels is necessary for success.

Sport Nutrition Supplementation: Evidence-based options include creatine, caffeine, beta-alanine, nitrates, and protein. These supplements improve body composition, athletic performance, and recovery. When combined with a healthy diet, these tools can enhance endurance, strength, and energy metabolism. Key supplements are frequently grouped by effectiveness, with significant support for those that support fatigue control, energy, and fuel synthesis.

Transparency-Based Trust Framework: A framework explaining how scientific transparency builds credibility and trust by providing evidence and reducing uncertainty, ultimately driving adoption intention and perceived product effectiveness

Chapter 5

Strategic Nutritional Interventions for Enhancing Recovery and Reducing Exercise-Induced Inflammation

Udit Mamodiya
http://orcid.org/0000-0002-8022-4252
Poornima University, India

Indra Kishor
http://orcid.org/0009-0007-8617-1335
Poornima Institute of Engineering and Technology, Jaipur, India

Sukumporn Sanguandeegul
http://orcid.org/0009-0004-7897-1496
Chiang Mai University, Thailand

ABSTRACT

Exercise-induced inflammation is an essential yet tightly regulated component of physiological adaptation. While acute inflammatory signaling supports tissue remodeling and performance gains, excessive or prolonged responses may impair recovery and increase susceptibility to overtraining. This chapter synthesizes contemporary evidence on strategic nutritional interventions aimed at enhancing recovery while preserving adaptive mechanisms. Current literature indicates that omega-3 fatty acids modulate membrane composition and promote inflammation resolution, whereas curcumin and polyphenol-rich foods attenuate cytokine amplification and

DOI: 10.4018/979-8-3373-9544-9.ch005

oxidative stress. Probiotics contribute to gut-mediated immune stability, and adequate protein—whether plant-based or dairy-derived—supports structural repair and systemic inflammatory balance. Carbohydrate availability further influences metabolic–inflammatory interactions. Emphasis is placed on periodized and individualized implementation, recognizing inter-individual variability in inflammatory phenotype and training demands.

1. INTRODUCTION

It is a fact that exercise has become one of the pillars of human health, functional capacity, and longevity of performance. From elite sport to clinical rehabilitation and active aging, structured exercise improves metabolic efficiency, cardiovascular health, neuromuscular coordination, and psychological health. However, the same stimulus that triggers mechanical overload also triggers metabolic stress, transient muscle injury, oxidative perturbation, and inflammatory signaling. This is a paradox in a major problem in sports nutrition and exercise physiology: how to hasten recovery and reduce excess inflammation without undermining adaptive training effects. Another area of research has identified strategic nutritional interventions as a promising pathway to bridge this tension and to regulate molecular pathways in muscle repair, immune regulation, and oxidative balance.

Muscle damage related to exercise (EIMD) involves structural disruption of myofibrils, alterations in sarcolemmal permeability, Ca2+ dysregulation, and ensuing inflammatory cascades. Manifold manifestations include delayed-onset muscle soreness (DOMS), decreased force production, elevated creatine kinase, and elevated systemic inflammatory markers. Although a moderate level of inflammation is necessary for tissue remodeling, excessive or persistent inflammation will hamper future performance and predispose the organism to overtraining or injury. Rehabilitative dietary interventions have thus been studied over a long period (Sousa et al., 2014). Timing of macronutrients and protein intake was the focus of early studies, though more recent studies are questioning the role of bioactive substances and lipid mediators, as well as the use of functional foods that can modulate immune-metabolic cross-talk.

An emerging body of evidence indicates that nutritional supplementation may mitigate indicators of muscle injury and oxidative stress after vigorous exercise (Harty et al., 2019). Carbohydrate-protein co-ingestion, essential amino acids, and branched-chain amino acids have been found to promote glycogen resynthesis and muscle protein synthesis. However, the issue of inflammatory dysregulation is not met completely by macronutrient adequacy. The systematic reviews highlight the potential for complementary effects among polyphenols, omega-3 fatty acids, antioxidants, and novel bioactives (Bongiovanni et al., 2020; Talebi et al., 2023). Although there are promising results, a lack of unifying protocols and dosing schedules, along with a heterogeneous population, precludes the development of a unified practice guideline.

Recovery Biology is a complex field of study that requires a complex approach. Exercise triggers inflammatory reactions, which are coordinated by means of cytokine signaling, the production of reactive oxygen species (ROS), mitochondrial responses to stress, and the infiltration of immune cells. The regulatory effects of antioxidative stress and muscle inflammation have been studied in vitamins C and E and naturally derived antioxidants (MacGregor, 2024). Although antioxidant supplementation can decrease lipid peroxidation and inflammatory biomarkers, there is still controversy about whether it interferes with endogenous redox-sensitive responses. The difficulty is not in the unselective inhibition of oxidative stress, but in the selective adjustment.

Recent umbrella reviews synthesizing randomized studies indicate that nutritional interventions can reduce the severity of EIMD; however, effects vary by nutrient type, training status, and exercise modality (Talebi et al., 2023). Notably, the literature is no longer based on isolated supplement paradigms; rather, comprehensive dietary frameworks are being developed. Enriched functional foods containing bioactive compounds are being promoted as viable alternatives to high-dose supplementation, with sustainability as a key advantage (Wang et al., 2024). Such a shift indicates the overall acceptance that dietary matrices affect bioavailability, metabolic integration, and adherence in the long run.

Omega-3 fatty acids have been of particular interest as a lipid-based strategy. Eicosapentaenoic acid (EPA) and docosahexaenoic acid (DHA) regulate the fluidity of membranes, the synthesis of cytokines, and specialized pro-resolving mediator (SPM) synthesis. A review has postulated that omega-3 supplementation may limit the extent of muscle damage and inflammatory markers during exercise (Rasińska et al., 2025). Besides, exercise and omega-3-enriched, high-protein staples have been shown to modulate inflammatory gene expression and serum biomarkers, especially in older individuals (Hass et al., 2023). These results suggest the possibility of synergy between lipid-mediated immunomodulation and mechanical loading.

In addition to conventional fish oil preparations, there has been recent interest in SPM-containing marine oils. These substances do not suppress inflammation but promote its resolution. Narrative analyses suggest that these interventions can enhance and accelerate recovery through specific pro-resolving pathways (de Souza et al., 2025). Transforming the traditional anti-inflammatory to the pro-resolving nutrition is an excellent evolution in the science of recovery.

Foods rich in polyphenols also contribute to this changing picture. Olive polyphenols have been investigated for anti-inflammatory and antioxidant effects during exercise (Lillis et al., 2025). In a similar vein, coenzyme Q10 has been tested for its ability to alleviate oxidative stress and inflammatory conditions associated with intense activity (Yasul et al., 2024). These compounds have potential effects on mitochondrial bioenergetics and redox balance, providing a mechanistic basis for performance and recovery advantages.

Carbohydrate plans remain the cornerstone, especially for endurance athletes. Recent randomized crossover studies investigating the effects of maltodextrin-fructose supplementation on inflammatory biomarkers and lipidomic profiles after a long-term running session (Righetti et al., 2024). Carbohydrate supply affects cortisol dynamics, glycogen depletion patterns, and cytokine release, suggesting that substrate supply is inherently linked to inflammatory control.

Functional foods based on protein are another example of the overlap between nutrition and systemic inflammation. A combination of resistance training and Greek yogurt consumption has been linked to modulation of inflammatory markers in healthy young men (Fraschetti et al., 2025). The findings emphasize the significance of whole-food sources of protein, which can provide not only amino acids but also micronutrients and probiotic components that can affect immune function.

Despite these developments, critical gaps remain. First, most of the literature analyses stand-alone nutrients rather than combined eating habits. Second, research tends to focus on short-term biomarkers without examining recovery patterns or long-term functional adaptation. Third, there is the issue of population specificity, i.e., sex differences, aging physiology, or training status that are under-researched. In addition, the effects of nutritional intervention and exercise mode (eccentric resistance training, endurance training, or high-intensity interval training) are to be systematically clarified.

The other question, which has not yet been answered, concerns the maintenance of inflammation required for adaptation to change, with excessive inflammation harming the recovery process. Inflammatory signaling can be blunted at random, thereby suppressing hypertrophic or mitochondrial responses. Hence, the interventions applied in strategies should be timed accurately and be dosed adequately, not to suppress but to help resolve. This subtlety is often not given due consideration in applied sports nutrition.

Moreover, systematic reviews present the cumulative evidence, although no clear-cut conclusion can be drawn due to variability in methodological rigor, supplementation duration, and biomarker selection (Talebi et al., 2023; Bongiovanni et al., 2020). New paradigms promote personalized nutrition systems based on the models of molecular phenotyping and metabolic profiling (Ihsan et al., 2024). The customized recovery plan can be based on dietary lipids, antioxidants, carbohydrate timing, and protein ratios, adjusted to the training load and body response.

Against this background, this chapter advances a strategic approach to nutritional interventions to improve recovery without disrupting adaptive signaling. Instead of tabulating the evidence for the supplements individually, it integrates evidence on macronutrients, lipid mediators, polyphenols, antioxidants, and functional foods. The rationale is to put the nutritional strategies into perspective within the broader immunometabolic context of exercise recovery.

There are three contributions in this chapter. First, it theorizes recovery nutrition as a dynamic adjustment of inflammatory resolution mechanisms and not a static anti-inflammatory supplementation. Second, it is an approach that combines lipidomics, cytokine biology, and mitochondrial redox regulation into a single explanatory framework. Third, it focuses on translational alignment, bridging randomized controlled evidence and practical implementation strategies, an approach applied to both athletic and clinical groups.

The systematic incorporation of recent discoveries - omega-3-mediated changes in gene expression (Hass et al., 2023), SPM-enriched marine oil mechanisms (de Souza et al., 2025), and nutritional recovery strategies are placed in the framework of precision-oriented paradigms (Lillis et al., 2025). It critically analyzes antioxidant supplementation in the context of adaptive redox signaling (MacGregor, 2024).

Overall, exercise-induced inflammation is an adaptive driver and a potential obstacle to achieving high performance in its uncontrolled form. Nutritional interventions are scientifically based, strategic approaches that can address this duality. Nevertheless, its effectiveness is context and time-specific, dose-dependent, and variable. An all-encompassing evidence-based strategy is thus needed.

This introduction provides the scientific basis of the systematic study of recovery-oriented nutritional strategies. The following paragraphs will discuss mechanistic pathways, assess intervention effectiveness across nutrient classes, identify methodological shortcomings, and suggest an integrative framework that should optimally improve recovery outcomes without undermining physiological adaptation. It is through this that nutrition is not only supportive but also strategically transformative in managing inflammation, supporting exercise, and restoring performance.

2. LITERATURE REVIEW

The discussion on scientific knowledge on exercise recovery has changed significantly in the last ten years. Protein timing and carbohydrate replenishment have often been discussed, and recovery has been viewed as mostly a metabolic refueling process. Today, the lens is much wider. The concept of recovery is increasingly recognized as a multifaceted interplay among immune signaling, oxidative stress, muscle remodeling, intestinal integrity, and neuroendocrine responses. However, nutrition is at the core of this network. The types of food an athlete eats before, during, and after exercise can influence cytokine activity, redox homeostasis, membrane composition, and even gene expression.

Simultaneously, the literature is still disjointed. Other studies examine individual nutrients such as omega-3 fatty acids or curcumin; others examine probiotics, vegetarian proteins, or polyphenols derived from spices. These findings are increasingly being synthesized in more and more reviews, but they are frequently complicated by variations in dosage, population characteristics, and exercise protocols. It is also a stable conflict between the need to reduce excessive inflammation and the need to maintain the inflammatory cues required for adaptation.

Against this background, the literature review below critically analyzes recent evidence on nutritional measures that could be implemented to promote recovery and counteract the effects of exercise-induced inflammation. The section is divided into themes, which begin with immune physiology and proceed to functional foods, covering specific nutrient groups and approaches. Instead of introducing individual findings, it attempts to establish patterns, strengths, weaknesses, and findings in the area.

2.1 Exercise, Immune Function, and the Inflammatory Response

Exercise induces a strong coordinated body response that occurs at the minute, hour, and even day levels. The post-exercise changes are immediate, as circulating leukocyte count, pro-inflammatory cytokine production, and oxidative stress markers are elevated immediately after intense/prolonged activity. This is not necessarily a detrimental acute response. It is actually a stage of tissue remodeling as required. But as training loads build up, and the recovery is not sufficient, the inflammatory response can be sustained, immune surveillance can be changed, and susceptibility to disease or performance stalemate.

Recent physiological studies indicate that immune modulation during exercise is a situational phenomenon (Via et al., 2024). Acute endurance exercise can temporarily suppress certain immune parameters, whereas resistance training elicits local inflammatory responses associated with muscle repair. The contribution of adaptive and innate immunity is particularly significant for athletes who undergo frequent training sessions. Recovery nutrition, in its turn, should consider both the systemic immune balance and local processes in a muscle.

In a broader context of clinical applications, surgical recovery protocols also offer useful insights. Enhanced Recovery After Surgery (ERAS) models show that specific nutritional and metabolic approaches can lead to substantial reductions in inflammatory biomarkers and accelerated tissue healing (Alves Bersot et al., 2024).

Though exercise does not match the extent and pathology of surgical trauma, there are similarities in these two events with regard to cytokine signaling and oxidative stress regulation. These results support the notion that nutrition may alter inflammation in a systematic and quantifiable manner.

2.2 Omega-3 Fatty Acids and Lipid-Mediated Resolution

Omega-3 fatty acids, among the nutritional measures, are one of the most researched. Synthetic randomized controlled trials included in systematic reviews indicate that omega-3 supplementation can mitigate indicators of post-exercise inflammation, lessen muscle soreness, and even aid performance recovery (Fernández-Lazarillo et al., 2024). Mechanistically, EPA and DHA modify the phospholipid composition of membranes and serve as precursors to anti-inflammatory lipid mediators.

Notably, the literature tends to distinguish between anti-inflammatory suppression and the active resolution of inflammation. In contrast to preventing cytokine synthesis, omega-3 derivatives can stimulate the production of specific pro-resolving mediators that direct the inflammatory response toward resolution. This minor difference has consequences for long-term adaptation, with full suppression of inflammation potentially having the theoretical effect of turning off training-induced signaling.

There is also evidence of variations in dose-response relations. Moderate supplementation seems to have a positive effect, but when it is too high, the effect has not always been superior (Fernández-Lazaro et al., 2024). The inter-individual variability also makes interpretation more difficult. Responsiveness is likely to be affected by baseline dietary intake, training status, and genetic polymorphisms. Such subtleties help emphasize the significance of the accuracy-based approach over standardized doses.

2.3 Curcumin and Turmeric-Derived Compounds

Curcumin, a polyphenolic compound in turmeric, has attracted considerable interest in sports nutrition. Reviewing the literature, it is possible to suggest that curcumin supplementation can decrease the creatine kinase, perceived muscle soreness, and inflammatory cytokines levels after strenuous exercise (Popescu et al., 2024; Rosińska-Lewandoska et al., 2024). The compound also exerts its effects by regulating nuclear factor-κB (NF-κB) signaling and antioxidant pathways.

Additional information can be seen through recent dose-response studies. It seems that hydrolyzed curcumin preparations help to increase bioavailability, and recovery indicators improve as the dose increases (Helder et al., 2025). This implies that the form and absorption kinetics of bioactives are vital factors of effectiveness.

The conventional form of curcumin has low systemic availability, which has led to the development of nanoparticle and hydrolyzed curcumin.

They have also been investigated in practical use in athletic populations. A pilot study of elite male footballers has indicated that recovery indices improve after turmeric supplementation during periods of competition (Clayton et al., 2023). Such findings are promising but should be interpreted with caution due to small sample sizes. However, there are growing indications that curcumin could offer a specific means of controlling exercise-induced inflammation, especially when taken in bioavailable form.

2.4 Probiotics and Gut–Immune Interactions

Probiotic supplementation has been considered as one of the possible strategies to control cytokine responses following exercise. A recent meta-analysis finds that probiotics can affect post-exercise inflammatory profiles, but the effect varies with strain specificity and duration of supplementation (Aparicio-Pascual et al., 2025).

In parallel, systematic reviews indicate that probiotic supplementation may suppress the effects of certain inflammatory markers in physically active individuals (Fernández-Lazar et al., 2023). The mechanisms can include enhanced protection of the intestinal barrier, decreased endotoxemia, and regulation of immune cell signaling. High-intensity endurance exercise transiently increases gut permeability, allowing lipopolysaccharides to enter the circulation and thereby enhancing inflammation. Portobiotics can overcome this effect.

The literature remains heterogeneous, even though interest has increased. Variations in strains, colony-forming units, and athletes make it difficult to directly compare studies. In addition, the evolutionary history of the microbiota suggests that short-term interventions may play a small role. To determine whether sustained use of probiotics has a significant effect on recovery trajectories, longitudinal designs are necessary.

2.5 Plant-Based Proteins and Recovery Dynamics

Protein consumption continues to underpin muscle repair, but the focus has shifted away from conventional animal-based sources. A systematic review of the literature on plant-derived protein supplementation has shown that these proteins may aid in the recovery from muscle injury caused by resistance exercise in healthy young adults (Govindasamy et al., 2025). Plant proteins seem to promote muscle protein synthesis when consumed in appropriate amounts and with the right proportions of essential amino acids.

Nevertheless, some restrictions still remain. Plant proteins are likely to have low leucine content and are not as readily digested as whey or casein. These concerns can be allayed by mixing protein sources or fortifying with constraining amino acids. In addition to amino acid composition, plant-based diets contain phytochemicals that may provide ancillary anti-inflammatory benefits.

The increased responsibility of nutrition professionals comes into play at this point. Dietary planning, macronutrients, and micronutrients adequacy are to be planned and monitored by a professional (Filho, 2024). A single supplement is unlikely to be effective in recovery strategies, and such strategies are formed through coordinated dietary frameworks.

2.6 Overtraining Syndrome and Nutritional Countermeasures

Constant stress on the training load relative to the recovery period may lead to chronic overtraining syndrome, characterized by persistent fatigue, mood swings, and changes in hormonal and immune levels. Protective factors for the prevention and mitigation of this condition have been proposed, including nutritional interventions (Pereira et al., 2024). An adequate energy supply, appropriate macronutrient proportions, and anti-inflammatory elements in the diet can all help lower the risk.

Muscular issues are not the only ones, and overtraining involves neuroendocrine and immune dysregulation. Inflammatory parameters are usually not lowered, and oxidative stress increases. Nutritional interventions that maintain energy balance and provide antioxidant-rich diets can help stabilize homeostasis. However, the evidence is mostly observational, underscoring the need for controlled longitudinal trials.

2.7 Functional Marine Foods and Bioactive Lipids

In addition to traditional fish oil supplements, whole-food marine supplements have been assessed for recovery. The recovery of muscle tissue was also shown to involve New Zealand Greenshell™ mussel powder as a supplement in untrained male rats subjected to eccentric exercise-induced muscle injuries (Lomiwes et al., 2023). Not only omega-3 fatty acids but also unique bioactive lipids that can enhance anti-inflammatory signaling are present in such products.

These results indicate that food matrices may affect efficacy. Whole-food interventions can provide a range of compounds in synergistic form that cannot be isolated in supplements. Scalability and cost may, however, be constraints to widespread use. Additional studies are needed to compare whole-food and purified-lipid strategies to determine their relative efficacy.

2.8 Spices, Polyphenols, and Anthocyanin-Rich Foods

Compounds of plant origin are increasingly being considered ergogenic aids. Systematic reviews indicate that some spices can affect muscle performance and recovery rates, as well as inflammatory responses (Chodador et al., 2025). These effects are probably caused by the content of polyphenolics and antioxidants.

They have also focused on an anthocyanin-rich purple plant food as a method of redox regulation and exercise recovery (Nuszkiewicz et al., 2025). Anthocyanins exhibit bioavailability sufficient to act on cellular antioxidant mechanisms. Of particular interest is their ability to modulate oxidative stress without completely inhibiting adaptive signaling. Food-derived polyphenols do not have the strong physiological effects of high-dose synthetic antioxidants and may have weaker, more integrated effects.

Curcumin and turmeric, among the spices, are included in this broader category, indicating that ingredient systems in the traditional diet can be accessible for quantifiable functional value when carefully researched.

2.9 Integrated Nutritional Strategies for Injury Prevention and Recovery

In the context of injuries, literature on injury prevention and recovery emphasizes the importance of thorough nutritional planning (Moreira et al., 2024). Sufficiency of macronutrients, hydration, and micronutrient adequacy, as well as selective supplementation, affect tissue repair. The active ingredient is also a limited approach that may fail to account for interactions among various components of a diet.

Athlete-based models focus on periodizing nutrition in accordance with training periods. The need to provide high-intensity blocks with greater anti-inflammatory support may be influenced by the need to adjust the adaptation phases to support protein synthesis and mitochondrial biogenesis. This dynamic methodology aligns with emerging perspectives on precision nutrition.

2.10 Synthesis and Emerging Themes

In the literature, there are several common themes. To begin with, inflammation is not a bad thing; it is an essential part of the adaptation. The goal of the nutritional interventions is to be modulatory rather than eliminatory. Second, bioavailability and dose are important. Formulations of hydrolyzed curcumin and omega-3 are stronger compared to generic preparations (Helder et al., 2025; Fernandez-Lazararo et al.,

2024). Third, whole-food methods have the potential to exhibit synergistic effects compared with individual compounds (Lomiwes et al., 2023).

However, there are still serious gaps. Most studies have small sample sizes, short intervention periods, or all-male participants. Sex-specific reactions have not been properly examined. Also, there are not many studies that combine two or more nutritional strategies. Future studies need to incorporate integrated interventions (e.g., omega-3 and probiotics, or curcumin and anthocyanin-rich foods) to reflect eating habits in the field.

To sum up, the literature demonstrates that nutritional interventions have strong potential to improve recovery and reduce exercise-induced inflammation. The efficacy of omega-3 fatty acids, curcumin, probiotics, plant-based proteins, marine bioactives, and anthocyanin-rich foods varies. Nevertheless, it has to be implemented with contextual knowledge, personal planning, and an understanding of how to use the fine line between inflammation and adaptation effectively. The following section will use this as the starting point to suggest an integrated, strategy-based recovery nutrition framework grounded in existing evidence and physiological understanding.

2.11 Mechanistic Basis of Exercise-Induced Inflammation and Nutritional Modulation

The inflammation brought about by exercise is not accidental and is not entirely harmful. It is a carefully controlled biological reaction to mechanical stress, metabolic disruption, and acute cellular damage. Exposure of skeletal muscle fibers to eccentric contractions or chronic endurance stress results in microstructural damage, disruption of calcium homeostasis, and mitochondrial dysfunction. Such events trigger intracellular signaling cascades that recruit immune cells, activate cytokine networks, and induce tissue remodeling (Via et al., 2024). Recovery nutrition lies in the difficulty of not inhibiting this cascade, but rather modulating its magnitude and extent to promote more rapid repair without disrupting adaptation.

Pathophysiology of Exercise-Induced Muscle Damage

Muscle tissue damage after strenuous activity encompasses structural, biochemical, and immunological aspects. Disruption of sarcomeres increases membrane permeability, allowing the efflux of intracellular enzymes such as creatine kinase. Simultaneously, the accumulation of reactive oxygen species (ROS) results from cellular inflammatory processes and mitochondrial electron transport chain flux. Inflammatory processes trigger the infiltration of neutrophils and macrophages into the injured tissue, leading to the release of cytokines such as interleukin-6 (IL-6) and tumor necrosis factor-alpha (TNF-α). Although this inflammatory stage is necessary for clearing debris and activating satellite cells, a prolonged inflammatory response might slow functional restoration (Sousa et al., 2014; Talebi et al., 2023).

At this point, nutritional modulation starts. A proper amount of protein intake assists in muscle protein synthesis and repair (Harty et al., 2019). The systematic assessment shows that, when consumed in adequate amounts and in balanced amino acid foods, plant-based proteins can mitigate damage caused by resistance exercise (Govindasamy et al., 2025). In addition, functional dairy products such as Greek yogurt have been shown to help regulate systemic inflammatory indices during resistance training (Fraschetti et al., 2025). These results emphasize that structural restoration and inflammatory control are not independent processes.

Oxidative Stress and Redox Regulation

Cytokine patterns shift dynamically following exercise, and this is the inflammatory response. IL-6 is an agglomerated cytokine in endurance exercise and functions as a pro- and an anti-inflammatory cytokine. This is followed by the resolution of inflammation, with the production of anti-inflammatory cytokines such as IL-10. Nevertheless, the long-term increase in pro-inflammatory mediator levels can precondition athletes to overtraining and immune imbalance (Pereira et al., 2024).

Omega-3 fatty acids have been shown to affect cytokine production and gene expression. The summary of randomized trials included in systematic reviews suggests a decrease in inflammatory indicators and oxidative stress with supplementation (Fernández-Lazaro et al., 2024; Rasińska et al., 2025). The action of EPA and DHA, in a mechanistic manner, incorporates into cell membranes and competes with arachidonic acid, which changes eicosanoid production. Moreover, high-protein diets enriched in omega-3 have been found to modulate the expression of inflammatory genes in peripheral blood mononuclear cells (Hass et al., 2023).

Another source of immune modulation is probiotics. It may be indicated that exercise can trigger an increase in cytokines, which can be mitigated by supplementing with probiotics, achieved by maintaining gut barrier integrity and regulating endotoxins (Aparicio-Pascual et al., 2025; Fernandez-Lazar et al., 2023). Thus, the gut-immune axis becomes one of the most important mediators of systemic inflammatory tone.

Lipid Mediators and Inflammation Resolution

The role of oxidative stress in exercise adaptation is two-fold. ROS is a signaling mediator that enhances mitochondrial biogenesis and the activity of antioxidant enzymes. However, excessive ROS can damage lipids, proteins, and DNA. The antioxidant strategies should therefore be balanced.

The regulatory effects of vitamin C, vitamin E, and natural antioxidants on the exercise-induced oxidative stress have been studied (MacGregor, 2024). Bioactive antioxidants, such as polyphenol-rich foods, compounds derived from olives, and anthocyanin-containing purple plants, can be used to help in recovery without fully inhibiting adaptive redox signaling (Lillis et al., 2025; Nuszkiewicz et al., 2025).

Curcumin is another compound with an increasing evidence base, which is an antioxidant and anti-inflammatory compound. The systematic reviews suggest that curcumin supplements lower the indicators of muscle damage and inflammation (Daniel Vasile et al., 2024; Rosińska-Lewandoska et al., 2024).

Carbohydrate Availability and Metabolic–Inflammatory Interaction

The recent conceptual changes are not only centered on inhibiting inflammation but also on resolving it. Omega-3 fatty acids are converted into specialized pro-resolving mediators (SPMs), which facilitate the termination of inflammation. Narrative analyses suggest that SPM-enriched marine oils can accelerate recovery by promoting the polarization and clearance of inflammatory debris by macrophages (de Souza et al., 2025).

Figure 1. Mechanistic Pathways Linking Exercise-Induced Muscle Damage and Nutritional Modulation

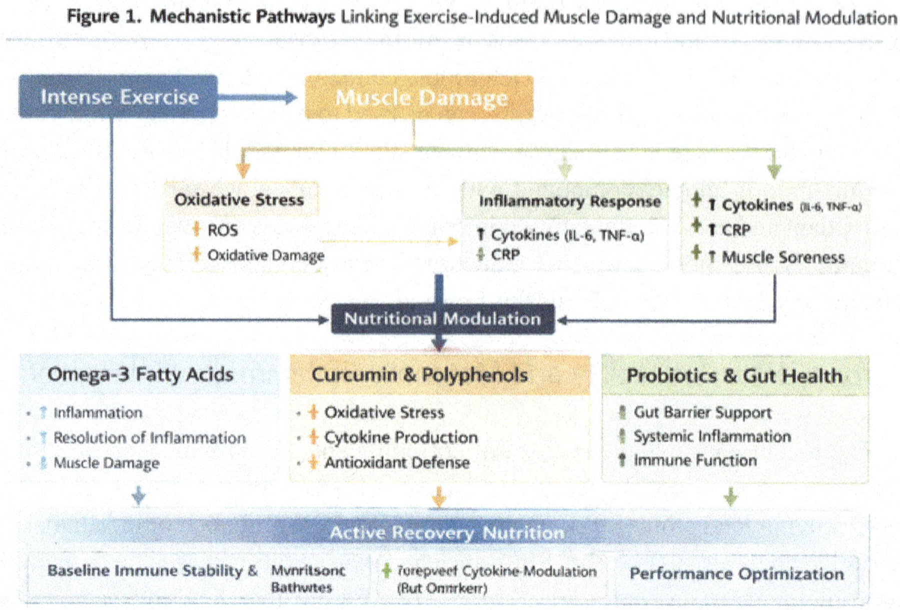

Figure 1 replicated, The Conceptual schematic representation of the effects of mechanical stress on the muscle and its key consequences on cytokine release, oxidative stress formation, and immune activation, and the possible pathways of nutritional regulation (omega-3 fatty acids, curcumin, probiotics, antioxidants, and protein sources). Conceptually adapted based on the mechanisms that were described by Sousa et al. (2014), Fernandez-Lazaro et al. (2024), Aparicio-Pascual et al. (2025), and de Souza et al. (2025).

Table 1 presents a mechanistic classification of nutritional interventions that address exercise-induced inflammation and recovery, synthesized from systematic reviews and randomized trials (Bongiovanni et al., 2020; Talebi et al., 2023).

3. METHODOLOGY

3.1 Integrative Perspective

The concept of recovery nutrition is increasingly understood as a systems-level intervention. It overlaps with immune biology, redox signaling, lipid mediator dynamics, and metabolic regulation. The nutrition professional is necessary for personalizing strategies to training loads and physiological responses (Filho, 2024).

Notably, no evidence favors the unselective use of high-dose supplementation. In its place, moderate, context-specific interventions seem to be the most effective in preserving adaptation and reducing excessive inflammation. The literature highlights the importance of balance, i.e., between ROS signaling and oxidative damage, cytokine activation and resolution, nutrient adequacy, and over-supplementation.

The information obtained from surgical recovery models supports the overall idea that the adaptability of inflammatory pathways can be altered through organized nutrition planning (Alves Bersot et al., 2024). To translate such a notion into sports, there should be accuracy and longitudinal analysis.

The mechanistic data suggest that strategic nutritional interventions affect multiple layers of biology, including cellular membrane composition, gene transcription, cytokine signaling, gut integrity, and mitochondrial redox balance. Each of the above-mentioned foods targets specific, though linked, pathways since omega-3 fatty acids, curcumin, probiotics, plant-based proteins, marine bioactives, and polyphenol-rich foods have different targets.

3.2 Data Collection and Analysis

This chapter follows a systematic, evidence-based approach to assessing the effectiveness of nutritional interventions in reducing muscle damage during exercise and promoting recovery. A systematic review of peer-reviewed literature was conducted to gather data, thereby ensuring the scientific relevance of the foundational and current studies. A systematic review was adopted, following Siripipatthanakul et al. (2025; a, b & c).

The search was conducted across the largest academic databases, focusing on exercise-induced muscle damage, recovery nutrition, modulation of inflammation, omega-3 supplementation, and antioxidants in athletes. High-quality study designs were prioritized in the selection process, particularly randomized controlled trials, systematic reviews, and meta-analyses.

In order to remain consistent and relevant, studies were included when they: (i) included physically active people or athletes, (ii) tested the nutritional interventions that were associated with recovery or inflammation, and (iii) provided physical or performance outcomes that were measurable. Articles that were not methodologically clear or did not apply to the exercise context were filtered out. The outcomes of this screening process were an edited list of scientifically sound and thematically corresponding studies.

Important information was systematically selected and organized into an orderly structure. The information extracted included the nature of the nutritional intervention (e.g., omega-3 fatty acids, curcumin, probiotics, protein supplementation), participant variables, exercise regimens, inflammatory and oxidative biomarkers, and recovery outcomes (e.g., muscle soreness, muscle performance) related to the intervention.

The analysis method was a synthesis of qualitative and comparative analyses. Research papers were categorized by nutrition type, allowing cross-comparison of results within and between intervention types. In addition to the outcome-based assessment, a mechanistic approach was added to link the observed effects to underlying physiological processes, including cytokine regulation, oxidative stress, muscle protein synthesis, and interactions between the gut and the immune system.

Even though fluctuations in research design and intervention regimens represent limitations in themselves, the focus was on patterns of similar evidence and biological plausibility. On the whole, this combined analytical model guarantees a well-balanced and scientifically based interpretation of the existing literature about nutritional recovery strategies.

4. RESULTS

Table 1. Summary of Key Nutritional Interventions and Mechanistic Targets

Nutritional Strategy	Primary Mechanism	Key Outcomes Reported	Representative References
Omega-3 Fatty Acids	Modulation of eicosanoids; SPM production; membrane incorporation	Reduced inflammatory markers; improved recovery	Fernández-Lázaro et al. (2024). Rasińska et al. (2025); Hass et al. (2023)
Curcumin/ Turmeric	NF-κB inhibition; antioxidant activity	Decreased CK levels; reduced soreness	Daniel Vasile et al. (2024); Helder et al. (2025); Clayton et al. (2023)
Probiotics	Gut barrier integrity; endotoxin reduction; cytokine modulation	Improved inflammatory profile post-exercise	Aparicio-Pascual et al. (2025); Fernández-Lázaro et al. (2023)
Plant-Based Proteins	Amino acid support for muscle repair; phytochemical synergy	Enhanced muscle recovery	Govindasamy et al. (2025)
Anthocyanin-Rich Foods	Redox regulation; antioxidant pathways	Reduced oxidative stress markers	Nuszkiewicz et al. (2025)
Marine Bioactives	SPM generation; lipid mediator regulation	Accelerated resolution phase	de Souza et al. (2025); Lomiwes et al. (2023)

4.1 Strategic Nutritional Interventions: Evidence-Based Applications and Practical Framework

Mechanistic knowledge leads to biological plausibility, but putting it into practice requires an evidence-based organization. Sportspeople and professionals do not act at the molecular level; they act within training programs, performance programs, and the dietary limitations imposed by the real world. Therefore, understanding the effects of nutrients on inflammation is no longer the question; rather, it is how the nutrients can be implemented to contribute to better recovery without hampering the adaptation process.

Recent literature emphasizes that recovery nutrition needs to be periodized, individualized, and context-sensitive (Ihsan et al., 2024; Bongiovanni et al., 2020). Instead of blanket supplementation, targeted deployment in accordance with training load, exercise modality, and athlete physiology seems to be the most suitable. In this section, existing evidence is synthesized to make application models.

4.2 Timing and Periodization of Anti-Inflammatory Nutrition

The process of inflammation is not harmful at all times. Early inflammatory signaling is needed to stimulate satellite cell activation and muscle remodeling during hypertrophy phases or adaptation-oriented blocks. Thus, post-exercise aggressive anti-inflammatory measures are not necessarily good across the board.

The use of omega-3 supplementation, in particular, seems more effective in the long term than in the acute phase (Fernândez-Lazar et al., 2024; Rasińska et al., 2025). Progressive incorporation of the membranes helps slow the inflammatory tone rather than suddenly suppress it. In the same vein, hydrolyzed curcumin has been found to be dose-dependent in its usefulness during heavy training (Helder et al., 2025), indicating that its strategic application during competition congestion may be most effective in the short term.

Co-intake of carbohydrates with endurance training suppresses the effects of stress hormones and changes inflammatory biomarkers (Righetti et al., 2024). Thus, carbohydrate plans are still at baseline, especially during long sessions or those that drain glycogen stores.

Practical implication:

- Chronic omega-3 for baseline modulation
- Acute curcumin or polyphenol use during congested schedules
- Carbohydrate availability is maintained during high-volume endurance

4.3 Functional Foods Versus Isolated Supplements

This shift from supplement-focused models toward functional foods is becoming more widespread (Wang et al., 2024). Whole foods are sources of complex matrices that affect absorption kinetics and synergistic bioactivity.

The use of Greek yogurt during resistance training has been linked to changes in systemic inflammatory markers (Fraschetti et al., 2025). Plant proteins show recovery benefits when consumed in adequate amounts and in appropriate proportions (Govindasamy et al., 2025). On the same note, Greenshell™ mussel powder is an excellent source of bioactive marine lipids not found in conventional fish oil preparations (Lomiwes et al., 2023).

Foods containing olive-derived polyphenols and anthocyanins provide antioxidant benefits to natural food matrices (Lillis et al., 2025; Nuszkiewicz et al., 2025). Food-based compounds, compared with synthetic antioxidants, can have less intense but more physiologically integrated effects, which will minimize the risk of disrupting redox-sensitive adaptation.

Clinical translation: prioritize whole-food strategies before high-dose isolated supplementation when possible.

4.4 Gut-Targeted Strategies and Immune Stability

High-intensity exercise undermines intestinal barrier integrity, leading to endotoxin leakage and systemic inflammatory amplification. Probiotic supplementation has also been found to regulate cytokine activity after exercise (Aparicio-Pascual et al., 2025; Fernandez-Lazaro et al., 2023).

Nevertheless, probiotic effectiveness appears to be both strain-specific and time-dependent. Short-duration interventions might help little, whereas long-term supplementation could stabilize immune function over time. Hence, endurance athletes who undergo recurring gastrointestinal stress are particularly at risk of using gut-targeted methods.

4.5 Lipid-Mediated Resolution and Marine Bioactives

Recent research shows the relevance of biology at the resolution stage. Marine oils containing SPMs stimulate the resolution of inflammation rather than its inhibition (de Souza et al., 2025). It is also critical during intense training, when inflammation must resolve effectively to avoid chronic low-grade immune activation.

The fact that omega-3 supplementation lowers indicators of muscle injury and inflammation is supported by systematic reviews and randomized trials (Fernández-

Lazaro et al., 2024; Rasińska et al., 2025). Elite athletes thus go beyond energy provision to include structural and signaling roles in lipid nutrition (Toledo et al., 2025).

Figure 2. Evidence-Based Strategic Framework for Nutritional Recovery

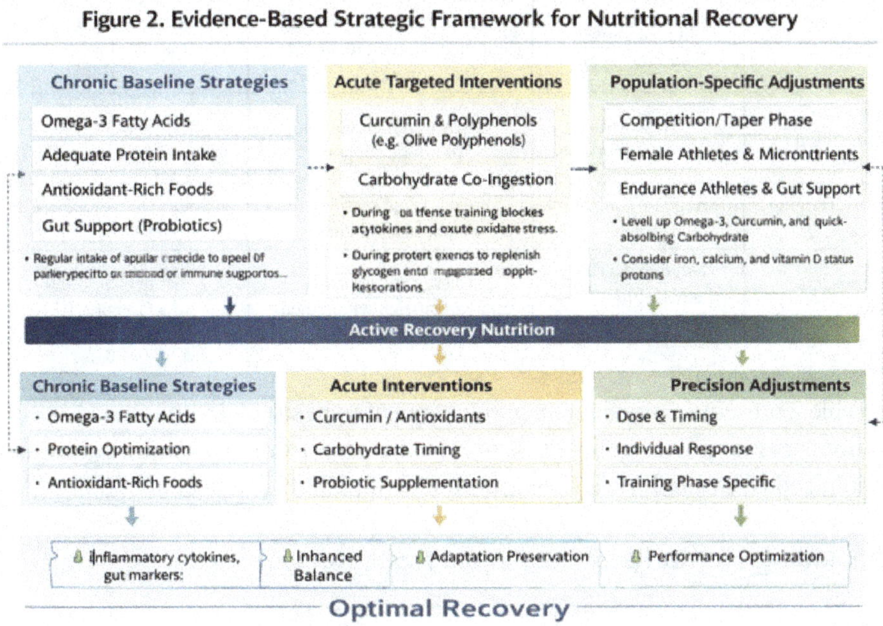

Figure 2, Integrated framework demonstrating periodized nutritional strategies that are consistent with training intensity and training inflammatory load. Membrane and immune stability is maintained by chronic baseline interventions (incorporation of omega-3, balanced protein consumption), whereas acute interventions (curcumin, carbohydrate co-ingestion, probiotics during heavy load) regulate cytokine amplitude and oxidative stress. Synthesis: Conceptual synthesis based on Fernandez-Lazar et al. (2024), Helder et al. (2025), Aparicio-Pascual et al. (2025), Wang et al. (2024), and de Souza et al. (2025).

Table 2. Applied Nutritional Strategies Across Training Phases

Training Context	Primary Physiological Stress	Recommended Nutritional Focus	Supporting Evidence
High-Volume Endurance	Glycogen depletion, oxidative stress	Carbohydrate co-ingestion; anthocyanin-rich foods	Righetti et al. (2024); Nuszkiewicz et al. (2025)
Resistance Hypertrophy Phase	Microtrauma, cytokine surge	Adequate protein (animal or plant-based); moderate omega-3	Govindasamy et al. (2025); Fernández-Lázaro et al. (2024)
Congested Competition Schedule	Repeated inflammatory peaks	Hydrolyzed curcumin; probiotic support	Helder et al. (2025); Aparicio-Pascual et al. (2025)
Heavy Training Block	Chronic inflammatory tone	SPM-enriched marine oils; balanced lipid intake	de Souza et al. (2025); Toledo et al. (2025)
Overreaching Risk	Neuroendocrine stress; immune suppression	Energy sufficiency; antioxidant-rich whole foods	Pereira et al. (2024); MacGregor (2024)

Table 2 presents a practical mapping of nutritional strategies to training-specific inflammatory and metabolic stressors, synthesized from systematic reviews and randomized controlled trials (Bongiovanni et al., 2020; Talebi et al., 2023).

Concluding Remarks of the Applied Section

Recovery nutrition is gradually evolving toward a more precision-oriented model rather than a generalized one. Conventional recommendations usually offer uniform doses of omega-3 fatty acids, antioxidants, or protein, depending on the average population reaction. However, inflammatory processes that arise from exercise are highly personal. Training condition, heredity, intestinal microbiota composition, regular diet, age, sex, and metabolic flexibility all influence the extent of inflammation and recovery dynamics. What is a win-win strategy to one athlete can be a win-lose strategy to another.

5. DISCUSSIONS

Precision recovery nutrition is thus based on three pillars, namely (1) individual inflammatory phenotype, (2) training load and adaptation phase, and (3) nutrient-genes-microbiome interaction. Instead of blindly acting on inflammation, the goal is narrowed to fine-tuning regulation in the direction of adaptive interests.

5.1 Inter-Individual Variability in Inflammatory Response

The responses of cytokines to exercise vary significantly among individuals (Via et al., 2024). There are cases of athletes with high levels of IL-6 and TNF-α who resolve their inflammation after training, and others who retain it. This response is affected by genetic polymorphism of inflammatory mediators, predisposing dietary patterns, and omega-3 status habits.

Supplementation with omega-3 fatty acids has shown heterogeneous effects across randomized trials (Fernández-Lázaro et al., 2024; Rasińska et al., 2025). Base level EPA/DHA status seems to exclude responsiveness. Professional athletes who do not eat fish regularly might benefit more than those who already eat fish-rich diets. Additionally, dietary patterns that combine high protein and omega-3 intake have been shown to modulate gene expression in peripheral immune cells (Hass et al., 2023), suggesting personalized metabolic adjustments.

Likewise, probiotic supplementation does not consistently affect cytokine reorganization in all athletes (Aparicio-Pascual et al., 2025; Fernandez-Lazar et al., 2023).

5.2 Nutrigenomics and Molecular Signaling

Recent studies identify such encounters between the nutrients and genes as a key frontier in the recovery science. Lipid mediators mediate the action of transcription factors, including NF-κB and peroxisome proliferator-activated receptors (PPARs), thus affecting the expression of inflammatory genes (de Souza et al., 2025). Curcumin also regulates intracellular signaling cascades, and dose-response studies support the bioavailability of curcumin preparations (Helder et al., 2025; Popescu et al., 2024).

Purple plant foods rich in anthocyanins have antioxidant and redox-regulatory roles at the cellular level (Nuszkiewicz et al., 2025). In contrast to high-dose synthetic antioxidants, these compounds seem to act on endogenous antioxidant enzyme systems rather than dominate them. This low-pass modulation could conserve positive adaptation information.

Practically, nutrigenomic profiling, though in its infancy, potentially will inform nutrient choice and dose in the future. Athletes with a tendency toward excessive inflammatory amplification may benefit from lipid-mediated resolution strategies, in particular, while others may be best served by a strategy of predominant structural protein support.

5.3 Training Phase–Specific Modulation

Different roles of inflammation are dependent on the training stage. Inflammatory signaling helps in muscle remodeling during hypertrophy or in response to forces that drive adaptation. Adaptation could be flattened by aggressive repression at this stage. On the contrary, in the periods of strained competition schedules, the speed of recovery takes center stage.

There is scientific evidence supporting the use of omega-3 supplementation to reduce markers of muscle damage during intensified training (Fernández-Lazar et al., 2024). Hydrolyzed curcumin exhibits acute recovery effects when exposed to high-stress levels (Helder et al., 2025; Clayton et al., 2023). Resistance programs can provide combined anti-inflammatory and protein benefits from functional dairy proteins, including Greek yogurt (Fraschetti et al., 2025).

Inflammatory outcomes are also influenced by carbohydrate availability, especially when undertaking endurance exercise (Righetti et al., 2024). Glycogen adequacy reduces increases in stress hormones and inflammatory responses. As such, the accuracy strategies must align training requirements with nutrient timing.

Figure 3. Conceptual Model of Precision Recovery Nutrition

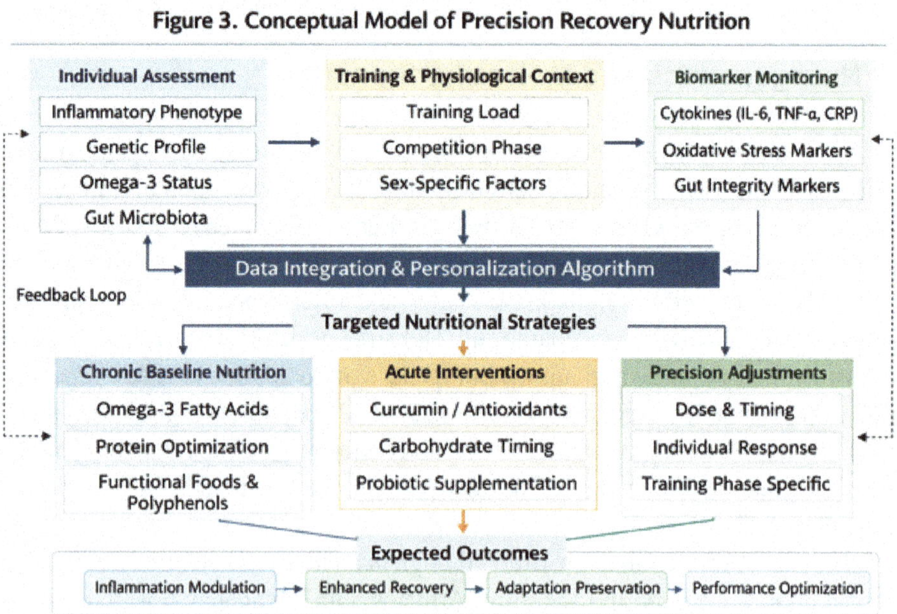

As shown in Figure 3, the precision recovery nutrition model combines personal inflammatory phenotype, training phase, gut microbiota status, and nutrigenomic response. The acute targeted interventions (curcumin, probiotics, anthocyanins) in combination with chronic baseline interventions (balanced protein intake, omega-3 incorporation) can be used to regulate cytokine amplitude and resolution pathways.

Theoretical model based on Hass et al. (2023), Fernandez-Lazaro et al. (2024), Aparicio-Pascual et al. (2025), Helder et al. (2025) and Nuszkiewicz et al. (2025).

5.4 Microbiome-Informed Recovery Strategies

The gut-muscle axis is a very vital point of diet-immune interaction. Gastrointestinal permeability exercise could augment systemic inflammatory signaling. There is moderate evidence supporting cytokine modulation post-exercise with probiotic supplementation (Aparicio-Pascual et al., 2025; Fernandez-Lazar et al., 2023). Nevertheless, strain specificity is an important determinant.

Individualized probiotic prescriptions, informed by microbiome sequencing, can improve recovery. Although it is a new discipline, it fits into the wider paradigm of precision nutrition.

5.5 Functional Foods as Long-Term Precision Tools

Functional foods provide a viable way of applying personalized tactics. Layered bioactive compounds are found in the natural matrices of olive-derived polyphenols, marine bioactives, and fruits with high concentrations of anthocyanins (Lillis et al., 2025; Lomiwes et al., 2023; Nuszkiewicz et al., 2025). Whole-food strategies can be a better part of long-term dietary patterns than isolated supplements.

Experiences with improved recovery models in the surgical setting show that coordinated nutritional frameworks can attenuate inflammatory variables and improve outcomes (Bersot et al., 2024). Applying this systematic mechanism to sport needs to be translated into one-on-one appraisal rather than strict supplementation guidelines.

Figure 4. Dynamic Interaction Between Nutrient Classes and Inflammatory Phases

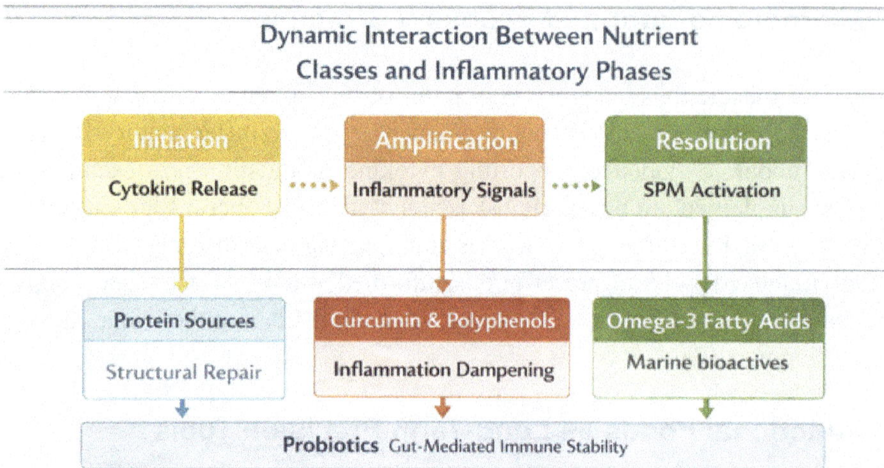

Figure 4, depicting Temporal interaction between periods of inflammation (initiation, amplification, resolution) due to exercise and nutrient-specific modulation. Marine bioactives and omega-3 fatty acids promote resolution; curcumin and polyphenols inhibit amplification; protein sources promote structural repair; probiotics stabilize gut-mediated immune activation. Theories are conceptualized based on de Souza et al. (2025), Fernandez-Lazarillo et al. (2024), Popescu et al. (2024), Aparicio-Pascual et al. (2025), and Govindasamy et al. (2025).

Precision nutrition reconceptualizes anti-inflammatory interventions as adaptive rather than blanket. There is evidence and practice supporting the use of omega-3 fatty acids, curcumin, probiotics, polyphenol-rich foods, functional proteins, and marine bioactives to modulate pathways to recovery. Their efficacy, however, depends on a person's physiology, the training environment, and time.

The combination of biomarker-based personalization, multi-nutrient synergy trials, and sex-specific research should be incorporated into future studies. With advances in recovery science, the incorporation of nutrigenomics, microbiome profiling, and training analytics will likely become the next frontier in performance nutrition.

5.6. Integrated Translational Model and Future Directions in Strategic Recovery Nutrition

The above sections have explored the biological basis of exercise-induced inflammation, discussed specific nutritional interventions, and explored the possibilities of precision-based interventions. Integration is the logical next step. Even good research can be disjointed - isolated studies on omega-3 fatty acids, small-scale probiotic studies, and short-term studies of curcumin. However, athletes do not take nutrients separately. They consume food, observe patterns, and seasons change. Translational recovery nutrition should thus work on the system level.

This part offers a combined model that integrates mechanistic understanding, applied tactics, and individual modulation, organizing them into a consistent framework applicable to both high-performance and clinical groups.

5.7 From Isolated Nutrients to Coordinated Systems

The previous recovery models paid much attention to macronutrient replenishment -protein to repair the muscle, and carbohydrate to restore glycogen (Sousa et al., 2014; Harty et al., 2019). Although critical, this model did not give the complexity of inflammatory signaling and immune modulation due to its foundational nature. In recent reviews, it has been noted that omega-3 fatty acids, polyphenols, probiotics, marine bioactives, and functional proteins interact in several physiological areas (Talebi et al., 2023; Bongiovanni et al., 2020).

For example, omega-3 supplementation affects membrane lipid composition and the production of inflammatory mediators (Fernández-Lazar et al., 2024; Rasińska et al., 2025). Curcumin also regulates transcription factors associated with cytokine expression (Popescu et al., 2024; Helder et al., 2025). Upon probiotics, gut permeability is stabilized, and the amplification of inflammatory systems in the body is minimized (Aparicio-Pascual et al., 2025; Fernandez-Lazar et al., 2023). These interventions act on different but related biological processes.

Their synergy can be even greater than the effect of each intervention when used wisely. This, however, may lead to excessive overlap, especially in antioxidant activity, thereby blunting beneficial redox signaling (MacGregor, 2024). As such, integrated systems should be able to reconcile synergy and restraint.

5.8 Translational Recovery Across Training Cycles

The dynamics of inflammation vary in macrocycles, mesocycles, and microcycles. When the exercise is high-intensity, cytokine levels are elevated, and recovery intervals are minimized. Inflammatory signaling is involved in structural remodeling during periods of adaptation.

There is systematic evidence supporting the use of omega-3 supplementation to prevent post-exercise inflammation and muscle injury (Fernández-Lazar et al., 2024; Rasińska et al., 2025). However, all these effects are most evident with chronic intake rather than acute dosing. The acute recovery effect of Curcumin has been observed during increased training periods (Helder et al., 2025; Clayton et al., 2023).

Structural repair is supported by functional proteins (such as those in plant foods and dairy matrices), including Greek yogurt, and has a moderate effect on inflammatory markers (Govindasamy et al., 2025; Fraschetti et al., 2025).

Carbohydrate diets have been found to be critical for endurance recovery, particularly due to their effects on stress hormone and inflammatory biomarker responses (Righetti et al., 2024).

These findings suggest a layered periodization model:

- **Chronic baseline support:** omega-3 incorporation, adequate protein distribution
- **Acute stress response management:** curcumin, polyphenol-rich foods
- **Endurance stabilization:** carbohydrate sufficiency
- **Gut resilience:** targeted probiotics

Figure 5. Integrated Translational Framework for Strategic Recovery Nutrition

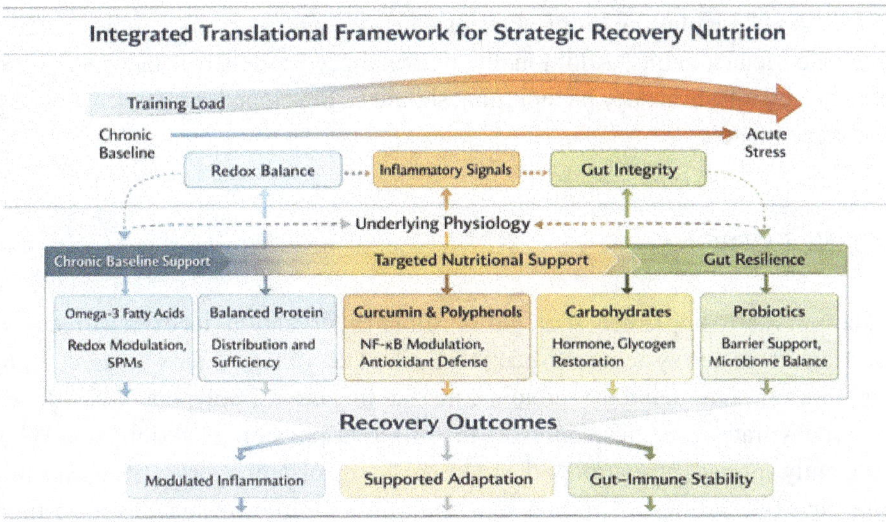

The multilevel translational model, as illustrated in Figure 5, connects training load, inflammatory amplitude, gut integrity, redox balance, and nutrient-specific interventions. Baseline nutrition (omega-3 fatty acids, balanced protein) is needed to ensure membrane and immune system stability; acute targeted strategies (curcumin, anthocyanins, probiotics) can be used to regulate cytokine peaks; carbohydrate availability may adjust the metabolic-inflammatory balance. The synthesis of the concepts was based on Talebi et al. (2023), Fernandez-Lazaro et al. (2024), Aparicio-Pascual et al. (2025), Helder et al. (2025), and Wang et al. (2024).

5.9 Future Research Priorities

Despite promising evidence, important limitations remain:

1. **Short-Term Study Designs:** Many trials evaluate acute biomarker changes rather than long-term adaptation outcomes (Talebi et al., 2023).
2. **Male-Dominated Samples:** Female athlete physiology remains underrepresented.
3. **Single-Nutrient Focus:** Combined intervention trials are rare.
4. **Limited Biomarker Integration:** Multi-omic approaches—lipidomics, transcriptomics, microbiomics—are still emerging.

Future studies will have to involve an integrated panel of biomarkers to measure not only inflammatory suppression but also the dynamics of resolution and the preservation of adaptation. Multi-nutrient synergy trials can be more representative of real-life dietary habits. Additionally, personalized models that incorporate microbiome and inflammatory phenotyping should be developed to enhance precision in recovery models.

6. CONCLUSIONS

The best way to implement strategic nutritional interventions for exercise recovery is from an integrated systems perspective. Each of the omega-3 fatty acids, curcumin, probiotics, plant and dairy proteins, marine bioactives, polyphenol-rich foods, and carbohydrate strategies addresses the different physiological domains. When intelligently applied, in relation to the training phase, inflammatory profile, and individual physiology, they provide a potent framework for improving recovery without jeopardizing adaptation. It is a critical crossroad in the field. These strategies are set to be further developed through advances in nutrigenomics, microbiome science, and molecular biomarker profiling. The future goal is not to decrease inflammation but to maximize its resolution, timing, and engagement with adaptation. Recovery is not an idle period between training sessions; it is a dynamic process in the body that is either positive or negative, and it determines whether exercise stress leads to adaptation or maladaptation. In this chapter, exercise-induced inflammation is no longer considered an enemy to be destroyed, but rather a controlled physiological indicator to be managed carefully. The issue with sports nutrition science is that it must strike a balance between supporting tissue repair and immune stability and inhibiting processes that can lead to long-term increases in performance. The synthesized evidence presented in the mechanistic, applied, and precision-oriented sections reveals several consistent themes. To begin with, exercise-induced inflammation is complex, involving cytokine cascades, oxidative stress, membrane lipid remodeling, and gut-mediated immune signaling. All these layers are affected by nutritional interventions. The omega-3 fatty acids also alter membrane composition and support resolution-phase biology. Curcumin has been shown to regulate transcriptional processes related to the amplification of inflammation. Probiotics help maintain the integrity of gut barriers and may reduce inflammatory spillover in the system. Redox balance is maintained by polyphenol compounds, such as olive derivatives and anthocyanin-containing plants. Plant- and dairy-based functional proteins are also involved in structural repair and in regulating inflammatory markers.

There are some areas of research that should be given priority. First, more natural trials that examine synergistic combinations, e.g., omega-3 with probiotics or curcumin with anthocyanins, would more closely reflect natural dietary habits. Second, the use of biomarkers to personalize in order to improve the dosing strategy. Third, it may be more inclusive and applicable by exploring sex-specific inflammatory and recovery responses. Lastly, performance adaptation and inflammatory modulation measures must be evaluated in long-term studies to ensure that short-term recovery benefits do not undermine long-term improvement.

To sum up, strategic nutritional interventions provide an effective, biologically based approach to improving recovery and regulating exercise-induced inflammation. The best strategies are those that do not ignore the duality of inflammation, which is an agent and a limit. With a mechanistic understanding, periodized implementation, and personal evaluation, recovery nutrition can be transformed from a generic prescription into a specific performance-management approach. The future of this field is not to eliminate inflammation, but to coordinate the timing, magnitude, and resolution of training adaptation with inflammation.

REFERENCES

Alves Bersot, C. D., Ferreira Gomes Pereira, L., Goncho, V. G. V., Pereira, J. E. G., & Falcão, L. F. D. R. (2024). Enhancing recovery and reducing inflammation: The impact of enhanced recovery after surgery recommendations on inflammatory markers in laparoscopic surgery—A scoping review. *Frontiers in Surgery*, *11*, 1450434. DOI: 10.3389/fsurg.2024.1450434 PMID: 39717352

Aparicio-Pascual, D., Clemente-Suárez, V. J., Tornero-Aguilera, J. F., & Rubio-Zarapuz, A. (2025). The effect of probiotic supplementation on cytokine modulation in athletes after a bout of exercise: A systematic review and meta-analysis. *Sports Medicine - Open*, *11*(1), 58. https://link.springer.com/article/10.1186/s40798-025-00860-7. DOI: 10.1186/s40798-025-00860-7 PMID: 40402402

Bongiovanni, T., Genovesi, F., Nemmer, M., Carling, C., Alberti, G., & Howatson, G. (2020). Nutritional interventions for reducing the signs and symptoms of exercise-induced muscle damage and accelerate recovery in athletes: Current knowledge, practical application and future perspectives. *European Journal of Applied Physiology*, *120*(9), 1965–1996. DOI: 10.1007/s00421-020-04432-3 PMID: 32661771

Clayton, D. J., Burbeary, R., Hennis, P. J., James, R. M., Saward, C., Colledge, A., Scott, R., Gilpin, S., McMahon, R., & Varley, I. (2023). Turmeric supplementation improves markers of recovery in elite male footballers: A pilot study. *Frontiers in Nutrition*, *10*, 1175622. DOI: 10.3389/fnut.2023.1175622 PMID: 37293669

Daniel Vasile, P. R., Patricia, M. L., Marta, M. S., & Laura, E. (2024). Evaluation of curcumin intake in reducing exercise-induced muscle damage in athletes: A systematic review. *Journal of the International Society of Sports Nutrition*, *21*(1), 2434217. DOI: 10.1080/15502783.2024.2434217 PMID: 39623590

de Souza, L. C., Moris, J. M., Gordon, P. M., Heileson, J. L., & Funderburk, L. K. (2025). From fish oil to resolution: A narrative review on the potential of SPM-enriched marine oil for exercise-induced muscle damage recovery. *Nutrients*, *17*(12), 2014. DOI: 10.3390/nu17122014 PMID: 40573125

Fernández-Lázaro, D., Arribalzaga, S., Gutiérrez-Abejón, E., Azarbayjani, M. A., Mielgo-Ayuso, J., & Roche, E. (2024). Omega-3 fatty acid supplementation on post-exercise inflammation, muscle damage, oxidative response, and sports performance in physically healthy adults—A systematic review of randomized controlled trials. *Nutrients*, *16*(13), 2044. DOI: 10.3390/nu16132044 PMID: 38999792

Fernández-Lázaro, D., Sánchez-Serrano, N., Rabail, R., Aadil, R. M., Mielgo-Ayuso, J., Radesca Fabiano, K., & Garrosa, E. (2023). Is probiotics supplementation an appropriate strategy to modulate inflammation in physically active healthy adults or athletes? A systematic review. *Applied Sciences (Basel, Switzerland)*, *13*(6), 3448. DOI: 10.3390/app13063448

Filho, E. M. A. A. (2024). O papel do nutricionista no acompanhamento de atletas: como a nutrição pode auxiliar na melhora do desempenho atlético e na recuperação pós-exercício. 12–13. https://doi.org/DOI: 10.69849/revistaft/fa10202408241812

Fraschetti, E. C., Abdul-Sater, A. A., Perry, C. G., & Josse, A. R. (2025). Resistance exercise training and Greek yogurt consumption modulate markers of systemic inflammation in healthy young males—A Secondary Analysis of a Randomized Controlled Trial. *Nutrients*, *17*(17), 2816. DOI: 10.3390/nu17172816 PMID: 40944203

Govindasamy, K., Parpa, K., Katanic, B., Clark, C. C., Elayaraja, M., Kambitta Valappil, I. N., Dulceanu, C., Geantă, V. A., Tolan, G. A., & Zouhal, H. (2025). Effect of Plant-Based Proteins on Recovery from Resistance Exercise-Induced Muscle Damage in Healthy Young Adults—A Systematic Review. *Nutrients*, *17*(15), 2571. DOI: 10.3390/nu17152571 PMID: 40806155

Harty, P. S., Cottet, M. L., Malloy, J. K., & Kerksick, C. M. (2019). Nutritional and supplementation strategies to prevent and attenuate exercise-induced muscle damage: A brief review. *Sports Medicine - Open*, *5*(1), 1. DOI: 10.1186/s40798-018-0176-6 PMID: 30617517

Helder, T. A., Condon, S., Grant, I., Lewis, N. A., Hill, J., Pedlar, C. R., & Hughes, L. (2025). The dose–response effects of hydrolyzed curcumin on recovery, inflammation, and oxidative stress following exercise-induced muscle damage in males. *Physiological Reports*, *13*(15), e70504. DOI: 10.14814/phy2.70504 PMID: 40781899

Ihsan, F., Nasrulloh, A., Kozina, Z., Hidayat, R. A., Perdana, S., & Sukendro, S. (2024). Nutritional strategies for rapid recovery in sport: A literature review. *Retos: nuevas tendencias en educación física, deporte y recreación*, (57), 153–164. https://doi.org/DOI: 10.47197/retos.v57.105622

Lillis, J. B., Willmott, A. G., Chichger, H., & Roberts, J. D. (2025). The application of olive-derived polyphenols on exercise-induced inflammation: A scoping review. *Nutrients*, *17*(2), 223. DOI: 10.3390/nu17020223 PMID: 39861354

Lomiwes, D., Barnes, M., Shaw, O., Ngametua, N., Sawyer, G., Burr, N., Hedderley, D., Kanon, A., Bear, T., Carroll, A., Bentley-Hewitt, K., Tian, H. S., & Miller, M. R. (2023). The Efficacy of New Zealand Greenshell™ Mussel Powder Supplementation in Supporting Muscle Recovery Following Eccentric Exercise-Induced Muscle Damage in Healthy, Untrained Adult Males. *Nutrients*, *15*(10), 2316. DOI: 10.3390/nu15102316 PMID: 37242198

MacGregor, E. A. (2024). The Regulatory Effects of Vitamin C, Vitamin E, and Natural Antioxidants on Oxidative Stress and Muscle Inflammation Induced by High-Intensity Exercise. *Studies in Sports Science and Physical Education*, *2*(4), 1–5. DOI: 10.56397/SSSPE.2024.12.01

Moreira, Y. S., de Carvalho Simões, M. A., & Borba, É. L. (2024). O uso de estratégias nutricionais na prevenção e recuperação de lesões em atletas: Uma revisão de literatura. *Research. Social Development*, *13*(5), e6813545807–e6813545807. DOI: 10.33448/rsd-v13i5.45807

Nuszkiewicz, J., Wróblewska, J., Wróblewski, M., & Woźniak, A. (2025). Anthocyanin-Rich Purple Plant Foods: Bioavailability, Antioxidant Mechanisms, and Functional Roles in Redox Regulation and Exercise Recovery. *Nutrients*, *17*(15), 2453. DOI: 10.3390/nu17152453 PMID: 40806038

Pereira, D. M., Dos Santos, V. T., Vilela, M. M., De Oliveira, T. M., Oliveira, D. C., & Junior, J. K. K. (2024). *Contribuição da nutrição para a prevenção e recuperação da Síndrome do Overtraining em atletas*. Brazilian Journal of Health Review., DOI: 10.34119/bjhrv7n1-560

Popescu, R. D.-V., Martínez-López, P., Massip-Salcedo, M., & Esquius, L. (2024). Evaluation of curcumin intake in reducing exercise-induced muscle damage in athletes: A systematic review. *Journal of the International Society of Sports Nutrition*, *21*(1), 2434217. Advance online publication. DOI: 10.1080/15502783.2024.2434217 PMID: 39623590

Rasińska, A., Jachimczak, J., Rzyczniok, P., Bala, P., Matusik, J., Rostkowska, A., Grydź, F., Filipow, J., Kupisiak, S., Pasierb, N., & Kopczyński, M. (2025). The impact of omega-3 fatty acids supplementation on reducing exercise-induced muscle damage: A review. *Archiv EuroMedica*, *15*(3). Advance online publication. DOI: 10.35630/2025/15/3.321

Righetti, S., Medoro, A., Graziano, F., Mondazzi, L., Martegani, S., Chiappero, F., Casiraghi, E., Petroni, P. A., Corbi, G., Pina, R., Scapagnini, G., Davinelli, S., & Ricordi, C. (2024). Effects of Maltodextrin–Fructose Supplementation on Inflammatory Biomarkers and Lipidomic Profile Following Endurance Running: A Randomized Placebo-Controlled Cross-Over Trial. *Nutrients, 16*(18), 3078. DOI: 10.3390/nu16183078 PMID: 39339678

Rosińska-Lewandoska, D., Lewandowska, D., Morawska, M., Jarosz, K., Wolff, A., Kożuchowska, K., Gruszka, S., Szewczyk, M., Pilarz, D., & Ufnal, J. (2024). The impact of curcumin supplementation on inflammatory processes and recovery in athletes. *Journal of Education, Health and Sport, 76*, 56583. DOI: 10.12775/JEHS.2024.76.56583

Siripipatthanakul, S., Phuangsuwan, P., & Jaipong, P. (2025, a). Mobile application security: A case study of Bank of Ayudhya PCL.(KMA), Thailand. In *International Conference on Data Processing and Networking* (pp. 479–493). Springer, Singapore. https://link.springer.com/chapter/10.1007/978-981-96-3102-5_36

Siripipatthanakul, S., Rungsiyanont, S., & Siripipattanakul, S. (2025, c). Sustainable dentistry using artificial intelligence (AI) for digital education and business among university dental hospitals. In *Sustainable development for hospitals and clinics* (pp. 33–64). IGI Global Scientific Publishing. DOI: DOI: 10.4018/979-8-3693-9800-5.ch002

Siripipatthanakul, S., Phuangsuwan, P., Jaipong, P., & Muthmainnha. (2025,b, September). Wi-Fi Networks and Security: A Systematic Review. In *International Conference on Artificial Intelligence and Networking* (pp. 81–92). Singapore: Springer Nature Singapore. https://link.springer.com/chapter/10.1007/978-981-96-2015-9_6

Sousa, M., Teixeira, V. H., & Soares, J. (2014). Dietary strategies to recover from exercise-induced muscle damage. *International Journal of Food Sciences and Nutrition, 65*(2), 151–163. DOI: 10.3109/09637486.2013.849662 PMID: 24180469

Talebi, S., Zeraattalab-Motlagh, S., Arab, A., Ghoreishy, S. M., Amiri Khosroshahi, R., & Djafarian, K. (2023). Nutritional interventions for exercise-induced muscle damage: An umbrella review of systematic reviews and meta-analyses of randomized trials. *Nutrition Reviews*. Advance online publication. DOI: 10.1093/nutrit/nuad078 PMID: 37460208

Toledo, M. C. B., Brustoloni, J. G. F., Rocha, I., Faleiro, A. M. A., Costa, A. M., Dourado, A. R., Nunes, F., Takahagassi, R. H., Castro, A. V., & Rodrigues, M. S. (2025). A influência da nutrição lipídica em atletas de alto rendimento: Uma revisão sistemática. *Revista CPAQV, 17*(2), 9. DOI: 10.36692/V17N2-76R

Via, J., Reid, J., & Oehlert, G. (2024). Pedalling toward a deeper understanding of exercise effects on immune function. *The Journal of Physiology, 602*(19), 4705–4707. Advance online publication. DOI: 10.1113/JP287173 PMID: 39167713

Wang, L., Meng, Q., & Su, C.-H. (2024). From Food Supplements to Functional Foods: Emerging Perspectives on Post-Exercise Recovery Nutrition. *Nutrients, 16*(23), 4081. DOI: 10.3390/nu16234081 PMID: 39683475

Yasul, Y., Yılmaz, B., Yasul, M. E., Şenel, Ö., & Çinar, V. (2024). *Recovery response of coenzyme Q10 to exercise-related physiological muscle damage, inflammation and oxidative stress: A systematic review*. Turkish Journal of Kinesiology., DOI: 10.31459/turkjkin.1429014

Chapter 6

Balancing Natural Nutrition for Athletic Performance, Recovery, and Well-Being

Shuvasree Banerjee
http://orcid.org/0000-0001-5255-2489
Amity University, Mumbai, India

Mohammad Badruddoza Talukder
http://orcid.org/0009-0008-1662-9221
International University of Business Agriculture and Technology, Bangladesh

Tathagata Banerjee
http://orcid.org/0009-0002-9586-9907
International Institute of Hotel Management, India

Tamonwan Sitthipon
http://orcid.org/0009-0008-9939-5546
GlobalNxt University, Malaysia

ABSTRACT

An effective and well-balanced nutritional plan is essential for optimum athletic performance and recovery. This chapter will evaluate the concept of dietary balance from the perspective of functionality to support athletes by increasing the availability of energy, enhancing the regeneration of muscle tissue, reducing oxidative damage, and promoting sustenance over the long term. The demands on an athlete's body are greater than a non-athlete's due to the excessive amount of training and competition, thus having sufficient energy available is crucial to avoid fatigue and decreased

DOI: 10.4018/979-8-3373-9544-9.ch006

ability to recover from exercise and perform at a high level. Finally, the chapter will discuss how the use of plant-based foods has become increasingly important for those who lead active lifestyles, as these foods provide proteins, carbohydrates, and micronutrients as well as contain bioactive compounds to aid in recovery and decreasing the inflammatory process.

1. INTRODUCTION

Athletes are not only effective, competitive, and efficient, but also more than just training intensity and skill training; recovery from such events is closely related to their nutrition and thus heavily depends on it. Athletes have greater physiological demands than non-athletes; therefore, nutrition is paramount for energy metabolism, tissue repair, immune response, and, in addition, long-term health. Poor dietary habits can limit performance, slow recovery, compromise injury prevention, and increase injury risk; on the other hand, better nutrition can improve endurance, strength, and adaptability. Energy balance is a fundamental tenet in sports nutrition, representing the correlation between energy intake and expenditure.

Fatigue, hormonal imbalance, and lean mass loss can result from chronic energy deficit, while overconsumption can lead to poor body composition and metabolic inefficiency. Micronutrients such as iron, magnesium, calcium, zinc, and B-complex vitamins are essential for oxygen delivery, muscle contraction, and neuromuscular coordination. Athletic recovery involves exercise-induced oxidative damage. Antioxidants in plant-based meals protect cells from harm and reduce inflammation, helping athletes cope with training stress. Plant-based nutrition is now regarded as an alternative for improving athletic performance and supporting global health and environmental goals. It is becoming clear that athletes' performance and recovery depend on balanced nutrition, training intensity, and skill development. Athletes have higher physiological demands than non-athletes, so nutrition is crucial for energy metabolism, tissue repair, immune function, and long-term health. Poor Nutrition or a poorly planned Nutrition Program can hurt an athlete's performance, slow recovery, and increase the risk of injury and illness. Optimised Dietary Practices boost endurance, strength, and adaptability (Dima-Cozma et al., 2014).

Energy Balance is a basic principle in sports nutrition: the balance between Energy Intake from dietary sources and Energy Expenditure from Basal Metabolism, Physical Activity, and Recovery. Energy Deficiencies Over Time in Athletes have been shown to result in Fatigue, Hormonal Disturbance, Decreased Lean Body Mass, and Impaired Performance; meanwhile, excessive Energy Intake leads to Body Composition and Metabolic Efficiency Issues (Bryndin & Bryndina, 2017). As a result, Athlete Nutrition must be Individualized, Dynamic and Proactive in accordance with Training Loads and Competitive Cycles. Beyond energy intake, micronutrients play a decisive role in athletic recovery and performance. Minerals and vitamins such as iron, calcium, magnesium, zinc, and B-complex vitamins are essential for oxygen transport, muscle contraction, protein synthesis, and neuromuscular coordination. Deficiencies in these micronutrients have been linked to reduced exercise capacity, delayed muscle repair, and increased fatigue, particularly in endurance athletes and those following restrictive or plant-based diets (Lasya, 2022; Li et al., 2019). Intensive physical activity also induces oxidative stress by increasing the production of reactive oxygen species. While moderate oxidative stress is necessary for physiological adaptation, excessive levels can damage muscle tissue and impair recovery. Dietary antioxidants derived from natural foods have been shown to support cellular defence mechanisms and reduce inflammation associated with strenuous exercise, thereby improving recovery and training resilience (Suzuki et al., 2016; Yang & Landau, 2000).

The use of plant-derived foods provides Energy via Complex Carbohydrates Long and Sustained, and provides many Bioavailable Micronutrients, as well as Antioxidants and Phytochemicals to aid in Recovery and Overall Health, when combined strategically and properly, Plant-Based nutrition is a viable way to meet the Functional needs of Active Individuals while at the same time Supporting Cardio-Respiratory Health and Metabolic health for an indefinite Timeframe (Singletary, 2018; Schneider & Segre, 2009). This Chapter Provides a Functional Perspective on the Balance of Nutrition for the Athlete in Training and Recovery by Integrating the Evidence Surrounding Energy Balance, Micronutrient adequacy, the management of Oxidative Stress, and the Strategies of Plant-Based Nutrition As Such, We Present a Perspective that Will Help Us Align Nutritional Science with the Physiology of Athletic Training so as to Provide a Holistic Approach to Enhancing Performance, speeding Up Recovery, and Supporting the Long-Term Development of an Athletes.

Collaboration is necessary across all sectors of society, at the national, regional, and local levels, to achieve the 17 Sustainable Development Goals (SDGs) and their 169 corresponding targets. The 3rd Sustainable Development Goal is to ensure the attainment of good health and well-being for people of all ages. Enhancing individuals' well-being and overall standard of living is seen not only as one of the three fundamental principles of sustainable development, but also as a necessary condition for achieving the other two objectives. There is a widely held idea that health is both a necessary condition for and an outcome of successful sustainable development, and that these three concepts are closely interconnected. (Ionescu et al. 2020).

The globe, individuals, economic well-being, and the intricate and distinct challenges they confront now produce enduring issues, varying perspectives, and pioneering initiatives aimed at transforming and advancing. An enduring society for the future, given the current circumstances of fluctuation and re-evaluation of the manner in which things are done

As society progresses, we discover alternative courses of action that require government participation. Civil society, multinational businesses, governmental and private players, NGOs, and other groupings. Through a "global partnership," countries work together towards achieving the common objectives of the Sustainable Development Goals. The concept of sustainable development encompasses the environmental, social, and economic aspects.

The concept of the "global partnership" emerged following the events of September 25, 2015. When the 193 member states of the United Nations officially adopted the Sustainable Development Goals (SDGs), it signified not only their acceptance but also their commitment to align with them. The Sustainable Development Goals (SDGs) offer a significant opportunity to fundamentally transform and redefine society's approach to sustainable development for two main reasons. Firstly, they include areas that are open to exploration, examination, reinterpretation, and innovative concepts. Secondly, the United Nations and its member states' dedication to achieving the SDGs by 2030 has emphasised the urgent requirement for both quantitative and qualitative research. The expectation is that these investigations will prompt action across all domains of society, including politics, economics, and the environment.

The results should inspire prompt action in all economic, political, and social spheres. The rationale for this aspect lies in the fact that, even in the contemporary era, nations exhibit imbalances and disparities. This is primarily due to the diverse influences of multinational corporations, public and private entities, resources, and market positions, which reflect various facets of society and the economy. These elements undeniably influence the objectives set out in the 2030 Agenda.

The explicit commitment of each member state to eliminate poverty, enhance health and education, diminish inequality, and foster economic growth further emphasises this issue, particularly given the prominent status of the 17 Sustainable Development Goals as global benchmarks (Gavurova & Megyesiova, 2022).

One goal of sustainable development is to ensure the well-being and happiness of the population. The COVID-19 epidemic has threatened billions of lives, disrupted economies, and harmed numerous nations. The nation's readiness to address health issues and fund important public services was clear during this crisis. Several scientific studies and literature promoted global health before COVID-19. Increased life expectancy, lower newborn and maternal mortality rates, and other indicators indicate improved individual health. Given the increasing prevalence of chronic diseases, lifestyle changes, and societal improvements, health policies that improve access to and quality of healthcare are crucial. Financial resources for healthcare are essential to the sustainability and accessibility of the health system.

For years, researchers, economists, and international organizations have tried to assess a nation's health and welfare. The methodological and procedural concerns of these examinations are covered in several papers. The same technique applies to understanding the determinants of the global healthcare system. National health systems are heavily influenced by economic and social factors, politics, technology, and other factors. A sustainable health system must be universally accessible, collaborative between patients and doctors, and adaptable to changing demographics and finances. Healthcare systems must improve their efficacy and quality through creative innovation to survive (Fernandez, 2019).

Sustainable Development Goal 3 promotes lifelong health and well-being. The WHO charter was formed in 1948. The International Organization for Standards defines health as "a state of complete physical, mental, and social well-being, and not simply the absence of disease." SDG 3 has nine goals that can be broadly categorized into distinct but interconnected areas: reducing morbidity and mortality rates among vulnerable populations (such as newborns, the elderly, children, and mothers), lowering the prevalence of communicable and non-communicable diseases, mitigating risk factors (such as tobacco use, substance abuse, road traffic injuries, hazardous chemicals, and pollution), and ensuring universal access to heal. The SDG 3 targets do not mention socioeconomic factors affecting health and well-being. Health and well-being depend on a safe and supportive environment, which is achieved by minimizing climate change (SDG 13) and sustainably using water and land (SDGs 14 and 15). Systems thinking and the contemporary focus on planetary health recognize the close relationship between environmental and human health (Howden-Chapman et al., 2017). Hence, it can be noted that SDG goal no. 3, Health and Well-Being, aims to improve living conditions, thereby enhancing health and providing effective treatments for many diseases.

COVID-19 is expected to increase economic and social inequality. If people work toward the Sustainable Development Goals, human advancement could exceed pre-COVID levels. Green economic efforts, socially oriented innovation, alignment of business purpose with the SDGs, and political commitment from all levels of government must be prioritized. Family enterprises can contribute significantly to the SDGs in numerous ways. Many family business owners want to leave a legacy, and the SDGs align with that. The goals allow them to link their corporate activities to a larger purpose and to improve their local communities. Family businesses exist to leave a legacy through their mission. Thus, the firm's long-term prospects are prioritized over its short-term ones (Hales & Birdthistle, 2023).

2. LITERATURE REVIEW

The development of sports nutrition has occurred alongside scientific research in academia on the importance of nutrition to performance, recovery time, and long-term health. The gruelling pace of training and competition schedules puts considerable physiological stress on athletes, so they must eat a balanced diet with enough calories, micronutrients, and antioxidants to reduce oxidative stress. Nutrition has been shown to play an important role in metabolic efficiency, health, and overall performance, particularly in the context of overall health. Energy balance is key in sports nutrition, defined as the ratio of energy intake to energy expenditure. It is crucial for regularized energy levels to avoid fatigue, hormonal changes, and depleted exercise potential (Dima-Cozma et al., 2014). Relative energy deficiency in sport (RED-S) is a condition that may affect athletes experiencing chronic energy deprivation. It decreases bone density, disrupts metabolic balance, and attenuates immune response. In contrast, one must have a personalized meal plan and consider it important, as excess calories can negatively affect agility and body composition. In sports nutrition, micronutrient adequacy has been extensively investigated. Vitamins and minerals are important for tissue repair, neuromuscular coordination, and oxygen transport. While iron is needed for haemoglobin production and oxygen carriage, calcium and magnesium help build strong bones and muscles. Deficiencies of critical micronutrients might result in decreased physiological resilience and an increased propensity for harm and illness (Bryndin & Bryndina, 2017). This importance is even more salient among endurance athletes and those following restricted or vegetarian diets, due to a possible increased risk of vitamin deficiencies. People who engage in a lot of physical activity produce more reactive oxygen species (ROS), which increases oxidative stress. This phenomenon is a focus of research. An excess of reactive oxygen species (ROS) can harm a cell's structure and make it less effective in recovering, while a moderate oxygen stress contributes to physiological flexibility. (Suzuki et al.,2016; Yang & Landau, 2000) emphasized the benefits of dietary antioxidants, including flavonoids and polyphenols, in mediators of anti-inflammatory and free radical scavenging. As these findings suggest, adding antioxidant-rich foods to athletes' diets would improve recovery and immune function. Based on this, the high nutritional content and sustainability of plants have received significant attention in sports nutrition for their nutrient-dense nature and environmental benefits. They reveal that well-structured plant-based diets provide adequate macronutrients and micronutrients to enhance athletic performance, as well as anti-inflammatory and antioxidant benefits. Bioactive substances in herb- and plant-derived diets can impact metabolic pathways and cardiovascular health (Singletary, 2018).

Schneider & Segre (2009) also observed similar metabolic benefits, including a decreased risk of chronic disease, in their study of plant-based diets. Academic interest has been drawn to the health and sport recovery benefits of natural components, including Bok choy, basil, spinach, and tea. Much research on the effects of tea consumption has been driven by tea's high polyphenol content. Li et al. (2019) reported a positive interaction between tea intake and bone health in adults, while Pan et al. (2017) confirmed that habitual tea consumption is associated with improved health-related quality of life. Yang & Landau (2000) reported that spinach, a green vegetable, is rich in essential nutrients. Spinach, due to its high levels of vitamins, iron, and antioxidants, supports oxygen transport and muscle recovery.

Jovanovski et al. (2015) suggest that spinach nitrate may improve endurance athletes' performance by promoting vascular function through dietary and nutritional decreases in arterial stiffness. Kanabur & Reddy (2014) highlighted that spinach itself contains bioactive constituents that induce anti-inflammatory and antioxidant responses, which are supported by several studies on its antioxidant properties. Despite its widespread recognition for its food and medicinal uses, basil's medicinal potential has a scientific basis for research. Basil, as mentioned in Singletary (2018), offers anti-inflammatory and cardioprotective essential oils and flavonoids. Romano et al. (2022) similarly highlighted the presence of bioactive substances, e.g., caffeic and ferulic acids, which exhibit notable antioxidant and immunomodulatory effects. Due to these characteristics, basil may also help active individuals cope with stress and reduce recovery time after physical activity. Some nutritional studies were conducted on bok choy, a leafy, vitamin- and glucosinolate-rich cruciferous vegetable. Gattani and Kumari (2023) claim that bok choy contains phytochemicals, some of which have anticancer and metabolic activities.

Petpiamsiri et al. (2018) studied this phenomenon. Discussions about sports nutrition are not limited to physical health; they have expanded to include lifestyle behaviors, sustainable health paradigms, and customized dietary elements (Liu & Liu, 2019). The third Sustainable Development Goal 3 is to make people healthier and better able to live well and contribute to the global community by addressing the health and well-being of all. Macassa (2022) identified that sustainable health behaviors (e.g., a sustainable diet and physical activity) are key to achieving this goal. Houlden et al. (2021) found that time spent in natural settings and in the presence of biodiversity has beneficial effects on both mental and physical health. It is another indicator of how diet, lifestyle, and general well-being are intertwined. The literature stresses the importance of long-term health and livelihoods systems in improving nutrition-based health. Chambers & Conway (1991) introduced the concept of sustainable livelihoods, which promote long-term flourishing by increasing resilience and conserving resources. Nutrition-based health promotion can contribute to general social development, as emphasised by Fernandez (2019), thereby linking SDG 3 to other sustainability aims. The information analyzed shows that plant-based diets, antioxidant concentration, and diet balance are highly impactful on our performance in sports and on our recovery. The functions of native products go beyond nutrition, as their functional benefits may also enhance metabolic, cardiovascular, and immune system function. This impact is evident in sustainable frameworks, where sports nutrition contributes to health and wellness and to public health in ways not seen elsewhere. In conclusion, the current evidence demonstrates the importance of applying functional, natural nutritional interventions to achieve optimal athletic performance and rapid recovery. More empirical studies are required, but so far, no research has examined athlete-specific interventions or individual diet. This study is based on the assumption of sustainable well-being and considers the possible effects of natural nutrition on sports health.

3. METHODOLOGY

The systematic review and thematic content analysis are typically used in a review article that draws on related topics and keywords from scholarly papers (Siripipatthanakul et al., a, b, & c).

This chapter employs a comprehensive literature review to examine how a natural diet improves athletic performance, recovery, and well-being, thereby supporting sustainable health and Sustainable Development Goal 3. Instead of collecting primary data, the study synthesized scholarly information using a systematic review design. Systematic literature discovery, review, search, selection, and thematic synthesis guarantee rigor and transparency in research. A qualitative literature review of parallels, theoretical considerations, and areas for improvement in sports nutrition, antioxidant consumption, micronutrient absorption, and plant-based diets guided the exploratory and descriptive study design. It concentrated on tea, spinach, basil, and bok choy, which have been examined for their bioactive qualities and sports health benefits.

Sports nutrition/lifestyle, and sustainability create a health-promotion and well-being-based paradigm. The scientifically relevant scholarly papers are thoroughly reviewed. Search Scopus, Web of Science, PubMed, Google Scholar, and ScienceDirect for relevant peer-reviewed papers. This chapter searched this list for sports nutrition and recovery, natural ingredients and athletic performance, antioxidants and exercise stress, plant-based diet and athletes, and tea, spinach, basil, or bok choy and health benefits using keywords and Boolean operators. Other health promotion and SDG 3 were added to provide transdisciplinary perspectives on nutrition, public health, and sustainability.

To ensure consistency in analysis and interpretation, only English-language papers were searched. To ensure study relevance and credibility, inclusion and exclusion criteria were created. Valid peer-reviewed journal articles, book chapters, or reports on nutrition, natural ingredient use, dietary habits, physical health, sports performance, health recovery, or results were accepted. Micronutrients, antioxidants, and the sustainability of health need more research. Non-academic sources with questionable methodology, articles that only reported pharmacologic interventions unrelated to nutrition, and pharmacologic intervention-focused studies. These were removed due to academic unreliability, weak evidence, and theory-based opinions. Studies were selected using multi-stage screening. First, titles and abstracts were reviewed for research literature. Full-text reviews of shortlisted studies and research and theoretical reviews showed methodological rigor and thematic value. The final collection contained sports science, nutrition, public health, and sustainability studies.

Filtering for relevant, reputable data sources was crucial. Thematically screened data. For all selected studies, nutritional data and physiological and performance objectives were organized by research objective and methodological approach. Results on energy balance, micronutrient adequacy, antioxidant activity, and plant-based diets were prioritized. Data analysis using 'thematic synthesis' methodologies revealed recurrent patterns and conceptual linkages to other studies.

The energy balance in athletic performance and metabolic efficiency, as well as micronutrients in muscle regeneration, immune response, and physiological resilience, are crucial. The antioxidant mechanisms that reduce exercise-related oxidative stress, and the functional effects of natural ingredients and a plant-based diet to promote recovery and optimal health. These themes guided the literature analysis and influenced the results and the debate. Various academic databases to eliminate selectivity and obtain evidence from over 1 peer-reviewed, well-cited source. A clear inclusion standard and a rigorous review approach ensured methodological consistency, while thematic investigation ensured the application of content across disciplines. No formal quality evaluation methods were utilized; quality control tools selected publications from high-quality journals with good methodology. Source citation and academic honesty were ethical. It used secondary data from the literature; ethical approval was not sought. This study presented the original findings in APA format for evidence. However, its use is flawed. The secondary literature's focus favors publishing strong results. The review's English-language articles may not adequately contextualize regional research. Organized and credible, this chapter's theme methodology summarizes knowledge of natural nutrition and sports health. Science allows systematic investigation of natural nutrition, athletic performance, and sustainable well-being. A systematic assessment of sports science, nutrition, and public health literature shows that natural dietary practices improve performance, recovery, and overall health and are crucial for holistic health.

4. RESULTS

A natural diet has been shown to improve athletic performance and recovery in rigorous studies. The research theme reviews encompassed energy balance, micronutrient adequacy, antioxidant effects, and the functional efficacy of natural components and plant-based diets. Diet affects athletes' physiological resilience and performance in three ways. Metabolic homeostasis and athletic performance require energy equilibrium. In field tests, insufficient energy intake leads to fatigue, sluggish training adaptation, and injury, while high energy intake reduces body composition and agility. Customized diets match competitive exercise. This routine replenishes glycogen, regulates hormones, and strengthens muscles to increase endurance and strength. Micronutrient restoration. Vitamins heal muscles. Iron, calcium, magnesium, zinc, and B-complex vitamins support oxygen production, neuromuscular coordination, and immunity. These findings suggest that endurance athletes and plant-based eaters are deficient in certain vitamins. Green vegetables and herbs include micronutrients that regenerate tissue, alleviate fatigue, and speed recovery. Antioxidants lower oxidative stress. Dietary antioxidants addressed exercise-related oxidative damage. Vitamins, flavonoids, and polyphenols reduce reactive oxygen species during intense exercise. Plant non-steroidal antioxidants reduced inflammation, discomfort, and immune responses. Research shows that antioxidant-rich diets improve cellular adaptation and cause less oxidative damage than high-concentration synthetic supplements. Healthy Plant-Based Foods and Materials. Tea, spinach, basil, and bok choy boost athletes, the review stated. High tea-to-water ratios improved cardiovascular, anti-inflammatory, and metabolic health. Spinach nitrate improved vascular function and endurance. Basil reduces stress and inflammation, while bok choy provides vitamins, fiber, and glucosinolates to support immunological and metabolic health. Minerals rejuvenate and prolong life. Plant-based diets improved athletic performance through nutrient density, antioxidants, and anti-inflammatory effects. Fit plant-based diets balance macronutrients and support cardiovascular and metabolic health. These findings link sports nutrition, sustainability (e.g., animal-based meals), and healthy natural diets. Athletic performance relies on a balanced natural diet to maintain long-term well-being, improve recuperation, and provide constant energy without supplements. The best approach is a nutrient-dense, whole-food diet adjusted for workout intensity and macronutrient timing.

5. DISCUSSIONS

5.1 Athletic Health, Performance Optimization, and Recovery Support

A crucial and transformative element in achieving sustainability is health promotion, which involves enabling individuals to assume responsibility for and improve their own health. Significance in promoting the progress of public health goal 3: Ensure the well-being of individuals of all ages by promoting good health. Health promotion aims to modify the social, institutional, economic, and environmental contexts in which decisions about health and well-being are made, with a focus on justice and sustainability. On the contrary, sustainable development considers the needs of both the current generation and future generations. The economic, environmental, and social sectors are mutually reliant and must undergo this shift. By uniting them and leveraging their collective progress in practical settings, our aim is to establish a sustainable society capable of accommodating the entire human population and providing benefits to all its residents. Economic sustainability refers to the ability to maintain a consistent level of economic production over an extended period. When making decisions in this economy, sustainability is constantly taken into account alongside other factors. Furthermore, it is suggested that combining sustainable economic practices with social and environmental factors yields a significantly more advantageous outcome.

Yang & Landau (2000) reported that spinach, a green vegetable, is rich in essential nutrients. Spinach, due to its high levels of vitamins, iron, and antioxidants, supports oxygen transport and muscle recovery. Whereas Jovanovski et al. (2015) suggest that spinach nitrate may improve endurance athletes' performance by promoting vascular function through dietary and nutritional decreases in arterial stiffness. Kanabur & Reddy (2014) highlighted that spinach itself contains bioactive constituents that induce anti-inflammatory and antioxidant responses, which are supported by several studies on its antioxidant properties. Despite its widespread recognition for its food and medicinal uses, basil's medicinal potential has a scientific basis for research.

Singletary (2018) presents essential oils and flavonoids with anti-inflammatory and cardioprotective properties. Romano et al. (2022) similarly highlighted the presence of bioactive substances, e.g., caffeic and ferulic acids, which exhibit notable antioxidant and immunomodulatory effects. Due to these characteristics, basil may also help active individuals cope with stress and reduce recovery time after physical activity. Some nutritional studies were conducted on bok choy, a leafy, vitamin- and glucosinolate-rich cruciferous vegetable. Gattani and Kumari (2023) claim that bok choy contains phytochemicals, some of which have anticancer and metabolic activities.

Petpiamsiri et al. (2018) studied this phenomenon in discussions about sports nutrition that go beyond physical health, expanding to include lifestyle behaviors, sustainable health paradigms, and customized dietary elements. Liu & Liu (2019) discuss Sustainable Development Goal 3, which is to make people healthier and better able to live well and contribute to the global community by addressing the health and well-being of all.

Macassa (2022) identified that sustainable health behaviors (e.g., a sustainable diet and physical activity) are key to achieving this goal.

Houlden et al. (2021) found that time spent in natural settings and in the presence of biodiversity has beneficial effects on both mental and physical health. It is another indicator of how diet, lifestyle, and general well-being are intertwined. The literature stresses the importance of long-term health and livelihoods systems in improving nutrition-based health. Chambers and

Conway (1991) introduced the concept of sustainable livelihoods, which promote long-term flourishing by increasing resilience and conserving resources. Nutrition-based health promotion can contribute to general social development, as emphasised by Fernandez (2019), thereby linking SDG 3 to other sustainability aims. The information analyzed shows that plant-based diets, antioxidant concentration, and diet balance are highly impactful on our performance in sports and on our recovery. The functions of native products go beyond nutrition, as their functional benefits may also enhance metabolic, cardiovascular, and immune system function. This impact is evident in sustainable frameworks, where sports nutrition contributes to health and wellness, as well as to public health, in ways not seen elsewhere. In conclusion, the current evidence demonstrates the importance of applying functional, natural nutritional interventions to achieve optimal athletic performance and rapid recovery. More empirical studies are required, but so far, no research has examined athlete-specific interventions or individual diet. The sustainable well-being assumption considers the possible effects of natural nutrition on sports health. Furthermore, environmental sustainability refers to a condition of equilibrium, durability, and interdependence that enables human society to fulfil its requirements without surpassing the ability of its underlying ecosystems to consistently renew the essential services needed to meet those requirements, nor by its actions reducing biological diversity. The main objectives of environmental sustainability are to mitigate the adverse impacts of human activities on the environment and to advocate for the conservation and rehabilitation of natural areas.

On the other hand, social sustainability is linked to efforts to improve society as a whole. This aspect of sustainability supports the concept of intergenerational fairness, which holds that future generations should enjoy a standard of living comparable to or better than that of the current generation. The social sustainability factor encompasses several aspects, such as labour rights, equitable access to healthcare, community development through public participation and social cohesion, support for justice and accountability, community resilience, cultural competence, and human adaptation. Health is an integral part of the social dimension of sustainable development and is equally important to the environmental and economic dimensions (Macassa, 2022).

Efforts to enhance global health have seen limited progress in recent years. For instance, the Sustainable Development Goal (SDG) target to reduce child mortality has been achieved or is anticipated to be achieved in 146 of 200 countries or territories. Effective treatment has led to the eradication of at least one neglected tropical ailment in 47 countries, and globally, the incidence of AIDS-related mortality has reduced by 52% since 2010. However, progress in many areas, such as expanding universal health care and reducing maternal mortality, has been insufficient. In 2019, a total of 381 million people were pushed into or further into severe poverty due to the need to personally cover their medical expenses. Additionally, in 2020, an average of 800 women lost their lives each day as a direct consequence of pregnancy or childbirth. Progress towards Goal 3 has been limited because of the COVID-19 pandemic and other obstacles. The immunisation rate for youngsters has reached its lowest level in three decades, while the mortality rates due to tuberculosis and malaria have surged to levels not witnessed since before the outbreak (SDG-Report-2023).

Government health policy measures over the past few years have prioritised promoting health and well-being. Multiple goals, objectives, and performance evaluations require more actions to tackle problems that are commonly perceived as persistent, stubborn, deeply rooted, and challenging to fix. This subject is sometimes called a "wicked issue" because it defies straightforward, universally applicable solutions, if any exist. The issues associated with a wicked edge have intricate roots and require complex solutions. Obesity, alcoholism, poor mental health, environmental degradation, and other public health challenges possess several attributes, with the most apparent ones being the ones that society confronts directly. Unlike "tame" problems that may be simply articulated and solved, wicked problems do not have a linear, analytical solution (Hunter, 2009).

Ecosystem services typically support the maintenance of a healthy, habitable environment. Access to nature in urban green spaces can improve overall well-being by replenishing depleted attention, reducing stress, and promoting positive emotions. Additionally, these greenspaces facilitate participation in health-promoting activities such as social interactions and physical exercise. One way natural regions may provide ecosystem services, particularly cultural benefits, is through biodiversity, which refers to the diversity of plant and animal species (Houlden et al., 2021).

5.2 Benefits of consuming natural ingredients

There has been a significant increase in the stated health benefits and overall appeal of botanicals and dietary supplements manufactured from natural components in the United States. The ultimate source of therapeutic skill is in nature, rather than in doctors. Therefore, it is imperative that the doctor adopt a receptive mindset and begin exploring nature. Due to the prevailing belief in their potential health benefits, botanicals and their derived products are gaining popularity worldwide as culinary ingredients. Moreover, these goods are occasionally referred to as "natural" as they originate from natural sources. Occasionally, the botanical or herbal origin serves as an ingredient in food, while in other instances it requires extensive purification before it can be utilised in food (Abdel-Rahman et al., 2011).

Ecosystem services refer to the diverse array of social benefits derived from natural habitats and the physical characteristics and processes originating from non-human sources. These services encompass the supply of goods such as food and raw materials, the regulation of pollution, water, and climate systems, the support of essential processes such as pollination and habitat development, and the provision of cultural human services, including scientific, spiritual, recreational, and therapeutic connections. Cultural services may significantly impact individuals' overall well-being and contentment. While some writers argue that it is difficult to fully integrate biophilic design into the built environment, the notion of biophilia asserts that people feel most at ease and flourish in settings that reflect the natural environments in which the species developed. To mitigate the stresses of modern urban living, cities should incorporate parks and other designated natural spaces into their urban development strategies (Houlden et al., 2021).

Table 1. Connection of the Ingredients with Athletic Outcome

Ingredient	Current Focus	Needed Athletic Framing
Tea	Cardiovascular health, disease	Antioxidants for recovery, fatigue reduction, and inflammation control
Spinach	Anemia, BP, and general nutrition	Iron for oxygen transport, nitrates for endurance & blood flow
Basil	Stress, immunity	Stress modulation, cortisol balance, recovery support
Bok choy	Vitamins, digestion	Micronutrients for muscle repair & immune resilience

Table 1 highlights the role and importance of consuming natural ingredients, which are beneficial for health and have been proven effective in treating many diseases. This paper highlights natural ingredients such as tea, spinach, basil, and bok choy that support the SDG 3-Health & Well-Being goal.

a.) Impact Upon Consuming Tea

Consuming tea, derived from the dehydrated foliage of the Camellia sinensis plant, is a widespread custom worldwide. Approximately 3 billion kilograms of tea are produced and consumed annually. Many individuals have a keen interest in further exploring the potential health benefits of tea, prompting academics to investigate this topic. Several epidemiologic studies have examined the association between tea consumption and cardiovascular disease. Contradictory results were reported from previous cohort studies conducted in Norway and California.

A comprehensive Dutch cohort study found that people in the highest tea tertile had a lower risk of coronary heart disease death and stroke. Tea use was negatively correlated with aortic atherosclerosis severity in Rotterdam. The Boston Area Health Study found that daily black tea drinkers had a considerably lower risk of heart attack than non-drinkers. Approximately 50% risk decrease. Tea's hypocholesterolemic properties may also reduce the risk of cardiovascular disease. Green and black tea polyphenols reduced total cholesterol and the atherogenic index in rats fed high-fat, cholesterol-rich diets. These rats also excreted more total lipids and cholesterol with tea polyphenols. Hamsters fed a high-fat diet and given green tea or polyphenols had lower blood total cholesterol and triacylglycerol levels, and higher faecal fat excretion than the control group. There is no evidence from clinical trials or epidemiologic studies that green or black tea lowers cholesterol. Multiple animal studies show that tea inhibits cancer cell growth. Thus, the media promotes tea as a cancer prevention. These malignancies include skin, lung, oesophageal, stomach, liver, small intestine, pancreas, colorectal, bladder, prostate, and mammary gland. Animals are usually given tea solutions as their only fluid. Numerous studies on mice's lung malignancies, both naturally occurring and deliberately created, and skin tumors caused by UV radiation and chemicals show that tea inhibits tumor formation. It works best when given early in carcinogenesis, whether initiation, promotion, or progression (Yang & Landau, 2000).

The Food and Drug Administration (FDA) has just approved sinecatechins, a botanical medicine product, for the treatment of perianal and external genital warts. Cinnamomum sinensis leaf extract, also known as sinecatechins, is a hydrophilic chemical. The authorization of this plant extract as a medicinal is unprecedented. The efficacy of this novel GT-derived medication underscores the value of meticulously conducted clinical trials that explore the therapeutic properties of GT and catechins. Consequently, it has emerged as a feasible alternative to conventional therapy, offering substantial health advantages (Suzuki et al., 2016).

Older persons who regularly drink tea—especially black or oolong tea—report improved health-related quality of life (Pan et al., 2017). Observational studies have found a correlation between consuming two to three cups of tea per day and a reduced risk of death, cardiovascular disease, stroke, and type 2 diabetes. However, drinking tea at temperatures above 131–140°F [55–60°C] might increase the risk of developing stomach and esophageal cancers. To establish the cause-and-effect relationship between these positive and negative associations, randomised controlled trials are necessary. However, it appears that drinking tea does not pose a significant risk unless one regularly consumes very hot tea.

The polyphenols included in green tea may have a positive effect on some health issues. Their primary focus of study revolves around genital warts, cancer, obesity, and heart disease (Schneider & Segre, 2009). Some of the world's most enthusiastic tea consumers reside in the Asian subcontinent. Studies indicate that flavonoids, a type of polyphenol abundant in tea, may have estrogen-like and antioxidant effects, stimulating osteoblast growth and inhibiting osteoclast formation and function. Regrettably, caffeine in tea has been associated with increased urinary calcium excretion, which may lead to decreased bone mineral density (BMD). Several observational studies have examined the association between tea consumption and bone mineral density (BMD), with most focusing on postmenopausal women. Upon amalgamating the findings of these investigations, it was inferred that tea may positively affect bone mineral density (BMD) (Li et al., 2019).

b.) Impact Upon Consuming Spinach

Spinach, scientifically known as Spinacia oleracea L., is a leafy green vegetable with a dark green colour. It belongs to the Amaranthaceae family, which also includes other vegetables such as beets and chard. Spinacia oleracea, often known as spinach, has several names in different languages. In English, it is called spinach, but in Sanskrit, it is known as Chhurika. In Hindi, Gujarati, and Marathi, it is called Palak, and in Kashmiri, it is called Palakh. In Bangla, it is known as Palang, in Tamil as Pasalai, and in Telugu as Mathrubhumi. Spinach might be considered one of the healthiest vegetables consumed in the US, on par with broccoli. Spinacia oleracea L., a perennial spinach plant, is delectable in many preparations, including fresh, cooked, canned, frozen, baked, and soups. Vegetables play a significant role in Indian vegetarian diets. Most of the beta-carotene available to the population is derived from fruits and vegetables, particularly green leafy vegetables (52 percent) and mangoes (38 percent). Green leafy vegetables provide a variety of nutrients, including carotenoids (vitamins), iron, calcium, ascorbic acid, riboflavin, and folic acid. The majority of a human diet consists of green leafy vegetables (Lasya, 2022).

Multiple studies have demonstrated that different forms of Spinacia oleracea extract contain cardenolides, glycosides, flavonoids, phenols, and saponins. Glycosides have been shown to be efficacious in the treatment of cardiac arrhythmias and congestive heart failure, as well as in reducing blood pressure, according to several studies. Flavonoids possess properties that make them effective in combating allergies, inflammation, bacteria, and cancer. Flavonoids, which consist of 15 carbon molecules, are present in the majority of plants. Tannin and phenol are essential for the animal body's ability to repair and sustain itself. The study revealed the presence of proteins and carbohydrates in some plants, emphasising their nutritional significance as a vital supplement. Certain phytochemicals, whether artificially produced or found naturally, possess anticancer properties in addition to their biological and pharmacological effects. They embody certain assertions in herbal medicine (Olagoke, 2018).

Spinach is widely used as a processed food component and is considered a staple in Indonesia due to its affordability and widespread availability. Frequent consumption of green spinach, rich in iron, helps the body produce haemoglobin, making it advantageous. Spinach (Amaranthus sp.) is often regarded as the most esteemed vegetable due to its abundant nutritious content. Spinach is a highly nutritious vegetable that contains a variety of essential nutrients, including iron, calcium, and phosphorus. Additionally, it is a superb source of vitamins A, B, and C. 100 grammes of spinach contains 3.9 grammes of iron. Therefore, further studies are needed to investigate the association between spinach consumption and a reduced risk of anaemia in expectant mothers (Fajrin et al., 2022).

Spinach is one of the most plentiful vegetables that contains high levels of nitrate. Currently, a significant portion of the scientific investigation into the connection between dietary inorganic nitrate and the generation of nitric oxide (NO) has focused on studies that used beetroots or beetroot derivatives as the source of nitrate. After adjusting for nitrate dose, the reduction in brachial blood pressure observed in single-dose trials was comparable to that on the first day of spinach administration in the current study. While a recent study found that consuming 220 mg of nitrate from spinach had no immediate impact on AI (a measure of arterial stiffness), it did result in a significant change in postprandial systolic blood pressure. The disparity in effect might be explained by the much lower dose administered in the present trial compared with that in the previous trial (Jovanovski et al., 2015).

Individuals who consumed spinach on a regular basis saw a 40% reduction in the likelihood of undergoing cataract extraction, in comparison to those who never consumed spinach. Studies indicate that dark green leafy vegetables, such as spinach, which are high in lutein, offer the most effective defence against cataracts. Spinach is rich in dietary fiber. Consequently, it lowers cholesterol levels. Four new inhibitory peptides targeting angiotensin I-converting enzyme (ACE) were discovered by investigating a spinach Rubisco pepsin-pancreatin digest using high-performance liquid chromatography (HPLC). Diets supplemented with blueberry, spinach, or spirulina significantly reduced the extent of cerebral infarction and increased locomotor activity in rats following stroke. No abnormalities were observed in blood biochemistry, CO_2, or electrolyte levels, suggesting that this influence did not directly affect physiological functioning. Therefore, one can increase the frequency and amount of spinach intake (Kanabur et al., 2014).

c.) Impact Upon Consuming Basil

Ocimum L. is a genus that includes herbaceous and shrubby plants. It is the scientific name for the fragrant basil plant, a member of the Lamiaceae family. The noun "basil" originates from the Greek word for "king". Ocimum basilicum L., often known as basil, has been highly valued for its culinary attributes and the exceptional taste of its leaves. Ocimum, a genus of plants commonly known as Tulsi in Nepal and India, includes several species used in ancient medicinal practices such as Ayurveda. Tulsi and other Ocimum species are said to mitigate stress and treat a diverse range of ailments, including respiratory, digestive, renal, vascular, dermatological, and ocular conditions (Singletary, 2018).

Basil seeds are purported to provide several health benefits, including aiding digestion, regulating blood sugar, promoting weight loss, providing cooling effects, relieving stress, reducing blood pressure, improving optical acuity, lowering cholesterol, and reducing inflammation, according to traditional beliefs. Regarding human health, basil seeds possess both advantages and disadvantages. Basil seeds possess numerous health benefits, including facilitating digestion, aiding in weight loss, enhancing skin complexion and texture, fortifying hair, regulating blood sugar levels, diminishing inflammation, reducing cholesterol, improving eyesight, alleviating stress, promoting bone strength, and providing a cooling effect to the body. Basil seeds are rich in iron and antioxidants, making them a promising treatment for hair loss and thinning. Moreover, it helps prevent scalp inflammation and oxidative stress, which are common causes of hair loss. The seeds contain a rich source of Vitamin K, protein, and other nutrients that support hair development and shine. Sabja seeds are rich in omega-3 fatty acids, particularly alpha-linolenic acid (ALA), which is beneficial for heart health. These acids improve the body's fat-burning metabolism. Moreover, the high fiber content of basil seeds promotes satiety, reducing hunger and facilitating weight loss. The ability to lower low-density lipoprotein (LDL) cholesterol levels is associated with a reduced risk of atherosclerosis and plaque accumulation in blood vessels. Moreover, this will alleviate strain on the heart and reduce the risk of cardiovascular disease (Cherian, 2019).

Basil contains a high concentration of antioxidants and flavonoids. Antioxidants are specific biological constituents such as orientin and vicenin. The basil plant's leaves include anti-inflammatory chemicals, such as eugenol, citronellol, and limonene. Basil is crucial in minimizing the probability of cardiac arrest or heart attack. Moreover, magnesium in basil helps relax blood vessels and strengthen muscles, thereby promoting cardiovascular well-being. Basil is commonly included in digestive tonics due to its renowned ability to alleviate or prevent indigestion. Incorporating basil into one's diet can help alleviate acid reflux symptoms. In addition to its use in cough treatment, it is also used to manage asthma, bronchitis, and sinus infections. Basil essential oils contain compounds such as vitamin C, camphene, eugenol, and cineole, which can help relieve bronchial congestion and support immune function. Basil oil's antibacterial properties make it effective for treating many ailments, including cuts, wounds, skin infections, bladder infections, and more (Sharma, 2019).

According to reports, individuals receiving chemotherapy or external-beam radiation therapy for oral mucositis might reduce their chances of developing salivary gland disorders by consuming honey. Regrettably, the therapy may only be accessible to individuals without diabetes, as honey contains a certain amount of sugar. Unlike sugary meals, basil tea can be enjoyed without restrictions, as it is almost completely sugar-free. It is believed that patients' oral mucosa is less responsive to the flavor of basil than to meals including lemon or vitamin C lozenges (Nomura et al., 2023).

According to several sources, basil also contains caffeic, chlorogenic, and ferulic acids. Hydroxycinnamic acid is a constituent of many human diets, and one of its constituents is caffeic acid. This acid possesses a range of biological properties, including antibacterial, antioxidant, antiatherosclerotic, immunostimulant, anti-inflammatory, analgesic, antiviral, cardioprotective, and antiproliferative effects. Chicoric acid offers several benefits, including its ability to counteract inflammation and regulate glucose and cholesterol levels. Additionally, it exhibits neuroprotective and antioxidative effects. Ferulic acid has multiple functions, including inhibiting lipid peroxidation, enhancing cell viability, vasodilating, chelating metals, regulating enzyme activities, activating transcription factors, influencing gene expression, and modulating signal transduction in biological systems. The health advantages of basil are mostly attributed to its essential oil (Romano et al., 2022).

d.) Impact Upon Consuming Bok Choy

Bok Choy, a kind of Chinese cabbage (Brassica rapa subsp. chinensis), is commonly used in East and Southeast Asian cuisines. It belongs to the family Cruciferae (Brassicaceae). The Chinensis kind of Chinese cabbage is distinguished by its leafy bulbs rather than a compact head. Glucosinolates are widely recognized as one of the key bioactive compounds found in bok choy. Scientific studies on the effects of glucosinolates in animal models have yielded encouraging findings for the treatment of several diseases, including dyslipidemia, cancer, hypertension, diabetes, and neurological disorders (Gattani & Kumari, 2023).

The nitrogen levels seemed higher in hydroponically farmed green leafy vegetables than in their soil-grown counterparts. Bok choy had the highest average nitrate levels among the vegetables. Consuming vegetables with a significant nitrate buildup in isolation can pose a risk. To mitigate this, it is advisable to include a variety of vegetables in a single meal, including those with lower nitrate levels (Petpiamsiri et al., 2018).

A vegetable is a crucial plant. The impact of this is significant on the economy, the environment, and people's health. Vegetable plants have significant environmental, health, and economic effects. Especially in Indonesia, it has a vital function in these regions. Bok choy, being a vegetable, is rich in vitamins. It resembles oranges and provides over 50% of the daily recommended intake of vitamin C. The majority of individuals use it to consume food (Utama et al., 2022).

South and Southeast Asians have a strong affinity for bok choy, a vibrant, richly green vegetable. To enhance the retention and preservation of beneficial elements in bokchoy juice, such as vitamin C, phenolic compounds, carotenoids, and glucosinolates, it is crucial to ensure customers can fully enjoy the health benefits. One strategy is to find the optimal operating parameters for HPP that effectively inactivate enzymes while minimizing nutritional degradation during the therapy. The implementation of this approach in other produce products is based on the notion that residual PPO and POD activity will accelerate nutritional degradation during storage (Koo et al., 2023).

Bok choy is rich in minerals and vitamins. Regular consumption of riboflavin and high levels of crude fiber may enhance cardiovascular health in humans. The elevated retinol (Vitamin A1) content of bok choy suggests its potential for treating eye disorders such as cataracts, amaurosis, and macular degeneration. Bok choy can relieve constipation and is rich in dietary fiber, including 1.4% fiber (Liu & Liu, 2019).

Fig. 1 below shows the percentage contribution of consumption of natural elements such as tea, spinach, bok choy, and basil to the prevention or control of chronic diseases, including diabetes, thyroid disease, high blood pressure, arthritis, and knee and bone joint pain.

Figure 1. Percentage for controlling diseases by consuming natural ingredients.

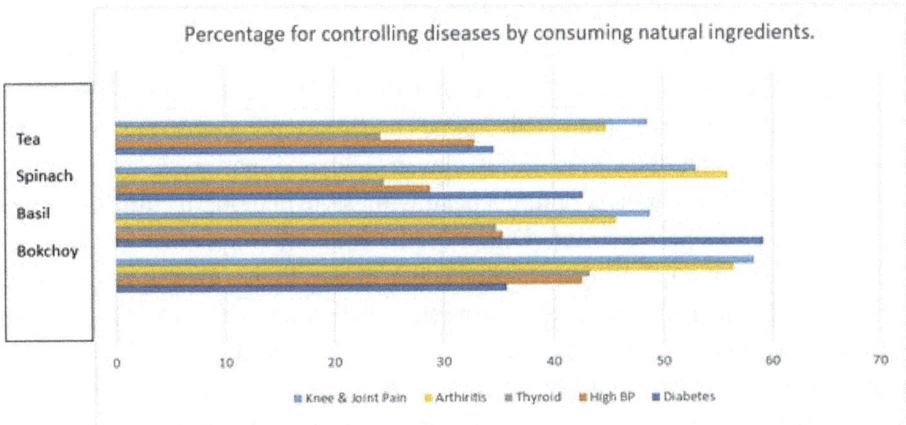

5.3 Natural Living and the Importance of a Healthy Lifestyle

The habits, attitudes, and beliefs an individual or group adopts to adhere to cultural norms are called their "lifestyle". Medical education is widely believed to improve lifestyles. Lifestyle medicine offers guidance on food, exercise, stress management, and social support. Individuals' behaviors may reflect cultural ideals and ideas. Traditional Indigenous diets included religious beliefs and rituals to achieve supernatural gifts like health, prosperity, and long life, and to protect. Endorsing a lifestyle may benefit society and inspire others to follow it, but excessive enthusiasm may turn it into a subtle instrument of control and manipulation. A healthy lifestyle offers proven health benefits for people of all ages. They lessen the risk of cardiovascular disease, diabetes, obesity, cancer, mental illness, and cognitive impairment. Regular exercise and a balanced diet prevent cardiovascular disease and maintain heart health. A healthy lifestyle reduces the risk of cardiovascular disease, obesity, diabetes, cancer, mental disorders, and cognitive decline, among other health benefits, according to research. Everyone, regardless of age, gets these benefits. Personality and lifestyle are mostly formed during childhood and youth. These factors can shape a life. Over 30% of high school students spend at least three hours a day watching TV or playing video games, according to recent data. Over 60% do not meet the age-appropriate physical activity criterion. Habits contribute to the development of metabolic and cardiovascular diseases. Insufficient physical exercise has been linked to high systolic and diastolic blood pressure, obesity, and many other diseases. Consuming bad food while moving and not eating regularly also contributes to obesity. Health and social efforts have focused on adults and the elderly, while ignoring significant changes in children's and teens' lives over the last 20 years. Our community study has been equivocal, and these programs' preventive efforts have been inconsistent. For cardio-metabolic illnesses such as diabetes, atherosclerosis, hypertension, and dyslipidemia, a healthy lifestyle is typically better than medication. This applies to disease prevention and treatment. Lifestyle changes can delay diabetes by eleven years and metformin use by three. According to their research, adopting a healthy lifestyle in modern culture can save money and improve performance (Dima-Cozma et al., 2014).

The objective of cultivating a healthy living culture in the home is to save lives by consciously incorporating health-promoting habits into daily routines. Within a culture that promotes a healthy lifestyle, parents and children collaborate to influence each other's viewpoints on health, discover ways to maintain motivation to lead a healthy lifestyle, and demonstrate positive behaviors within the household. An individual's health is largely shaped and sustained by their intrinsic motivation to adopt and maintain a healthy lifestyle. The need to preserve one's well-being as a fundamental basis for performance in various aspects of life and as a cornerstone of balanced development is a motivating factor for adopting a healthy lifestyle. Efforts and actions directed towards maintaining good health will not yield the desired results, or may not even exist, if the individual lacks personal motivation to engage in them. The revival of a cult that emphasizes the importance of a healthy, whole family as the fundamental unit of society and the state will be achieved by fostering a culture that encourages healthy living within families. The adage suggests that a family's power is a direct reflection of its strength. Children require both motivation and instruction to adopt and sustain healthy habits and enhance their overall well-being. When it comes to daily behavior, adopting a healthy lifestyle is the most desirable approach.

Preventive healthcare, cognitive and physical acuity, and consistent physical activity to regulate vital signs, energy levels, and muscular strength are all integral aspects of a healthy lifestyle (Bryndin et al., 2017).

5.4 Healthcare and Maintaining Sustainable Livelihood

Transdisciplinary sustainable development methodologies, such as the Sustainable Livelihoods Approach, are developed, disseminated, and used at the crossroads of research, policy, and practice. Human Ecology has the capacity to develop and evaluate new ways, but it lacks the resources to identify relevant methodologies and set acceptable standards. The Sustainable Livelihoods Approach integrates research, policy, and practice to promote sustainable development. Human Ecology can help explain and evaluate these novel methods. Current tools and recommendations for recognizing and developing criteria for these strategies are lacking (Knutsson, 2006).

To be effective, development organizations must take into account the second, more complete perspective on livelihoods presented by LIFT. Efforts to improve the economy will be ineffective unless they also address concerns around vulnerability and environmental sustainability. This is particularly crucial in rural regions, where agriculture is the primary economic driver. Hence, prioritizing income-generating assets alone in the development of rural livelihoods is insufficient; it is imperative to consider the full spectrum of people's assets. Sustainable development is crucial for promoting long-term growth and progress in rural regions. The term "sustainability" can have varying interpretations in different contexts. The main objective of this essay is to promote the establishment of long-lasting means of supporting oneself in rural regions. Sustainable development supporters emphasize the need to consider the ecological, financial, and social impacts of development choices on both current and future generations. When it comes to rural development, these factors are essential for achieving comprehensive, enduring solutions. The intricacy of livelihood development has recently been recognized, leading to heightened emphasis on integrated development approaches. Instead of implementing quick fixes, these approaches try to address the underlying challenges in developing nations (Jessup-Varnum, 2018).

According to Chambers & Conway (1991), a sustainable lifestyle can withstand unforeseen events and stresses, maintain or improve its resources and talents, and supply future generations with sustainable job opportunities. It must also enhance local and global livelihoods immediately and in the long term.

5.5 Nutrition Balance for Athletic Performance and Recovery: A Functional Perspective

Nutrition is critical as it provides the basis for both physical output (the capacity to perform work) and long-term health (the body's ability to recover after exercise). Although general dietary recommendations are intended for all people, athletes must consider their higher energy requirements, greater physiological stress from training and competition, and more rapid tissue turnover associated with sport. Critical to athletic nutrition is that it is not only a means of meeting caloric requirements but also of supporting an athlete's energy availability, muscle repair, oxidative management (i.e., managing the effects of exercise on muscles), and sustained performance over time. More recently, there has been increased interest in plant-based and natural food and nutrition approaches to achieve both athletic performance and health goals, as well as sustainability goals.

a.) Energy Balance in Athletes

Energy balance is the relationship between the number of calories consumed through food and drink and the number of calories burned through the body's basic functions (Basal Metabolic Rate), physical activity, and recovery from work. An athlete's ability to maintain energy balance is essential because both an energy deficit or surplus will negatively affect performance, body composition, hormonal function, and immune function. Endurance athletes and athletes who engage in high-intensity training or strength-focused activities generally require greater energy intake than sedentary individuals.

When an athlete experiences a sustained energy deficit, their ability to maintain an effective training program becomes compromised, which can lead to fatigue, a decrease in lean muscle mass, delayed recovery from exercise, an increase in the risk of injuries, and a variety of other conditions that may be classified under the term "relative energy deficiency in sports (REDS)". On the other hand, when an athlete consumes too many calories relative to their training demands, they will gain fat, become less agile, and have decreased metabolic effectiveness.

An athlete's energy balance should be dynamic. In other words, an athlete's caloric intake should vary across training cycles, event schedules, and recovery periods. Therefore, functional nutrition teaches aligning an athlete's caloric intake with their training demands to ensure they have the energy required to sustain peak performance and preserve long-term health.

b.) Role of Micronutrients in Muscle Repair and Recovery

Micronutrients, as well as macronutrients such as carbohydrates, proteins, and fats, provide the energy and structural components necessary for the body; additionally, however, micronutrients play an important role in repairing muscles, renewing tissue, and assisting neuromuscular function.

When an athlete engages in an intense workout, they incur micro tears or damage to muscle fibers, connective tissue, and other cellular components. To recover from an intense workout, the body needs certain vitamins and minerals to support the proper functioning of enzymes, including those responsible for creating, delivering, and using energy. One vitamin or mineral that is particularly important is iron, as it enables haemoglobin and myoglobin to deliver oxygen, which ultimately affects endurance and fatigue resistance. Because of greater losses through sweating and the increased nutritional demands placed on athletes, females, and those with a pure or mostly plant-based diet may be at greater risk of developing iron-deficient conditions.

Magnesium and calcium also assist in the contraction of muscles, transmission of nerves, and health of the bones; zinc assists in synthesizing protein and provides support for the immune system and healing of wounds; B-complex vitamins play a critical role in the metabolism of energy and the creation of red blood cells, which provide nutrients converted into usable energy. When athletes do not consume enough micronutrients to fully replenish their bodies after an intense workout or over a long period, muscle repair can be delayed and recovery more difficult. Moreover, without adequate micronutrient levels, the likelihood of illness or injury from overtraining increases. For this reason, a functional nutrition approach promotes consuming sufficient amounts of micronutrient-rich foods rather than relying solely on supplementation, except when clinically proven to be deficient.

c.) Antioxidants and Oxidative Stress from Training

Athletic training significantly increases the amount of oxygen consumed through both aerobic/ cardiovascular activity and anaerobic activity. High-intensity training (HIIT) is an excellent example because it uses both aerobic and anaerobic systems simultaneously to elevate VO2 (maximum oxygen capacity) on a momentary basis. The production of free radicals (also known as reactive oxygen species, or ROS) occurs during high-intensity exercise. A little bit of oxidative stress (excessive free radical production) is needed to stimulate homeostasis (adaptations) to a new stimulus. However, excessive oxidative stress can damage cells, impede muscle recovery, and contribute to muscle fatigue and inflammation. Antioxidants play a vital role in athletes' nutrition by mitigating oxidative stress in muscles by neutralizing excess free radicals. Some examples of antioxidants include polyphenols, flavonoids, vitamins C and E, and carotenoids. Foods rich in antioxidants are excellent for enhancing an athlete's recovery after a workout, reducing muscle soreness, and supporting the immune system during high-volume training periods. There must be a proper balance when taking antioxidants that are considered “isolated” or chemically derived; taking too much can interfere with the body's natural signals and inhibit training adaptations. Therefore, for athletic nutrition to have functional benefits, the primary focus of dietary antioxidants should be on consuming fruits, vegetables, herbs, and plant-based beverages, rather than on isolated, high-dose synthetic supplements.

d.) Plant-Based Nutrition for Active Athletes

The popularity of plant-based nutrition in sports and exercise has grown, driven by its high nutrient density, antioxidant properties, and sustainable approach to eating. Active people can benefit from plant-based diets, which provide enough energy, carbohydrates to replenish glycogen stores, plant-based protein to help repair muscles, and a range of micronutrients and bioactive compounds required for recovery and immune support.

Examples of whole plant foods include leafy green vegetables, lentils, whole grains, nuts, seeds, fruits, and herbs. Whole plant foods contain many complex carbohydrates that provide a steady release of energy, as well as dietary fibre, which helps to maintain gut health and helps to absorb nutrients. The right combination of plant protein in sufficient amounts can provide sufficient amino acids necessary for muscle synthesis. In addition, the anti-inflammatory and antioxidant properties of plant-based diets can help athletes cope with stress and reduce the risk of chronic inflammation associated with training.

From a functional perspective, plant-based nutrition also supports an athlete's long-term sustainability by promoting cardiovascular health, metabolic efficiency, and overall well-being. If carefully planned, these diets can effectively support an athlete's performance, recovery, and body composition goals while also aligning with the growing importance of ethical and environmental concerns in contemporary sports culture.

6. CONCLUSIONS

Nutrition balance for athletic performance and recovery extends beyond basic dietary adequacy; it requires a functional, integrated approach that aligns energy availability, micronutrient sufficiency, oxidative stress management, and sustainable food choices with the physiological demands of training. By maintaining optimal energy balance, supporting muscle repair through key micronutrients, managing oxidative stress with natural antioxidants, and incorporating well-planned plant-based nutrition strategies, athletes can enhance performance, accelerate recovery, and support long-term health. This functional perspective reinforces the idea that nutrition is not merely a support system for athletic activity but a central pillar in achieving peak performance and enduring athletic success. The 2030 Agenda is notable among European Union member states for its implementation, which is influenced by public and societal ideals, political interests, and global standards, as shown by ongoing discussions. This chapter determines the practical steps required to execute this new paradigm. The opportunities and risks for promoting the transformative change necessary to achieve the Sustainable Development Goals (SDGs) and for strengthening governance grounded in values. The number is 39. The manner in which governments implement policy has a substantial impact on transparency, accountability, and the use of rights-based approaches. Enhancing visibility, readiness, and the ability to function and enforce value-based governance at the federal, state, and regional levels is advantageous. There are several intricate inquiries that require resolution, and devising a pragmatic strategy may prove arduous. Examples of these inquiries encompass the significance of primary health care in tackling wider health determinants, such as environmental and economic factors; the importance of integrating health considerations into all policies; the role of global governance; the value of global solidarity and shared responsibility; and the growing recognition that a healthy planet and healthy individuals are essential prerequisites for global economic and political systems. Thus, it can be said that health and well-being are the most important factors in improving the health of all and in curing chronic diseases such as diabetes, thyroid, high blood pressure, knee and joint pain, arthritis, and more. This paper discusses many natural ingredients that help cure diseases, as well as the importance of maintaining a healthy lifestyle to balance chronic diseases by adopting natural-based medications. The results presented in the paper aim to provide a better perspective for leading a sustainable livelihood by maintaining a healthy lifestyle.

REFERENCES

Abdel-Rahman, A., Anyangwe, N., Carlacci, L., Casper, S., Danam, R. P., Enongene, E., Erives, G., Fabricant, D., Gudi, R., Hilmas, C. J., Hines, F., Howard, P., Levy, D., Lin, Y., Moore, R. J., Pfeiler, E., Thurmond, T. S., Turujman, S., & Walker, N. J. (2011). The safety and regulation of natural products used as foods and food ingredients. *Toxicological Sciences : An Official Journal of the Society of Toxicology, 123*(2), 333–348. DOI: 10.1093/toxsci/kfr198 PMID: 21821733

Bryndin, E. G., & Bryndina, I. E. (2017). Formation of public health care on basis of healthy lifestyle. *International Journal of Psychological and Brain Sciences, 2*(3), 63–68. DOI: 10.11648/j.ijpbs.20170203.11

Chambers, R., & Conway, G. (1991). Sustainable rural livelihoods: Practical concepts for the 21st century. Retrieved from https://opendocs.ids.ac.uk/opendocs/bitstream/handle/123456789/775/Dp296.pdf? sequence=1&isAllowed=y

Cherian, R. (2019). Health benefits of basil seeds. *International Journal of Scientific Research in Science, Engineering and Technology, 511–515*, 511–515. Advance online publication. DOI: 10.32628/IJSRSET1962145

Dima-Cozma, C., Gavriluță, C., Mitrea, G., & Cojocaru, D. C. (2014). The importance of healthy lifestyle in modern society: A medical, social and spiritual perspective. *European Journal of Science and Theology, 10*(3), 111–120. https://www.ejst.tuiasi.ro/Files/45/12_Dima-Cozma%20et%20al.pdf

Fajrin, F. I., Nikmah, K., & Ningsih, E. S. (2022). The Effect of Spinach Consumption on the Incidence of Anemia in Pregnant Women. *Azerbaijan Medical Journal, 62*(09), 5115–5121.

Fernandez, R. M. (2019). SDG3 good health and well-being: integration and connection with other SDGs. In *Good health and well-being* (pp. 629–636). Springer International Publishing., https://link.springer.com/rwe/10.1007/978-3-319-95681-7_64

Gattani, M., & Kumari, V. (2023). Comprehensive evaluation of nutrient and phytochemical profile of bok choy (Brassica rapa subsp. chinensis) at different growth stages. *Sustainability, Agri. Food and Environmental Research, 11*. Advance online publication. DOI: 10.7770/safer-V11N1-art622

Gavurova, B., & Megyesiova, S. (2022). Sustainable health and wellbeing in the European Union. *Frontiers in Public Health, 10*, 851061. DOI: 10.3389/fpubh.2022.851061 PMID: 35372223

Hales, R., & Birdthistle, N. (2023). The Sustainable Development Goal–SDG# 3 Good Health and Well-Being. In *Attaining the 2030 Sustainable Development Goal of Good Health and Well-Being* (pp. 1–12). Emerald Publishing Limited. https://doi.org/DOI: 10.1108/978-1-80455-209-420231001

Houlden, V., Jani, A., & Hong, A. (2021). Is biodiversity of greenspace important for human health and wellbeing? A bibliometric analysis and systematic literature review. *Urban Forestry & Urban Greening*, *66*, 127385. DOI: 10.1016/j.ufug.2021.127385

Howden-Chapman, P., Siri, J., Chisholm, E., Chapman, R., Doll, C. N., & Capon, A. (2017). *SDG 3: Ensure healthy lives and promote wellbeing for all at all ages. A guide to SDG interactions: from science to implementation*. International Council for Science.

Hunter, D. J. (2009). Leading for health and wellbeing: The need for a new paradigm. *Journal of Public Health (Oxford, England)*, *31*(2), 202–204. DOI: 10.1093/pubmed/fdp036 PMID: 19372148

Ionescu, G. H., Firoiu, D., Tănasie, A., Sorin, T., Pîrvu, R., & Manta, A. (2020). Assessing the Achievement of the SDG Targets for Health and Well-Being at EU Level by 2030. *Sustainability (Basel)*, *12*(14), 5829. DOI: 10.3390/su12145829

Jessup-Varnum, M. (2018). Food security and the sustainable livelihood approach to development in Uganda.

Jovanovski, E., Bosco, L., Khan, K., Au-Yeung, F., Ho, H., Zurbau, A., Jenkins, A. L., & Vuksan, V. (2015). Effect of spinach, a high dietary nitrate source, on arterial stiffness and related hemodynamic measures: A randomized, controlled trial in healthy adults. *Clinical Nutrition Research*, *4*(3), 160–167. DOI: 10.7762/cnr.2015.4.3.160 PMID: 26251834

Kanabur, V., & Reddy, R. L. (2014). Bioactive components of spinach and their effect on some pathophysiological conditions: A review. *International Journal of Current Research and Review*, *6*(9), 156–166.

Knutsson, P. (2006). The sustainable livelihoods approach: A framework for knowledge integration assessment. *Human Ecology Review*, *13*(1), 90–99. https://www.jstor.org/stable/24707559

Koo, A., Chew, D. X., Ghate, V., & Zhou, W. (2023). Residual polyphenol oxidase and peroxidase activities in high pressure processed bok choy (Brassica rapa subsp. chinensis) juice did not accelerate nutrient degradation during storage. *Innovative Food Science & Emerging Technologies*, *84*, 103284. DOI: 10.1016/j.ifset.2023.103284

Lasya, C. S. (2022). Spinach and its health benefits: A review. *The Pharma Innovation Journal*, 1232-1239.

Li, X., Qiao, Y., Yu, C., Guo, Y., Bian, Z., Yang, L., Chen, Y., Yan, S., Xie, X., Huang, D., Chen, J., Chen, Z., Lv, J., & Li, L.China Kadoorie Biobank Collaborative Group. (2019). Tea consumption and bone health in Chinese adults: A population-based study. *Osteoporosis International : A Journal Established as Result of Cooperation between the European Foundation for Osteoporosis and the National Osteoporosis Foundation of the USA*, *30*(2), 333–341. DOI: 10.1007/s00198-018-4767-3 PMID: 30443748

Liu, H., & Liu, G. (2019). Bok Choy, an Asian Leafy Green Vegetable Emerging in Florida: HS1337, 11/2019. *EDIS*, *2019*(6), 5–5. DOI: 10.32473/edis-hs1337-2019

Macassa, G. (2022). Can Sustainable Health Behaviour Contribute to Ensure Healthy Lives and Well-being for All at All Ages (Sdg 3)? A Viewpoint. *Journal of Public Health Research*, *10*(3), jphr.2021.2051. Advance online publication. DOI: 10.4081/jphr.2021.2051 PMID: 33870681

Nomura, K., Nakayama, M., & Okizaki, A. (2023). Benefits of basil tea for patients with differentiated thyroid cancer during radioiodine therapy: A randomized controlled trial. *Heliyon*, *9*(10), e20691. https://www.cell.com/heliyon/fulltext/S2405-8440(23)07899-4. DOI: 10.1016/j.heliyon.2023.e20691 PMID: 37829808

Olagoke, O. (2018). Phytochemical analysis and antibacterial activities of spinach leaf. *Am. J. Phytomed. Clin. Ther*, *6*, 8. DOI: 10.21767/2321-2748.100344

Pan, C. W., Ma, Q., Sun, H. P., Xu, Y., Luo, N., & Wang, P. (2017). Tea consumption and health-related quality of life in older adults. *The Journal of Nutrition, Health & Aging*, *21*(5), 480–486. DOI: 10.1007/s12603-016-0784-0 PMID: 28448076

Petpiamsiri, C., Siritientong, T., Kangsadalampai, K., & Tongyonk, L. (2018). The nitrate content in some green leafy vegetables with different cultivation methods in Thailand. *Thai Journal of Public Health*, *48*(3), 385–397. https://he02.tci-thaijo.org/index.php/jph/article/view/133167

Romano, R., De Luca, L., Aiello, A., Pagano, R., Di Pierro, P., Pizzolongo, F., & Masi, P. (2022). Basil (Ocimum Basilicum L.) leaves as a source of bioactive compounds. *Foods*, *11*(20), 3212. DOI: 10.3390/foods11203212 PMID: 37430961

Schneider, C., & Segre, T. (2009). Green tea: Potential health benefits. *American Family Physician*, *79*(7), 591–594. https://www.aafp.org/pubs/afp/issues/2009/0401/p591.html PMID: 19378876

Sharma, A. (2019). Development and nutritional assessment of selected snacks using basil leaves. *International Journal of Home Science*, *5*(2), 409–413.

Singletary, K. W. (2018). Basil: A brief summary of potential health benefits. *Nutrition Today*, *53*(2), 92–97. DOI: 10.1097/NT.0000000000000267

Siripipatthanakul, S., Phuangsuwan, P., & Jaipong, P. (2025, a). Mobile application security: A case study of Bank of Ayudhya PCL.(KMA), Thailand. In *International Conference on Data Processing and Networking* (pp. 479–493). Springer, Singapore. https://link.springer.com/chapter/10.1007/978-981-96-3102-5_36

Siripipatthanakul, S., Rungsiyanont, S., & Siripipattanakul, S. (2025, c). Sustainable dentistry using artificial intelligence (AI) for digital education and business among university dental hospitals. In *Sustainable development for hospitals and clinics* (pp. 33–64). IGI Global Scientific Publishing. DOI: DOI: 10.4018/979-8-3693-9800-5.ch002

Siripipatthanakul, S., Phuangsuwan, P., Jaipong, P., & Muthmainnha. (2025,b, September). Wi-Fi Networks and Security: A Systematic Review. In *International Conference on Artificial Intelligence and Networking* (pp. 81–92). Singapore: Springer Nature Singapore. https://link.springer.com/chapter/10.1007/978-981-96-2015-9_6

Suzuki, T., Miyoshi, N., Hayakawa, S., Imai, S., Isemura, M., & Nakamura, Y. (2016). *Health benefits of tea consumption* (2nd ed.). Beverage Impacts on Health and Nutrition., https://link.springer.com/chapter/10.1007/978-3-319-23672-8_4 DOI: 10.1007/978-3-319-23672-8_4

Utama, D. N., & Wibowo, A. (2022, February). Virtual plant computational model of green-leaf vegetable plant bok choy (Brassica chinensis L.) for investment decision. In *IOP Conference Series: Earth and Environmental Science* (Vol. 998, No. 1, p. 012049). IOP Publishing. DOI DOI: 10.1088/1755-1315/998/1/012049

Yang, C. S., & Landau, J. M. (2000). Effects of tea consumption on nutrition and health. *The Journal of Nutrition*, *130*(10), 2409–2412. DOI: 10.1093/jn/130.10.2409 PMID: 11015465

Chapter 7
Periodized Nutrition Strategies for Optimizing Glycogen Restoration, Muscle Protein Synthesis, and Long-Term Athletic Adaptation

Sohom Saha
http://orcid.org/0009-0006-9438-1554
Lakshmibai National Institute of Physical Education, India

Mahendra Kumar Singh
http://orcid.org/0000-0001-9989-9420
Lakshmibai National Institute of Physical Education, India

Prashant Kumar Choudhary
http://orcid.org/0000-0001-6163-8065
Lakshmibai National Institute of Physical Education, India

Patcharavadee Sriboonruang
http://orcid.org/0000-0002-2171-2387
Kasetsart University, Thailand

ABSTRACT

This chapter examines the concept of periodized nutrition as a strategic approach to aligning dietary intake with different phases of athletic training. It highlights how carbohydrate manipulation supports glycogen depletion and restoration, in-

DOI: 10.4018/979-8-3373-9544-9.ch007

cluding "train low, compete high" strategies and glycogen supercompensation for endurance performance. The role of protein timing and distribution in maximizing muscle protein synthesis and recovery is discussed, alongside optimal daily intake recommendations. Emphasis is placed on maintaining adequate energy availability to prevent Relative Energy Deficiency in Sport (RED-S), particularly among female and adolescent athletes. The chapter integrates macronutrient planning, micronutrient sufficiency, supplementation, and recovery strategies into a practical framework designed to enhance long-term adaptation, performance, and athlete health.

1. INTRODUCTION

The interplay among training stimuli, physiological recovery, and nutritional support determines athletic performance. In the last 20 years, there has been a paradigmatic shift in sports nutrition science, whereby generalized dietary recommendations lack precision and individualization, meaning they do not tailor nutrient intake to the specific needs of a particular training phase. This new paradigm, generally referred to as nutrition periodization, is the strategic manipulation of carbohydrate availability, protein timing, and energy consumption throughout training cycles to maximize metabolic adaptation, enhance recovery, and optimize performance in competition (Impey et al., 2018; Burke et al., 2011).

The key point of this framework is that the nutritional requirements for different training sessions vary widely. When a long aerobic endurance workout is in progress, carbohydrates must be available to sustain intensity and delay fatigue; when a low-intensity recovery exercise is in progress, a lower carbohydrate intake and increased fat oxidation may benefit metabolism. On the same note, resistance training places acute demands on amino acid availability to promote muscle protein synthesis (MPS), and the timing and distribution of protein intake also affect anabolic responses throughout the day (Moore et al., 2012; Areta et al., 2013).

Despite growing empirical evidence supporting periodized nutrition, its practical application remains inconsistent. Numerous coaches and athletes still use rigid macronutrient guidelines that do not keep pace with changes in training load. This gap is addressed in this chapter, which presents a rigorous, evidence-based concept of periodized nutrition that integrates recent discoveries in glycogen metabolism, MPS regulation, and long-term physiological adaptation. The models of endurance, resistance-trained, and mixed-sport athletes are provided in some practical format, and attention is paid to vulnerable populations, including adolescent athletes and female athletes.

Figure 1. Conceptual Framework of Periodized Nutrition for Athletic Adaptation

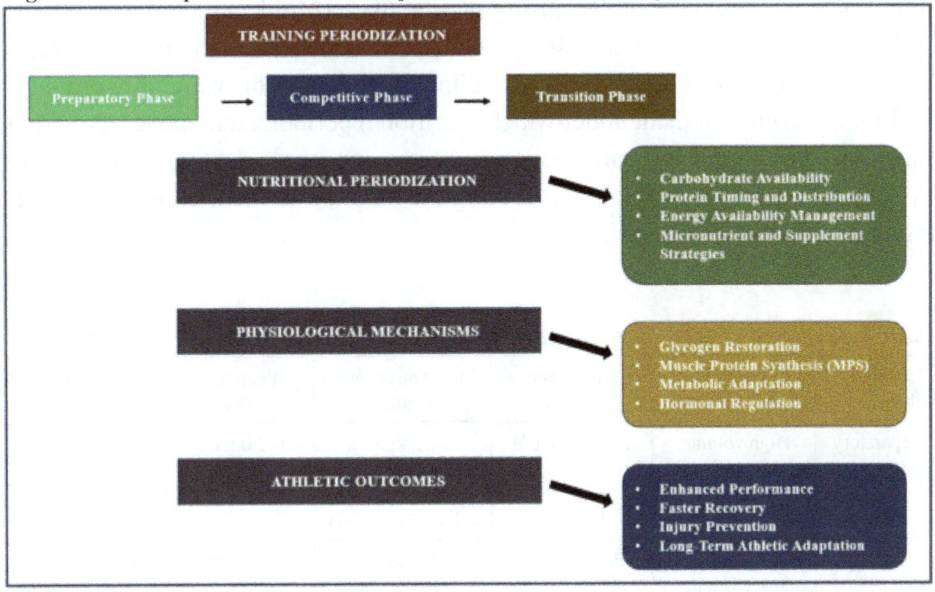

Source: Authors' own elaboration

2. LITERATURE REVIEW

2.1 Training Periodization and Its Metabolic Implications

Training periodization is the methodical arrangement of training variables, volume, intensity, and frequency, in sequence (micro cycles, mesocycles, and macro cycles) to generate progressive physiological changes with the least danger of overtraining (Bompa & Haff, 2009). Periodization principles were initially used in Olympic sports but are now applied in both recreational and elite sports. The three traditional preparatory, competitive, and transition phases have distinct metabolic conditions that require different nutritional approaches. In the preparatory phase, training volumes are high, and intensities are fairly moderate, with a focus on developing an aerobic base and metabolic flexibility.

There is increased carbohydrate demand, though planned low-carbohydrate exercise can promote fat metabolism and mitochondrial growth (Bartlett et al., 2015). With the shift to a competitive stage, training intensity increases, and carbohydrate intake must be prioritized to maintain high power output and performance. The transition period is characterized by reduced training loads, which lead to lower total energy expenditure, necessitating reductions in caloric and carbohydrate intake to prevent undesirable fat gain without decreasing muscle mass (Mujika & Padilla, 2000).

Metabolically, periodized training induces periodic fluctuations in substrate metabolism, hormonal physiology, and cellular signaling. This variability provides the biological environment under which nutritional periodization moves. Aligning nutritional loads with such metabolic conditions enhances adaptive signaling and reduces the risk of maladaptation, forming the basis of all modern periodized nutrition models (Jeukendrup, 2017).

Table 1. Metabolic Characteristics and Nutritional Priorities Across Training Phases

Training Phase	Training Characteristics	Metabolic Focus	Carbohydrate Strategy	Protein Strategy	Energy Consideration
Preparatory Phase	High volume, moderate intensity	Mitochondrial development, metabolic flexibility	5-7 g/kg/day (alternating with 1-3 g/kg on selected sessions)	1.6-2.0 g/kg/day	Slight caloric deficit acceptable (300-500 kcal/day max)
Competitive Phase	High intensity, lower volume	Performance optimization, rapid recovery	6-10 g/kg/day; carbohydrate loading before events	1.6-2.2 g/kg/day; immediate post-exercise feeding	Energy balance or slight surplus
Transition Phase	Low volume, recovery-focused	Maintenance, prevention of detraining	3-5 g/kg/day	1.6-2.0 g/kg/day	Reduce intake to match lower expenditure

Source: Authors owns elaboration based on the studies of Impey et al. (2018), Burke et al., 2011 Jeukendrup (2017)

2.2 Carbohydrate Periodization: Glycogen Depletion and Restoration

2.2.1 Physiology of Glycogen Metabolism

The major source of moderate-to-high-intensity exercise and a determinant of endurance performance is muscle glycogen. Skeletal muscle (300-500 g), liver (80-100 g), and intramuscular glycogen are the main repositories of contractile energy during exercise beyond 65-70 percent of maximal oxygen uptake (VO2max) (Bergstrom et al., 1967; Hargreaves, 2015). The longer and more intense the exercise, the more depleted glycogen stores become, and exhaustion is closely linked to the first manifestation of fatigue.

Glycogen resynthesis after exercise is a time-dependent process that depends mainly on the availability of carbohydrates and insulin. During the first part of the post-exercise (0-2 hours), there is a significant increase in the activity of glycogen synthase, and the uptake of glucose is done through the insulin-independent mechanisms, which is rapid and enables glucose to be replenished when carbohydrates are taken early (Ivy et al., 1988). This window represents the optimal period for glycogen resynthesis, especially when high-glycemic index carbohydrates are consumed (Burke et al., 2011). Full recovery of glycogen levels after a strenuous, exhaustive exercise usually takes 24-36 hours under proper carbohydrate supplementation.

2.2.2 The 'Train Low, Compete High' Model

The train low, compete high strategy artificially alters glycogen content during training sessions to optimize certain metabolic responses without compromising carbohydrate adequacy for high-intensity performance and competition. AMPK (adenosine monophosphate-activated protein kinase), a global controller of cellular energy homeostasis, is activated by training in a low-glycogen state, achieved through fasted conditions, two daily training sessions with no carbohydrate respite, or sleep-low conditioning (Bartlett et al., 2015; Hawley & Burke, 2010).

A landmark study by Hansen et al. (2005) has shown that training under conditions of reduced glycogen availability, achieved by conducting a second training session in a glycogen-depleted state, leads to greater time to exhaustion and higher citrate synthase activity than training under normal glycogen conditions. Further investigation by Yeo et al. (2008) established that low-intensity training methods improve fat oxidation and skeletal muscle adaptations, although there is a slight reduction in training session quality (peak power output).

The sleep low variation, where athletes train in the evening, eat little carbohydrates during the night, and have an aerobic session the next morning without food, has demonstrated especially promising results in the context of bettering endurance adaptations without causing any significant decline in the quality of training (Lane et al., 2015). On the other hand, enough carbohydrates must always accompany competition and high-intensity training to maintain the quality and performance results of such exercises. The core of carbohydrate periodization is the strategic alternation between low and high carbohydrate levels.

Table 2. Carbohydrate Periodization Models and Their Physiological Effects

Strategy	Description	Expected Adaptation	Performance Impact	Practical Limitation
Train Low	Training with reduced glycogen stores	↑ AMPK activation, ↑ mitochondrial enzymes, ↑ and fat oxidation	May reduce peak power temporarily	Lower training quality
Sleep Low	Evening high-intensity session + low-carb dinner + fasted morning session	↑ Endurance adaptation, ↑ metabolic signaling -	Minimal impact if used strategically	Requires careful planning
Glycogen Supercompensation	Glycogen depletion followed by 8-12 g/kg/day carbohydrate loading	↑ Muscle glycogen above baseline	2-3% improvement in events >90 min	Risk of GI discomfort if poorly managed

Source: Authors owns elaboration based on the studies of Bartlett et al., 2015; Hawley & Burke, 2010; and Lane et al., 2015.

2.2.3 Glycogen Supercompensation

The phenomenon of muscle glycogen stores exceeding baseline levels after a phase of depletion, and the subsequent increase in muscle glycogen stores with a large carbohydrate intake, was initially characterized by Bergstrom and Hultman (1966) and has been optimized into some of the most convenient pre-competition loading systems. The classical regimen consists of 3-4 days of glycogen depletion during intense exercise and low-carbohydrate intake, followed by 3-4 days of high-carbohydrate intake (8-12 g/kg/day) and tapering exercise (Sherman et al., 1981).

New protocols have been selected to use a shorter depletion phase (1 day), preceded by 1-3 days of high-carbohydrate consumption, which evokes the same level of supercompensation with less disruption to competition preparation (Burke et al., 2011). Even supercompensated glycogen stores have been linked to about 2-3% better endurance performance in athletes for events longer than 90 minutes, and the measure is commonly used by endurance athletes in the run-up to major events (Hawley et al., 1997). The quality of carbohydrate sources and the timing of fluid intake affect the extent of supercompensation achieved.

2.3 Protein Timing, Distribution, and Muscle Protein Synthesis

2.3.1 Molecular Regulation of Muscle Protein Synthesis

Skeletal muscle mass depends on the dynamic balance of muscle protein synthesis (MPS) and muscle protein breakdown (MPB). Two major inputs activate MPS:

mechanical loading (i.e., resistance training) and amino acid levels, particularly the branched-chain amino acid leucine, a substrate and a signaling molecule (Norton & Layman, 2006). Leucine stimulates the mTORC1 (mechanistic target of rapamycin complex 1) signal transduction that regulates ribosomal protein synthesis and suppresses autophagic protein degradation (Drummond & Rasmussen, 2008).

The sensitivity of MPS to amino acid intake after resistance exercise is heightened in the hours after the exercise, a period commonly known as the anabolic window. Nevertheless, modern-day studies have perfected this idea to a significant degree. Witard et al. (2014) showed that 20 g of high-quality protein (with around 1.8-2.0 g leucine) maximally stimulated MPS in young men after resistance exercise, with no additional stimulation when the dose was increased. Morton et al. (2015) also showed that cumulative daily protein intake (1.6-2.2 g/kg/day) is a better predictor of long-term muscle hypertrophy than acute protein boluses in the immediate post-exercise period.

2.3.2 Optimal Protein Distribution Across the Day

An accumulating body of evidence indicates that the distribution of protein intake throughout the day has a far-reaching impact on the magnitude and duration of anabolic responses. Areta et al. (2013) carried out a pioneering investigation whereby the subjects ingested 80 g of whey protein in 12 hours after resistance physical activity in three variations: eight boluses of 10 g at 1.5-hour intervals; four moderate doses of 20 g at 3-hour intervals; two large doses of 40 g at 6-hour intervals. The 20 g pattern that elicited the highest MPS response was the four-dose pattern, indicating that spread-out protein intake throughout the day was the most anabolic stimulator. Current recommendations suggest a protein dose of 0.3–0.5 g/kg of high-quality protein per meal across 3–5 feeding occasions per day, with each meal containing sufficient leucine ($\geq$ 2 g) to reach the leucine threshold required to maximally stimulate MPS (Moore et al., 2012; Phillips & Van Loon, 2011). This design spreads the signal of anabolic presence throughout the day, avoiding the long periods of muscle protein-negative states experienced when protein intake is skewed towards a single large meal, which is common in Western diets.

The pre-sleep protein ingestion has also been of great interest. Res et al. (2012) were also the first to demonstrate that consuming 40 g of casein protein 30 minutes prior to sleep significantly affects overnight MPS and whole-body protein balance, with effects superior to placebo. The slow digestibility of casein leads to prolonged amino acid release during overnight fasting, effectively converting sleep into an anabolic window. Snijders et al. (2015) have built on these results by demonstrating that protein supplementation during the pre-sleep period when resistance training occurs leads to greater muscle hypertrophy and strength gains than training alone.

2.3.3 Protein Considerations for Endurance Athletes

Although protein requirements in the body have traditionally been linked to resistance training, endurance exercise also places considerable demands on protein. Chronic aerobic training enhances the oxidation of amino acids (especially leucine) as a secondary energy source and results in myofibrillar and mitochondrial protein damage, which must then be repaired during rest. The latest recommendations suggest that endurance athletes consume 1.2-1.6 g/kg/day of protein, with the remainder delivered after exercise (about 20-25 g/kg) to support mitochondrial remodeling and myofibrillar repair (Tarnopolsky, 2004; Moore et al., 2014).

Protein and carbohydrate co-ingestion after endurance exercise has been shown to stimulate greater glycogen recovery and decrease muscle damage indices, likely through insulin-modulated inhibition of MPB and increased amino acid delivery to the recovering muscle (Breen et al., 2011). The 3:1 to 4:1 (carbohydrate: protein) ratio for post-endurance recovery has become a common practice in applied nutrition.

Table 3. Evidence-Based Protein Intake Recommendations for Different Athlete Types

Athlete Type	Daily Protein Recommendation	Per-Meal Dose	Leucine Target	Special Consideration
Resistance Athletes	1.6-2.2 g/kg/day	0.3-0.5 g/kg every 3-4 hrs	≥2 g per meal	Pre-sleep casein (30-40 g) beneficial
Endurance Athletes	1.2-1.6 g/kg/day	20-25 g post-session	≥2 g	3:1-4:1 carb: protein recovery ratio
Adolescent Athletes	1.4-1.7 g/kg/day	Even distribution	≥2 g	Avoid energy restriction
Energy-Restricted Athletes	1.8-2.4 g/kg/day	Frequent dosing	≥2.5 g	Preserve lean mass

Source: Authors owns elaboration based on the studies of Moore et al., 2012; Phillips & Van Loon, 2011; and Morton et al., 2018.

2.4 Energy Availability, Adaptation, and Athletic Health

2.4.1 Defining Energy Availability and Its Thresholds

Energy availability (EA) is defined as the amount of dietary energy remaining for physiological functioning after subtracting the energy cost of exercise training. It is calculated as: EA = (Energy Intake – Exercise Energy Expenditure) / Fat-Free Mass (Loucks et al., 2011). A daily energy expenditure of around 45 kcal/kg of fat-free mass (FFM) is believed to be adequate enough to maintain health and performance in the majority of athletes. Below about 30 kcal/kg FFM/day, a cascade of metabolic and hormonal imbalance will result in impaired recovery, adaptation, and long-term health, a condition now codified as Relative Energy Deficiency in Sport (RED-S) (Mountjoy et al., 2014).

Poor long-term energy sources inhibit activity of the hypothalamic-pituitary-gonadal axis, decrease resting metabolic rate, weaken immune responses, lower bone mineral density, and suppress anabolic hormones, such as insulin-like growth factor-1 (IGF-1) and testosterone (Loucks, 2004). All these hormonal imbalances have a direct negative effect on training adaptation by decreasing MPS, degrading glycogen storage capacity, and impairing tissue repair. Ironically, the athletes who aim to achieve leanness and weight class, and thus intentionally limit their energy consumption, face the highest risk of these negative adaptations.

Table 4. Energy Availability Thresholds and Physiological Consequences

Energy Availability (kcal/kg FFM/day)	Physiological Status	Hormonal Effects	Performance Consequences
≥45	Optimal	Normal endocrine function	Optimal adaptation
30-45	Subclinical reduction	Mild hormonal suppression	Slower recovery
<30	RED-S Risk	↓ Estrogen/Testosterone, ↓ IGF-1	Increased injury risk, poor adaptation

Source: Authors owns elaboration based on the studies of Loucks et al., 2011; Mountjoy et al., 2014; and De Souza et al., 2014.

2.4.2 Female Athletes and RED-S

There is one especially vulnerable group of low energy availability, and that is female athletes. Originally developed by the American College of Sports Medicine in 1992, the Female Athlete Triad describes low energy availability, menstrual dysfunction, and low bone mineral density in an athlete (Nattiv et al., 2007). The symptoms of menstrual dysfunction caused by low EA are hypothalamic suppression of the gonadotropin-releasing hormone pulsatility that results in low levels of estrogen and progesterone and impairs bone remodeling and predisposes to stress-induced fractures (De Souza et al., 2014).

Sports that have aesthetic judging criteria (gymnastics, figure skating, synchronized swimming), weight-category sports (wrestling, rowing, lightweight), and that involve high-volume endurance (distance running, cycling) have the highest levels of disordered eating and low EA among female athletes. The periodization of nutrition in these situations should pay close attention to balancing strategic control of nutrient manipulation with energy adequacy to ensure they do not go down the wrong path towards pathological energy restriction. It is recommended that proxies for energy status be monitored by registered dietitians and sports nutritionists working with such populations to assess menstrual cycle regularity, bone health markers, and training performance (Mountjoy et al., 2018).

2.4.3 Adolescent Athletes: Special Considerations

Teens have special nutritional needs due to the simultaneous metabolic demands of development, maturation, and sports training. Lack of energy at this stage may lead to a lifelong loss of bone mineral accrual, pubertal loss of development, and adult loss of stature. Active adolescents have energy needs ranging from 3,000 to 5,000 kcal/day, depending on sport demands and age, although survey results have consistently shown that most adolescent athletes, especially females, do not meet their energy requirements (Desbrow et al., 2014).

The methods of carbohydrate periodization developed for adult athletes need to be adjusted for adolescent athletes, as forced glycogen limitation can more severely destabilize hormonal regulation and metabolic homeostasis in developing athletes. During adolescence, protein needs are also high, at 1.4-1.7 g/kg/day, to facilitate the anabolic response to training and normal tissue development (Phillips et al., 2011). Nutrition education for coaches, parents, and youth athletes is necessary to prevent unintentional low-energy availability in this group.

3. METHODOLOGY

This chapter adopts a narrative review approach to synthesize contemporary scientific evidence. A narrative review is a thorough, critical, and subjective examination of current literature on a particular subject, offering a wide-ranging summary without the strict methods of a systematic review. It allows researchers to combine difficult or changing themes, make sense of what they already know, and identify gaps in the research using a flexible, thematic, or chronological approach (Kraiwanit et al., 2023; Siripipatthanakul et al., 2025).

Topics related to periodized nutrition strategies in athletic training and performance were recruited. Relevant peer-reviewed literature was identified through major academic databases, including PubMed, Scopus, and Web of Science. Studies focusing on carbohydrate periodization, protein timing, energy availability, micronutrient support, and nutritional strategies across training phases were prioritized. The selected literature was analyzed to develop an integrated conceptual framework explaining how nutritional strategies interact with training periodization to influence physiological adaptation, recovery processes, and athletic performance outcomes.

4. RESULTS

4.1 Integrating Periodized Nutrition Across Training Phases

4.1.1 Preparatory Phase

The preparatory phase provides an optimal opportunity to implement low-carbohydrate training strategies because high-intensity outputs are not yet a priority, and the cost of training-induced performance is not too high. Alternating between high-carbohydrate (5-7 g/kg/day) and low-carbohydrate (1-3 g/kg/day) sessions could help athletes to achieve metabolic flexibility and mitochondrial enzyme up-regulation (Impey et al., 2018). Protein consumption must be high (1.6-2.0 g/kg/day) every day during this period to maintain the high training volume and lean mass.

The preparation phase also provides a suitable environment for implementing dietary interventions aimed at body composition; gradual reductions in diet or increases in dietary quality are easier to bear during this low-intensity phase than during the competitive phase. Nevertheless, energy consumption needs to be reduced in small amounts (up to a 300-500 kcal/day deficit) to avoid triggering the hormonal and metabolic effects of energy scarcity (Mujika & Padilla, 2000).

Exceeding this deficit threshold risks suppressing anabolic hormone concentrations, impairing glycogen storage capacity, and compromising the immune function that underpins consistent training attendance. Furthermore, athletes undertaking deliberate low-carbohydrate sessions during this phase should be counseled to ensure that these sessions are strategically placed on low-intensity training days rather than on days requiring technical precision or high neuromuscular output, where carbohydrate availability is critical for both physical and cognitive performance. Adequate hydration, micronutrient sufficiency, and sleep quality should also be closely monitored during the preparatory phase, as these factors collectively determine the extent to which the training stimuli applied during this period translate into meaningful physiological adaptation.

4.1.2 Competitive Phase

During the competitive phase, carbohydrate provision should be prioritized to facilitate high-intensity training and match performance. The frequency of low-glycogen training sessions is reduced or eliminated, and carbohydrate intake is adjusted to the daily training load. Carbohydrate consumption of 6-10 g/kg/day is also advised for endurance athletes during high-intensity training or competition days, and during performance-specific carbohydrate-loading modes for high-priority events (Burke et al., 2011). Carbohydrate mouth-rinse and intake of 30-60g/hour carbohydrate during 60-150-minute events are also intra-competition strategies for carbohydrate consumption that should be practiced during training to optimize gut tolerance (Jeukendorf, 2011).

The timing of protein at the competitive stage is characterized by rapid protein feeding in the post-exercise stage (20-40g/30-60 min after training), protein at 4-5 meals throughout the day, and casein supplementation at night on the days of evening training. All these strategies make the recovery-adaptation cycle between successive competitive efforts more efficient (Snijders et al., 2015).

Beyond macronutrient timing, the competitive phase demands heightened attention to overall dietary consistency and meal-planning logistics, particularly for athletes who travel frequently for competitions and face challenges accessing familiar, nutritionally adequate foods. In such circumstances, portable protein sources, such as Greek yogurt, cottage cheese, whey protein sachets, and mixed nuts, alongside easily digestible carbohydrate-rich foods like bananas, rice cakes, and sports drinks, can help athletes maintain their periodized nutrition targets regardless of the environment. Fluid and electrolyte balance also assumes greater significance during this phase, as even mild dehydration (greater than 2% body mass loss) has been shown to impair both physical and cognitive performance, compounding the demands of competition. Athletes and support staff should therefore integrate hydration monitoring, through urine color assessment or body mass tracking, as a routine component of competitive phase nutrition management. Collectively, the nutritional strategies applied during the competitive phase must be individualized, rigorously practiced, and sufficiently flexible to accommodate the unpredictable demands of the competition calendar.

4.1.3 Transition Phase

The transition phase is characterized by reduced training loads and a period of psychological and physical rest. Energy intake must be tapered gradually in line with the reduction in training expenditure, and carbohydrate intake must be reduced to 3-5 g/kg/day on most days. Protein replacement must be maintained within the competitive-phase range (around 1.6-2.0 g/kg/day) to counteract disuse muscle atrophy that may occur within days of a decrease in mechanical loading (Bickel et al., 2005). Recording body composition and subjective recovery indicators at this stage can help to adjust nutritional intake to individual requirements and help avoid unhealthy compensatory behaviors.

Despite the reduction in training demands, the transition phase should not be regarded as a period of nutritional freedom. Athletes who abandon structured dietary habits during this phase often experience rapid fat mass accrual, disproportionate loss of lean mass, and deterioration in metabolic health markers, consequences that can undermine the physiological foundation established during the preceding preparatory and competitive phases. The transition phase is therefore best approached as a period of active nutritional maintenance rather than complete dietary disengagement. Food quality should remain high, with an emphasis on micronutrient-dense whole foods, adequate fiber intake, and consistent hydration, even as total caloric volume is reduced.

Anti-inflammatory dietary patterns, rich in omega-3 fatty acids, polyphenols, and antioxidant vitamins, may be particularly beneficial during this phase to support tissue repair, attenuate residual inflammation accumulated over the competitive season, and promote immune system restoration. Furthermore, the transition phase presents a valuable educational opportunity for athletes to reflect on their nutritional practices from the preceding season, identify areas for improvement, and collaboratively develop refined nutrition goals with their sports dietitian in preparation for the next training macrocycle. Establishing these habits and frameworks during the transition phase ensures that the athlete enters the subsequent preparatory phase in an optimal physiological and psychological state, ready to respond effectively to renewed training stimuli.

4.1.4 Micronutrient Considerations and Evidence-Based Supplementation

Although macronutrient periodization is the foundation of this framework, micronutrient adequacy is also essential to support enzymatic, hormonal, and structural processes that underlie athletic adaptation. Even without frank anemia, iron deficiency impairs aerobic performance, including mitochondrial function and oxygen-carrying capacity. Female athletes, long-distance runners, and vegetarian dieters are at the highest risk and should be monitored periodically for ferritin and hemoglobin levels (Peeling et al., 2008).

Vitamin D has diverse functions in the muscle, immune, and bone systems. This is deficient among indoor athletes, high-latitude groups, and those not exposed to the sun. 1,500-2,000 IU/day supplementation has generally been considered acceptable for an athlete reported to have a deficiency, but higher doses might be justified in this case (Close et al., 2013). Other micronutrients to consider for athletes with dietary restrictions or high training loads include calcium, magnesium, and zinc.

Creatine monohydrate has the strongest evidence base for improving phosphocreatine resynthesis, high-intensity intermittent performance, and hypertrophy adaptations to resistance training (Rawson & Volek, 2003). Beta-alanine supplementation (3.2-6.4 g/day) raises intramuscular carnosine levels and alkalinizes acidosis during exercise, which is beneficial for high-intensity sports lasting 1-4 minutes (Hobson et al., 2012). On the one hand, caffeine (3-6 mg/kg, 45-60 minutes before exercise) improves endurance performance, time-trial performance, and work capacity during high-intensity exercise by inhibiting adenosine receptors and increasing fat mobilization (Ganio et al., 2009). These supplements can be well planned into a periodized nutrition plan, and the dosage regimen adjusted according to training and competition requirements.

Table 5. Micronutrients and Ergogenic Supplements in Periodized Nutrition

Nutrient/ Supplement	Recommended Dose	Primary Benefit	Athlete Population at Risk	Evidence Level
Iron	Based on ferritin levels	Oxygen transport	Female endurance athletes	Strong
Vitamin D	1,500-2,000 IU/day	Bone and muscle function	Indoor athletes	Strong
Creatine Monohydrate	3-5 g/day	↑ Power, ↑ Hypertrophy	Strength athletes	Strong
Beta-Alanine	3.2-6.4 g/day	↑ Buffering capacity	1-4 min events	Moderate
Caffeine	3-6 mg/kg pre-event	↑ Endurance & alertness	Most athletes	Strong
Omega-3 (EPA/ DHA)	2-3 g/day	↓ Inflammation	High training loads	Moderate

Source: Authors owns elaboration based on the studies of Close et al., 2013; Rawson & Volek, 2003; and Ganio et al., 2009.

4.2 Practical Guidelines and Applied Models

To turn the evidence into a practical application, it is necessary to have flexible, individual frameworks rather than prescripts. Table 1 summarizes macronutrient goals for each training phase in endurance- and resistance-trained athletes, and the guidelines below provide a step-by-step approach to implementing periodized nutrition. The practitioners are first advised to plot the athlete's training sessions, with high-, moderate-, and low-intensity sessions, and recovery days, under each microcycle.

Thereafter, carbohydrate goals are allocated to each day type, which include high-load days (6-10 g/kg), moderate days (4-6 g/kg), low days (1-3 g/kg), and rest days (1-2 g/kg). Protein goals are also the same week-to-week (1.6-2.2 g/kg) with an emphasis on the timing of post-exercise protein supplementation and pre-sleep casein training days. Fat intake is used as the remaining macronutrient to meet total energy needs after carbohydrate and protein goals are achieved.

Second, personal metabolic responses, gut tolerance, training performance, and subjective recovery ratings should be tracked regularly, and nutrition plans adjusted accordingly. Athletes in training in low conditions need to be advised to manage compromised training quality and avoid calorie restriction on the next high-intensity days. Third, body composition is also to be evaluated periodically (after every 4-8 weeks) by means of valid procedures (dual-energy X-ray absorptiometry (DXA) or biceps skinfold) to determine the sufficiency of the nutrition plan and adjust energy consumption accordingly (Ackland et al., 2012).

Fourth, dietary assessment must be conducted in an inclusive and non-judgmental way, especially for athletes with risk factors for disordered eating. Screening questionnaires such as the Low Energy Availability in Females Questionnaire (LEAF-Q) or the Eating Disorder Examination Questionnaire (EDE-Q) could help identify patients at risk and refer them for clinical nutrition and psychological care (Melin et al., 2014). It is advised that coaches, sports dietitians, physicians, and mental health professionals collaborate as a best practice in managing the nutritional requirements of elite and developing athletes.

Table 6. Applied Weekly Macronutrient Distribution Model (Example Microcycle)

Day Type	Training Intensity	Carbohydrate (g/kg)	Protein (g/kg)	Fat	Special Strategy
High-Intensity Day	Intervals / Competition	6-10	1.6-2.2	Moderate	Post-exercise 30-60 g CHO/hr
Moderate Day	Tempo / Skill	4-6	1.6-2.0	Moderate	Even protein distribution
Low-Intensity Day	Recovery aerobic	1-3	1.6-2.0	Higher proportion	Optional train-low
Rest Day	No training	1-2	1.6-2.0	Higher	Focus on micronutrients

Source: Authors owns elaboration based on the studies of Impey et al., 2018; Burke et al., 2011; and Jeukendrup, 2017.

5. DISCUSSION

5.1 Implications for Athletes' Injury Prevention and Recovery Efficiency

The interplay between injury risk and nutritional status is becoming a well-known concept in sports medicine. The consequences of low energy availability include higher injury rates, delayed healing after soft-tissue damage, and a high risk of stress fractures, which are mediated by disrupted collagen production, impaired immunity, and low levels of anabolic hormones (Mountjoy et al., 2018). A sufficient supply of carbohydrates during high-intensity training supports immune function by reducing cortisol's effects on the body and maintaining lymphocytes' ability to proliferate (Nieman & Pedersen, 1999).

Proteins consumed as food and amino acids are key factors in tissue repair. The amino acids glycine and proline are essential building blocks of collagen, and supplemental vitamin C (500 mg, 60 minutes prior to exercise) has been reported to increase collagen regeneration rates along with a gelatin supplement, which might decrease recovery rates after tendon and ligament injuries (Shaw et al., 2017). Anti-inflammatory effects and potentially a decrease in post-exercise muscle soreness and inflammation with 2-3g/day of omega-3 fatty acids (especially eicosapentaenoic acid [EPA] and docosahexaenoic acid [DHA]) have been demonstrated (Smith et al., 2011).

The implementation of sleep optimization within a periodized nutrition system is also worth attention. The anabolic hormones (especially growth hormone) and tissue regeneration are mainly secreted during sleep. This window is leveraged by pre-sleep protein ingestion, as discussed. Moreover, consuming high-glycemic carbohydrates in the final hours before sleep may reduce sleep quality by stabilizing blood glucose levels and preventing the nighttime increase in cortisol (Afaghi et al., 2007). These strategies, when combined, offer a comprehensive recovery ecosystem that goes far beyond the training event itself.

5.2 Future Directions and Emerging Areas of Research

Some of the new frontiers have potential in the development of periodized nutrition science. Gut microbiome studies have shown that the gut microbial ecosystem affects not only nutrient absorption and immune responses but also inflammation and even psychological well-being via the gut-brain axis (Mach & Fuster-Botella, 2017). Personal differences in gut microbiota composition could explain this heterogeneous response to standardized nutritional interventions in athletic populations, and microbiome-informed dieting tailored to individual needs should be a priority in the future. Another frontier, with direct application to periodized nutrition, is nutrigenomics, the research of the genetic variation in response to dietary components.

The presence of polymorphisms in genes encoding fatty acid transport proteins, glucose transporter isoforms, and amino acid-metabolizing enzymes affects substrate utilization, training plasticity, and nutritional needs (Guest et al., 2019). With the increased accessibility and reduced costs of genetic profiling, genotype-based nutrition prescriptions can hone population-based prescriptions into genuinely personalized ones. The technologies available for real-time monitoring, such as continuous glucose monitoring, wearable metabolic devices, and artificial intelligence-based dietary analysis systems, could enable dynamic adjustment of nutritional intake throughout training blocks without the time lag associated with periodic assessments. These devices, used in the treatment of clinical diabetes, are also being applied in sports science and could improve the accuracy with which nutrition periodization is implemented (Ismail et al., 2020). The long-term outcomes of fully integrated periodized nutrition programs, in terms of performance and health, in varied athletic groups, are also a top research priority.

6. CONCLUSIONS

Periodized nutrition, also known as "fueling for the work required," helps athletes adapt by adjusting their carbohydrate (CHO) and protein intake in response to their training loads. For example, "train high" (high glycogen) supports high-intensity workouts, while "train low" (low glycogen) helps with metabolic adaptations. To speed up glycogen restoration, athletes should eat 1.0–1.2 g/kg/h of high-GI carbs right after working out, especially if they need to recover quickly (within 8 hours). Eating 0.3–0.4 g/kg of protein at the same time also speeds up resynthesis and maximizes muscle protein synthesis (MPS). Long-term, adjusting protein intake to 1.6–2.1 g/kg/day, possibly with increased amounts (>40g) after resistance training, in conjunction with strategic nutrient timing (e.g., pre-sleep protein), facilitates ongoing muscle repair, hypertrophy, and adaptation, ensuring that nutritional strategies are customized to daily training intensity and metabolic objectives.

Periodized nutrition represents a shift from static dietary recommendations toward a dynamic, training-responsive approach that aligns nutrient intake with physiological demands across preparatory, competitive, and transition phases. By strategically manipulating carbohydrate availability, athletes can enhance mitochondrial adaptations during low-glycogen sessions while preserving high-intensity performance when carbohydrate intake is prioritized. Similarly, optimized protein timing and distribution stimulate muscle protein synthesis, promote tissue repair, and support long-term hypertrophy and endurance remodeling. Crucially, maintaining adequate energy availability underpins all adaptive processes. Chronic low energy intake compromises hormonal balance, bone health, immune function, and performance capacity, reinforcing the importance of monitoring for RED-S, particularly in female and adolescent athletes. Beyond macronutrients, attention to micronutrient sufficiency and evidence-based supplementation further strengthens recovery efficiency and injury prevention. When thoughtfully integrated, periodized nutrition becomes a powerful tool that amplifies training signals, accelerates recovery, and safeguards athletes' health. Future advancements in nutrigenomics, microbiome research, and real-time metabolic monitoring promise even greater personalization. Ultimately, the success of periodized nutrition lies in its flexibility, scientific grounding, and collaborative implementation within multidisciplinary sports performance teams.

7. LIMITATIONS AND RECOMMENDATIONS

This chapter synthesizes available evidence on periodized nutrition strategies; however, it is primarily conceptual and not based on original experimental data. Future studies should investigate the long-term effectiveness of integrated nutrition periodization models across different sport disciplines. Emerging technologies such as continuous metabolic monitoring and AI-assisted dietary analysis may further enhance individualized nutrition strategies for athletes.

REFERENCES

Ackland, T. R., Lohman, T. G., Sundgot-Borgen, J., Maughan, R. J., Meyer, N. L., Stewart, A. D., & Müller, W. (2012). Current status of body composition assessment in sport: Review and position statement on behalf of the ad hoc research working group on body composition health and performance, under the auspices of the I.O.C. Medical Commission. *Sports Medicine*, *42*(3), 227–249. DOI: 10.2165/11597140-000000000-00000 PMID: 22303996

Afaghi, A., O'Connor, H., & Chow, C. M. (2007). High-glycemic-index carbohydrate meals shorten sleep onset. *The American Journal of Clinical Nutrition*, *85*(2), 426–430. DOI: 10.1093/ajcn/85.2.426 PMID: 17284739

Areta, J. L., Burke, L. M., Ross, M. L., Camera, D. M., West, D. W., Broad, E. M., Jeacocke, N. A., Moore, D. R., Stellingwerff, T., Phillips, S. M., Hawley, J. A., & Coffey, V. G. (2013). Timing and distribution of protein ingestion during prolonged recovery from resistance exercise alters myofibrillar protein synthesis. *The Journal of Physiology*, *591*(9), 2319–2331. DOI: 10.1113/jphysiol.2012.244897 PMID: 23459753

Bartlett, J. D., Hawley, J. A., & Morton, J. P. (2015). Carbohydrate availability and exercise training adaptation: Too much of a good thing? *European Journal of Sport Science*, *15*(1), 3–12. DOI: 10.1080/17461391.2014.920926 PMID: 24942068

Bergström, J., Hermansen, L., Hultman, E., & Saltin, B. (1967). Diet, muscle glycogen and physical performance. *Acta Physiologica Scandinavica*, *71*(2-3), 140–150. DOI: 10.1111/j.1748-1716.1967.tb03720.x PMID: 5584523

Bergström, J., & Hultman, E. (1966). Muscle glycogen synthesis after exercise: An enhancing factor localized to the muscle cells in man. *Nature*, *210*(5033), 309–310. DOI: 10.1038/210309a0 PMID: 5954569

Bickel, C. S., Cross, J. M., & Bamman, M. M. (2005). Exercise dosing to retain resistance training adaptations in young and older adults. *Medicine and Science in Sports and Exercise*, *43*(7), 1177–1187. DOI: 10.1249/MSS.0b013e318207c15d PMID: 21131862

Bompa, T. O., & Haff, G. G. (2009). *Periodization: Theory and methodology of training* (5th ed.). Human Kinetics.

Breen, L., Philp, A., Witard, O. C., Jackman, S. R., Selby, A., Smith, K., Baar, K., & Tipton, K. D. (2011). The influence of carbohydrate-protein co-ingestion following endurance exercise on myofibrillar and mitochondrial protein synthesis. *The Journal of Physiology*, *589*(16), 4011–4025. DOI: 10.1113/jphysiol.2011.211888 PMID: 21746787

Burke, L. M., Hawley, J. A., Wong, S. H. S., & Jeukendrup, A. E. (2011). Carbohydrates for training and competition. *Journal of Sports Sciences*, *29*(sup1, Suppl 1), S17–S27. DOI: 10.1080/02640414.2011.585473 PMID: 21660838

Close, G. L., Leckey, J., Patterson, M., Bradley, W., Owens, D. J., Fraser, W. D., & Morton, J. P. (2013). The effects of vitamin D3 supplementation on serum total 25[OH]D concentration and physical performance: A randomised dose-response study. *British Journal of Sports Medicine*, *47*(11), 692–696. DOI: 10.1136/bjsports-2012-091735 PMID: 23410885

De Souza, M. J., Nattiv, A., Joy, E., Misra, M., Williams, N. I., Mallinson, R. J., Gibbs, J. C., Olmsted, M., Goolsby, M., & Matheson, G. (2014). 2014 Female Athlete Triad Coalition consensus statement on treatment and return to play of the female athlete triad. *British Journal of Sports Medicine*, *48*(4), 289. DOI: 10.1136/bjsports-2013-093218 PMID: 24463911

Desbrow, B., McCormack, J., Burke, L. M., Cox, G. R., Fallon, K., Hislop, M., Logan, R., Marino, N., Sawyer, S. M., Shaw, G., Star, A., Vidgen, H., & Leveritt, M. (2014). Sports Dietitians Australia position statement: Sports nutrition for the adolescent athlete. *International Journal of Sport Nutrition and Exercise Metabolism*, *24*(5), 570–584. DOI: 10.1123/ijsnem.2014-0031 PMID: 24668620

Drummond, M. J., & Rasmussen, B. B. (2008). Leucine-enriched nutrients and the regulation of mammalian target of rapamycin signaling and human skeletal muscle protein synthesis. *Current Opinion in Clinical Nutrition and Metabolic Care*, *11*(3), 222–226. DOI: 10.1097/MCO.0b013e3282fa17fb PMID: 18403916

Ganio, M. S., Klau, J. F., Casa, D. J., Armstrong, L. E., & Maresh, C. M. (2009). Effect of caffeine on sport-specific endurance performance: A systematic review. *Journal of Strength and Conditioning Research*, *23*(1), 315–324. DOI: 10.1519/JSC.0b013e31818b979a PMID: 19077738

Guest, N. S., Horne, J., Vanderhout, S. M., & El-Sohemy, A. (2019). Sport nutrigenomics: Personalized nutrition for athletic performance. *Frontiers in Nutrition*, *6*, 8. DOI: 10.3389/fnut.2019.00008 PMID: 30838211

Hansen, A. K., Fischer, C. P., Plomgaard, P., Andersen, J. L., Saltin, B., & Pedersen, B. K. (2005). Skeletal muscle adaptation: Training twice every second day vs. training once daily. *Journal of Applied Physiology (Bethesda, Md.)*, *98*(1), 93–99. DOI: 10.1152/japplphysiol.00163.2004 PMID: 15361516

Hargreaves, M. (2015). Exercise, muscle, and carbohydrate metabolism. *Progress in Molecular Biology and Translational Science*, *135*, 129–152. DOI: 10.1016/bs.pmbts.2015.07.016

Hawley, J. A., & Burke, L. M. (2010). Carbohydrate availability and training adaptation: Effects on cell metabolism. *Exercise and Sport Sciences Reviews*, *38*(4), 152–160. DOI: 10.1097/JES.0b013e3181f44dd9 PMID: 20871231

Hawley, J. A., Schabort, E. J., Noakes, T. D., & Dennis, S. C. (1997). Carbohydrate-loading and exercise performance. *Sports Medicine*, *24*(2), 73–81. DOI: 10.2165/00007256-199724020-00001 PMID: 9291549

Hobson, R. M., Saunders, B., Ball, G., Harris, R. C., & Sale, C. (2012). Effects of β-alanine supplementation on exercise performance: A meta-analysis. *Amino Acids*, *43*(1), 25–37. DOI: 10.1007/s00726-011-1200-z PMID: 22270875

Impey, S. G., Hearris, M. A., Hammond, K. M., Bartlett, J. D., Louis, J., Close, G. L., & Morton, J. P. (2018). Fuel for the work required: A theoretical framework for carbohydrate periodization and the glycogen threshold hypothesis. *Sports Medicine*, *48*(5), 1031–1048. DOI: 10.1007/s40279-018-0867-7 PMID: 29453741

Ismail, H., McVicar, J., Lewandowski, A. J., Sherwood, A., Lwin, M. O., & Makin, S. (2020). Continuous glucose monitoring in sport: A systematic review. *Frontiers in Sports and Active Living*, *2*, 570324. DOI: 10.3389/fspor.2020.570324

Ivy, J. L., Katz, A. L., Cutler, C. L., Sherman, W. M., & Coyle, E. F. (1988). Muscle glycogen synthesis after exercise: Effect of time of carbohydrate ingestion. *Journal of Applied Physiology (Bethesda, Md.)*, *64*(4), 1480–1485. DOI: 10.1152/jappl.1988.64.4.1480 PMID: 3132449

Jeukendrup, A. E. (2017). Periodized nutrition for athletes. *Sports Medicine*, *47*(S1, Suppl 1), 51–63. DOI: 10.1007/s40279-017-0694-2 PMID: 28332115

Kraiwanit, T., Limna, P., & Siripipatthanakul, S. (2023). NVivo for social sciences and management studies: A systematic review. *Advance Knowledge for Executives*, *2*(3), 1-11. https://papers.ssrn.com/sol3/papers.cfm?abstract_id=4523829

Lane, S. C., Camera, D. M., Lassiter, D. G., Areta, J. L., Bird, S. R., Yeo, W. K., Jeacocke, N. A., Krook, A., Zierath, J. R., Burke, L. M., & Hawley, J. A. (2015). Effects of sleeping with reduced carbohydrate availability on acute training responses. *Journal of Applied Physiology (Bethesda, Md.)*, *119*(6), 643–655. DOI: 10.1152/japplphysiol.00857.2014 PMID: 26112242

Loucks, A. B. (2004). Energy balance and body composition in sports and exercise. *Journal of Sports Sciences*, *22*(1), 1–14. DOI: 10.1080/02640410310001405 18 PMID: 14974441

Loucks, A. B., Kiens, B., & Wright, H. H. (2011). Energy availability in athletes. *Journal of Sports Sciences*, *29*(sup1, Suppl 1), S7–S15. DOI: 10.1080/02640414.2011.588958 PMID: 21793767

Mach, N., & Fuster-Botella, D. (2017). Endurance exercise and gut microbiota: A review. *Journal of Sport and Health Science*, *6*(2), 179–197. DOI: 10.1016/j.jshs.2016.05.001 PMID: 30356594

Melin, A., Tornberg, Å. B., Skouby, S., Faber, J., Ritz, C., Sjödin, A., & Sundgot-Borgen, J. (2014). The LEAF questionnaire: A screening tool for the identification of female athletes at risk for the female athlete triad. *British Journal of Sports Medicine*, *48*(7), 540–545. DOI: 10.1136/bjsports-2013-093240 PMID: 24563388

Moore, D. R., Camera, D. M., Areta, J. L., & Hawley, J. A. (2014). Beyond muscle hypertrophy: Why dietary protein is important for endurance athletes. *Applied Physiology, Nutrition, and Metabolism*, *39*(9), 987–997. DOI: 10.1139/apnm-2013-0591 PMID: 24806440

Morton, R. W., Murphy, K. T., McKellar, S. R., Schoenfeld, B. J., Henselmans, M., Helms, E., Aragon, A. A., Devries, M. C., Banfield, L., Krieger, J. W., & Phillips, S. M. (2018). A systematic review, meta-analysis and meta-regression of the effect of protein supplementation on resistance training-induced gains in muscle mass and strength in healthy adults. *British Journal of Sports Medicine*, *52*(6), 376–384. DOI: 10.1136/bjsports-2017-097608 PMID: 28698222

Mountjoy, M., Sundgot-Borgen, J., Burke, L., Carter, S., Constantini, N., Lebrun, C., Meyer, N., Sherman, R., Steffen, K., Budgett, R., & Ljungqvist, A. (2014). The IOC consensus statement: Beyond the Female Athlete Triad, Relative Energy Deficiency in Sport (RED-S). *British Journal of Sports Medicine*, *48*(7), 491–497. DOI: 10.1136/bjsports-2014-093502 PMID: 24620037

Mountjoy, M., Sundgot-Borgen, J. K., Burke, L. M., Ackerman, K. E., Blauwet, C., Constantini, N., Lebrun, C., Lundy, B., Melin, A. K., Meyer, N. L., Sherman, R. T., Tenforde, A. S., Torstveit, M. K., & Budgett, R. (2018). IOC consensus statement on relative energy deficiency in sport (RED-S): 2018 update. *British Journal of Sports Medicine*, *52*(11), 687–697. DOI: 10.1136/bjsports-2018-099193 PMID: 29773536

Mujika, I., & Padilla, S. (2000). Detraining: Loss of training-induced physiological and performance adaptations. Part I. *Sports Medicine*, *30*(2), 79–87. https://link.springer.com/article/10.2165/00007256-200030020-00002. DOI: 10.2165/00007256-200030020-00002 PMID: 10966148

Nattiv, A., Loucks, A. B., Manore, M. M., Sanborn, C. F., Sundgot-Borgen, J., & Warren, M. P. (2007). American College of Sports Medicine position stand: The female athlete triad. *Medicine and Science in Sports and Exercise*, *39*(10), 1867–1882. DOI: 10.1249/mss.0b013e318149f111 PMID: 17909417

Nieman, D. C., & Pedersen, B. K. (1999). Exercise and immune function. *Sports Medicine*, *27*(2), 73–80. DOI: 10.2165/00007256-199927020-00001 PMID: 10091272

Norton, L. E., & Layman, D. K. (2006). Leucine regulates translation initiation of protein synthesis in skeletal muscle after exercise. *The Journal of Nutrition*, *136*(2), 533S–537S. DOI: 10.1093/jn/136.2.533S PMID: 16424142

Peeling, P., Dawson, B., Goodman, C., Landers, G., & Trinder, D. (2008). Athletic induced iron deficiency: New insights into the role of inflammation, cytokines and hormones. *European Journal of Applied Physiology*, *103*(4), 381–391. DOI: 10.1007/s00421-008-0726-6 PMID: 18365240

Phillips, S. M., & Van Loon, L. J. C. (2011). Dietary protein for athletes: From requirements to optimum adaptation. *Journal of Sports Sciences*, *29*(sup1, Suppl 1), S29–S38. DOI: 10.1080/02640414.2011.619204 PMID: 22150425

Rawson, E. S., & Volek, J. S. (2003). Effects of creatine supplementation and resistance training on muscle strength and weightlifting performance. *Journal of Strength and Conditioning Research*, *17*(4), 822–831. DOI: 10.1519/1533-4287(2003)017<0822:EOCSAM>2.0.CO;2 PMID: 14636102

Res, P. T., Groen, B., Pennings, B., Beelen, M., Wallis, G. A., Gijsen, A. P., Senden, J. M., & van Loon, L. J. C. (2012). Protein ingestion before sleep improves postexercise overnight recovery. *Medicine and Science in Sports and Exercise*, *44*(8), 1560–1569. DOI: 10.1249/MSS.0b013e31824cc363 PMID: 22330017

Shaw, G., Lee-Barthel, A., Ross, M. L., Wang, B., & Baar, K. (2017). Vitamin C-enriched gelatin supplementation before intermittent activity augments collagen synthesis. *The American Journal of Clinical Nutrition, 105*(1), 136–143. DOI: 10.3945/ajcn.116.138594 PMID: 27852613

Sherman, W. M., Costill, D. L., Fink, W. J., & Miller, J. M. (1981). Effect of exercise-diet manipulation on muscle glycogen and its subsequent utilization during performance. *International Journal of Sports Medicine, 2*(2), 114–118. DOI: 10.1055/s-2008-1034594 PMID: 7333741

Siripipatthanakul, S., Phuangsuwan, P., Jaipong, P., & Muthmainnha. (2025, September). Wi-Fi Networks and Security: A Systematic Review. In *International Conference on Artificial Intelligence and Networking* (pp. 81-92). Singapore: Springer Nature Singapore. https://link.springer.com/chapter/10.1007/978-981-96-2015-9_6

Smith, G. I., Atherton, P., Reeds, D. N., Mohammed, B. S., Rankin, D., Rennie, M. J., & Mittendorfer, B. (2011). Omega-3 polyunsaturated fatty acids augment the muscle protein anabolic response to hyperinsulinaemia-hyperaminoacidaemia in healthy young and middle-aged men and women. *Clinical Science (London, England), 121*(6), 267–278. DOI: 10.1042/CS20100597 PMID: 21501117

Snijders, T., Res, P. T., Smeets, J. S., van Vliet, S., van Kranenburg, J., Maase, K., Kies, A. K., Verdijk, L. B., & van Loon, L. J. C. (2015). Protein ingestion before sleep increases muscle mass and strength gains during prolonged resistance-type exercise training in healthy young men. *The Journal of Nutrition, 145*(6), 1178–1184. DOI: 10.3945/jn.114.208371 PMID: 25926415

Tarnopolsky, M. A. (2004). Protein requirements for endurance athletes. *Nutrition (Burbank, Los Angeles County, Calif.), 20*(7-8), 662–668. DOI: 10.1016/j.nut.2004.04.008 PMID: 15212749

Witard, O. C., Jackman, S. R., Breen, L., Smith, K., Selby, A., & Tipton, K. D. (2014). Myofibrillar muscle protein synthesis rates subsequent to a meal in response to small and large bolus doses of dairy proteins. *The American Journal of Clinical Nutrition, 99*(1), 86–95. DOI: 10.3945/ajcn.112.055517 PMID: 24257722

Yeo, W. K., Paton, C. D., Garnham, A. P., Burke, L. M., Carey, A. L., & Hawley, J. A. (2008). Skeletal muscle adaptation and performance responses to once a day versus twice every second day endurance training regimens. *Journal of Applied Physiology (Bethesda, Md.), 105*(5), 1462–1470. DOI: 10.1152/japplphysiol.90882.2008 PMID: 18772325

KEY TERMS AND DEFINITIONS

Carbohydrate Periodization: The planned variation of carbohydrate intake across training sessions to enhance metabolic adaptations and optimize performance.

Energy Availability (EA): The amount of dietary energy remaining for physiological functions after subtracting energy expended during exercise.

Glycogen Supercompensation: A process where muscle glycogen stores increase above normal levels following depletion and high carbohydrate intake, enhancing endurance performance.

Muscle Protein Synthesis (MPS): The biological process through which the body builds new muscle proteins, stimulated by resistance training and protein intake.

Narrative Review: A narrative review is a thorough, critical, and subjective look at the current literature on a certain subject. It gives a general picture without the strict rules of a systematic review. It lets researchers use a flexible, thematic, or chronological approach to put together complex or changing issues, make sense of what they already know, and find areas where more research is needed.

Nutrition Periodization: Nutrition periodization refers to the strategic manipulation of nutrient intake (especially carbohydrates and proteins) according to training phases to optimize performance and recovery.

Relative Energy Deficiency in Sport (RED-S): A condition caused by low energy availability that negatively affects metabolic, hormonal, and performance-related functions in athletes.

Chapter 8
Nutrition Balance for Females' Athletic Performance and Recovery Using AI Assistants

Astri Dwi Andriani
http://orcid.org/0000-0003-3951-4829
Universitas Putra Indonesia, Indonesia

Parichat Jaipong
http://orcid.org/0000-0002-9249-3169
GlobalNxt University, Malaysia

Shikha Khullar
http://orcid.org/0009-0000-5598-3145
Poornima University, India

ABSTRACT

Nutrition balance for female athletes is a specialized, data-driven approach focusing on maintaining high energy availability to support training, hormonal health, and menstrual cycle variations. This chapter utilizes a systematic review of literature indexed in Scopus, WOS, and Google Scholar from 2024 to 2026. The findings highlight that AI assistants and wearable technology are transforming the field by providing personalized, real-time insights for optimization. To maximize performance, nutritional balance is essential, ensuring adequate intake of carbohydrates for energy, protein for muscle repair, healthy fats for hormone regulation, and micronutrients

DOI: 10.4018/979-8-3373-9544-9.ch008

like iron and calcium to prevent common deficiencies. AI assistants play a significant role by offering individualized recommendations, monitoring hydration, and providing evidence-based guidance tailored to specific training regimens. With these tools, female athletes can maintain optimal nutrition, improving overall performance and facilitating more efficient recovery.

1. INTRODUCTION

Female athletes need high energy for exercise and hormone balance, which is linked to calorie consumption and hormone stability. Insufficient energy causes health concerns in sports. Energy intake must exceed activity output for bone remodeling and heart health in female athletes. Data should be utilized to regulate energy intake to avoid the physiological "shutdown" that occurs when athletes undereat. Diet substantially affects hormones. Nutrients affect female athletes' metabolism and reproduction. Healthy fats help female athletes produce hormones that support health and performance. Menstrual estrogen and progesterone may influence carbohydrate and protein digestion, according to research. Female athletes should occasionally change their diet.

Body composition affects nutrition and performance. Previous research has linked body composition to a mismatch between nutrient intake and requirements. However, this article examines how lifestyle factors like eating behavior and meal timing affect body composition. Due to hormone and growth factor imbalances, lifestyle factors might alter protein synthesis or breakdown, insulin resistance, and overeating. These factors consistently alter muscle and fat mass in juvenile and adult men and women. Sexual dimorphism of adiposity between men and women may influence dietary preferences. Chronic stress causes emotional eating, and proper sleep affects growth factors and hormone balances, but research is limited. Knowledge and lifestyle changes improve body composition regardless of gender or age (Feng, 2025).

Female athletes must maintain bone health to optimize performance, prevent injury, and support long-term health. Stress fractures, osteoporosis, and Relative Energy Deficiency in Sport (RED-S) can result from hormonal imbalances, dietary deficits, and overtraining. Adolescence and early adulthood are crucial for reaching optimum bone growth through weight-bearing and high-impact workouts, according to this analysis. The Female Athlete Triad, including poor energy, menstrual disruption, and low bone mineral density, is a risk factor for disordered eating. Bone health requires calcium, vitamin D, and balanced meals. Resistance exercise and plyometrics increase bone density, whereas planned training with recovery reduces bone stress. Menstrual irregularities influence bone health; thus, monitoring and hormonal therapies are needed. DEXA scans can detect early bone density abnormalities, especially in postmenopausal women. Education and multidisciplinary approaches help manage RED-S and raise awareness. Novel technologies such as biomarkers and genetic testing enable tailored care and monitoring. Sports physicians, dietitians, and psychologists work together to optimize bone health, reduce injury risks, and assist athletes throughout their lives (Rohilla & Therattil, 2024).

The female athlete triad (TRIAD) includes menstrual abnormalities, low bone mineral density, and low energy availability. The term "relative energy deficiency in sport" is frequently used to emphasize the widespread effects of low energy availability on the body. Female athletes across various sports are on the promise of a nutrition-focused approach to prevent or treat these diseases. Female athletes had several issues with energy, protein, and carbohydrate intake. All athlete groups evaluated had low vitamin D intake. The average requirements for Ca, Mg, Ca/P ratio, Zn, and Fe are likewise insufficient. A nutritional strategy is suggested to address such difficulties. Improved micronutrient absorption factors have also been explored. An increasing percentage of women with TRIAD/relative energy deficiency in sport require nutritional treatment, and physicians, dietitians, physiotherapists, and psychologists must collaborate (Grabia et al., 2024).

Understanding how endogenous and exogenous hormonal fluctuations affect exercise outcomes is essential for creating evidence-based training and dietary programs for female athletes. The effects of hormonal contraceptive (HC) use and eumenorrheic menstrual cycle physiology on sports performance, neuromuscular function, injury risk, and metabolic control in physically active women. Estradiol and progesterone fluctuations may modulate substrate utilization, connective tissue properties, central fatigue regulation, and symptom expression, but the modest magnitude of these physiological effects and methodological heterogeneity in menstrual cycle phase classification and verification across studies lead to small and inconsistent performance-related effects across menstrual phases. Although performance, injury prevention, and metabolic effects are mixed, HC reduces endogenous hormonal swings. Endocrine factors may affect energy expenditure, insulin sensitivity, hunger, inflammation, and recovery. Symptoms include pain, fatigue, sleep disruption, gastrointestinal discomfort, and fluid retention, all of which affect daily exercise tolerance. Nutrition affects metabolic reactivity, symptom severity, and performance consistency, but sex hormones set the baseline (Natalucci et al., 2026).

Well-planned nutrition helps female athletes manage hormones. It promotes regular activity and injury prevention. Female athletes can improve hormone levels with diet. Food and hormones are used to treat female athletes. AI technologies help female athletes track food and health. Female athletes receive individualized, real-time nutrition and training input with these revolutionary technologies. Wearables measure heart rate and temperature. It tracks female athletes' menstrual needs well.

AI systems can recognize weariness or recovery from this data. This allows female athletes to swiftly adjust their diet for performance and health. AI-driven insights and real-time body monitoring help female athletes manage food and health, advancing personalized sports science. Female athletes increasingly use AI assistants for personalized nutritional guidance tailored to their training and physical needs. These systems track athletes' food and drink intake, remind them to meet nutritional goals, and provide female athletes with evidence-based advice, such as on menstrual iron intake. Machine learning predicts athletes' diets depending on workout intensity and recovery. Last-minute diet changes are feasible. Female athletes who optimize diet for training and body cycles can better manage complex nutritional needs.

2. LITERATURE REVIEW: Nutritional Foundations for Female Athletic Performance

2.1. AI Assistants for Female Athletes Macronutrient (Carbohydrate, Protein, and Fat) Balance

The use of AI in precision exercise nutrition is changing how athletes optimize their diet for performance, recuperation, and well-being. AI technology can provide personalized dietary regimens for the specific physiological and metabolic needs of athletes. AI-based mechanisms such as real-time diet monitoring, continuous glucose monitoring, and nutrient optimization systems advance precision nutrition by analyzing complex datasets and integrating genetic, metabolic, and environmental factors to provide accurate dietary recommendations tailored to athletes' needs. However, AI presents challenges such as ethical concerns, data confidentiality, and the need for uniformity across varied populations. Employing AI can improve athletes' nutrition regimens, leading to improved performance and faster recovery from tiredness or injuries compared to traditional techniques. There is a potential for AI to enhance engagement in precision nutrition for athletes and fitness enthusiasts (Nasb et al., 2025).

Given the sport's rising competition and physical demands, female soccer players' performance and recovery must be optimized. Nutrition is crucial to athletes' physiological needs. However, nutritional requirements and their effects on performance and recuperation are unclear. This study examined female soccer players' dietary intake, physiological state, and training performance to address this crucial need. Athletic performance was strongly linked to protein, carbs, vitamin D, iron, and calcium. The experimental group improved in speed, endurance, skill tests, and physiological indices after implementing personalized nutrition strategies, proving that tailored nutrition plans improve sports performance, body composition, and health recovery (Guo et al., 2024).

Personalized, sport-specific training and nutrition with concurrent training to boost endurance, resilience, and efficiency. Nutrition techniques emphasize individualized calorie and macronutrient periodization, minimal energy availability hazards, and judicious supplement use. Female athletes were encouraged to monitor menstrual cycles and hormonal states, and to address knowledge gaps regarding hormonal effects on performance and injury risk. Rehabilitation should include criteria-based progression and multidisciplinary input to prevent tendon overuse and Achilles tendon ruptures, which can end athletic careers. Wearable sensors and multi-omics analysis could customize training and diet, but they need more testing in top settings. This consensus provides a practical, scientific framework to enhance elite athletes' performance and health, while emphasizing the need for ongoing research to address concerns and promote inclusive, evidence-based approaches (Bangsbo et al, 2025).

Endurance sports increasingly use AI to improve performance, recovery, nutrition, and supplement use. increase metabolic health monitoring, recovery prediction, and nutrition personalization. Glucose monitoring and AI algorithms improve performance during extended events by managing carbs. AI-driven supplementing techniques based on genetic polymorphisms and metabolic responses have improved ergogenicity. However, measurement validity and reliability of sensor-derived signals, dataset quality (noise, missingness, labeling error), model performance and generalizability, algorithmic transparency, and equitable access remain issues. Homogeneous training datasets limit applicability across varied athletic populations. AI in endurance sports can improve performance, recovery, and nutrition through tailored techniques. Model performance, generalizability, ethical transparency, and fair accessibility must be addressed to realize this promise (Grivas & Safari, 2025).

The Dietary Guidelines for Americans from 2025 to 2030 have changed a lot. They now feature new ideas about protein, dairy fat, and ultra-processed foods. This examination uses both government criteria and the most up-to-date peer-reviewed research to be useful. Cardiologists employ a holistic, evidence-driven dietary counseling framework. The 2025-2030 DGA encompasses meta-analyses, Mendelian randomization studies, and randomized controlled trials published up to January 2026. Dietary items based on their effect sizes, the strength of their causal inference, and how easily they could be changed at the population level. AI-assisted synthesis (Claude, Anthropic) enabled the amalgamation of cardiology, nutrition, epidemiology, and public health literature. Eating ultra-processed foods is the most important thing to do (RR 1.21 all-cause death). For diabetics, high-impact modifiable factors include eating meals with a lot of glycemic load, not getting enough omega-3s, and eating a lot of industrial trans fats. Evidence indicates that full-fat dairy rehabilitation, age-specific protein requirements (1.0-1.6 g/kg), and dietary pattern approaches are preferable to single-nutrient approaches (Lee, 2026).

Intense training and menstrual losses put female athletes at significant risk of iron, calcium, and vitamin D deficiencies. This can impair performance, hinder recovery, and even cause injuries. AI-powered nutrition systems and wearable devices can help with this by giving personalized, data-driven advice. For example, they can track female athletes' diet, sun exposure, and menstrual cycles to ensure you're getting the right nutrients at the right times. These technologies help athletes recover faster, reduce their risk of injury, and stay healthy in the long term by balancing magnesium and zinc, important micronutrients.

2.2. Essential Micronutrients in Iron and Calcium Deficiency Prevention using AI assistants for Female Athletes

Iron deficiency (ID), with or without anemia, is a common and complex health problem that affects female athletes more than male athletes. The molecular mechanisms regulating iron homeostasis, emphasizing the hepcidin-ferroportin axis, inflammation-induced sequestration (IL-6), and the effects of the menstrual cycle and Low Energy Availability (LEA). The exercise-induced mechanical stress (foot-strike hemolysis), metabolic alterations, and environmental influences contribute to a persistent negative iron balance. The effects on performance include lower VO_2max, less efficient mitochondria, and cognitive impairment. Advanced management measures, such as "hepcidin-aware" nutritional timing, the significance of Vitamin D, and periodized supplementation procedures, are crucial instruments for enhancing endurance and promoting long-term health in high-performance female populations (Paria et al., 2026).

Despite nutrition and health system gains, micronutrient deficiencies, or "hidden hunger," remain a global public health issue. Iron, vitamin A, iodine, zinc, and vitamin D deficiencies cause illness, cognitive impairment, poor pregnancy outcomes, and increased mortality, especially in vulnerable groups. The prevalence, determinants, and public health effects of global micronutrient deficiencies. Iron deficiency anemia, the most common micronutrient condition worldwide, is high in reproductive-age women and children. Vitamin A, iodine, zinc, and D deficits are common in low- and middle-income countries. Global trends indicate a changing frequency and a persistent public health burden due to insufficient dietary diversity, socioeconomic inequality, infectious diseases, and gaps in nutrition surveillance and intervention, despite some small gains. Micronutrient deficiencies remain a global health issue despite treatments. To reduce the long-term health and socioeconomic effects of these deficiencies and support global nutrition and health targets, integrated public health strategies, including food fortification, supplementation, dietary diversification, and routine screening in primary care, must be strengthened (Aurora, 2026).

Olympic victories are routinely highlighted, but Paralympic successes are sometimes forgotten. Disability and sport-specific energy consumption and nutrient needs present distinct dietary issues for Paralympic competitors. Hydration is essential for athletes with spinal cord injuries, who may have trouble regulating body temperature. Nutrition improves athletic performance, but the dietary needs of Paralympic competitors remain understudied. The energy, macronutrient, and micronutrient needs of Paralympic competitors aged 18 and older, including minerals, vitamins, supplements, and fluids. Paralympic athletes need customized nutritional preparation to perform well. Individual intake must be monitored to account for macronutrient and micronutrient supplements, as well as fluid changes. Developing appropriate dietary regimens for these athletes' unique needs requires ongoing research (Ghazzawi et al., 2025).

Iron is essential for female athletes’ cognitive function, metabolism, and performance, but intense training and menstruation increase their risk of deficiency. Calcium and vitamin D are crucial for bone strength and muscle function, with deficiencies raising the risk of injuries. AI-powered nutrition tools provide personalized guidance, helping female athletes optimize their intake of key micronutrients, adapt their diets to menstrual cycle changes, and improve nutrient absorption. This individualized approach helps prevent deficiencies, supports recovery, and enhances overall athletic performance and health.

2.3. Female Athletes' Specific Nutrition for the Menstrual Cycle Variations

Sports science has progressed by incorporating menstrual cycle irregularities into nutritional planning for female athletes. The hormonal changes during the follicular and luteal phases of the menstrual cycle affect metabolism, substrate use, thermoregulation, and fluid balance. Adjusting macronutrient intake and hydration according to these phases can enhance performance, recovery, and overall health. During the follicular phase, increased insulin sensitivity and carbohydrate utilization support high-intensity training, making carbohydrate intake crucial. As estrogen rises approaching ovulation, dietary modifications are needed to maintain ligament flexibility and reduce injury risk. In the luteal phase, high progesterone levels raise basal metabolic rate and protein breakdown, requiring increased calorie and protein intake to support muscle repair and lean tissue preservation, along with more healthy fats due to greater fat oxidation.

Ovarian steroids fluctuate during the menstrual cycle, affecting systemic metabolism and reproductive function. The menstrual cycle phase affects energy balance, macronutrient metabolism, micronutrient management, and bioactive chemical reactions. The mid-luteal phase has higher energy intake and lipid oxidation than the early follicular and peri-ovulatory phases. New metabolomics data show coordinated cyclical fluctuations in amino acids, B vitamins, and lipid species, suggesting time-sensitive windows during which low energy or micronutrient deficiency may worsen performance, recovery, or symptom load. Menstrual cycle-related metabolic variability encompasses oscillations in estradiol and progesterone and integrated adaptations across the hypothalamic–pituitary–adrenal axis, the autonomic nervous system, immunological signaling, and the gut microbiome. These interrelated mechanisms cause variability in metabolic phenotypes among individuals. The clinical and applied evidence supports "cycle-aware" but non-dogmatic nutritional regimens for metabolic dysfunction, high training loads, and reproductive problems. Recognition of the menstrual cycle as a biologically important metabolic variable may improve precision in women's nutrition, exercise, and metabolic risk assessment (García et al., 2026).

Winter sports training and wellness for female athletes. Puberty-related biological divergence in hemoglobin mass, heart dimensions, skeletal muscle mass, and body composition underlies sex variations in absolute performance. Many physiological differences are minimized when normalized to body mass or lean mass, although hemoglobin concentration and body fat % remain the key performance gap factors. Despite these disparities, modern evidence suggests that women and men physiologically adjust to training in ways that reflect their capacity after puberty. Thus, effective training principles apply to both sexes, highlighting the need for sport-specific, tailored training. Health is essential to performance. High rates of iron deficiency, relative energy deficiency in sport (REDs), and menstrual dysfunction in female athletes might impair adaptation, increase injury risk, and shorten careers. Monitoring and prevention must be integrated and sex-specific to address these issues. The evidence-based support to improve the performance and health of top female winter Olympians at Milano Cortina 2026 and beyond by converting biological insights into tailored training and health practices (Sandbakk et al, 2026).

Hormonal changes make hydration and electrolyte management especially important, particularly in the mid-luteal phase. AI assistants and wearable technologies can now track menstrual cycle stages and provide real-time guidance on diet, hydration, and supplements to improve performance, mood, and recovery. These systems help ensure adequate energy intake and nutritional balance, which are key to maintaining bone and cardiovascular health and to preventing conditions such as Relative Energy Deficiency in Sport (RED-S) and functional hypothalamic amenorrhea. Additionally, iron is vital before menstruation, while calcium and vitamin D are important during periods of high estrogen for endurance and bone strength. Since hormonal contraceptives can impact nutritional metabolism, female athletes need to tailor their diets accordingly. Overall, menstrual cycle tracking, personalized nutrition planning, and AI-driven tools enable female athletes and coaches to optimize training, recovery, and well-being throughout the cycle, leading to more consistent performance and health.

2.4. Integration of AI and Wearable Technology in Sports Nutrition for Female Athletes

AI-powered tools also offer timely reminders for nutrient intake, such as prompting a high-protein snack after exercise or suggesting increased carbohydrate intake before intense training. These reminders are dynamically timed based on the athlete's real-time activity and metabolic data, optimizing recovery and performance outcomes. Personalization is a key benefit of this technology, as AI-driven nutrition plans adapt to each athlete's training phase, physiological profile, and hormonal status. Research shows that these individualized plans are more effective than generic nutrition approaches for achieving performance goals and maintaining health. While these innovations greatly enhance access to elite-level sports science and empower female athletes with user-friendly, evidence-based nutrition guidance, they also raise important considerations around data privacy and the need for unbiased algorithms. Overall, the integration of AI and wearables is setting a new standard in sports nutrition for female athletes, enabling highly personalized, responsive, and effective support for their unique needs and long-term health.

AI and ML are being integrated into sports and fitness through wearable biosensing technologies that enable continuous monitoring and data-driven training adaptation. Their usefulness as coaches depends on biosensor data validity, analytical model robustness, and the conditions of empirical evaluation. To increase openness, an evidence map of essential empirical studies summarizes sensing modalities, cohort sizes, experimental settings (laboratory vs. field), model kinds, evaluation processes, and key outcomes. Field and laboratory studies show that wearable biosensors can reliably capture physiological (e.g., heart rate variability), biomechanical (e.g., inertial and electromyographic signals), and biochemical (e.g., sweat lactate and electrolytes) markers relevant to training load, fatigue, and recovery when provided with signal quality control and calibration. ML models trained on these data can estimate training adaptation and recovery better than standard workload measurements in endurance, strength, and team-sport contexts, when validated at the athlete level or longitudinally. Motion artifacts, inter-session variability, distribution shift between laboratory and field contexts, and overconfidence when contextual or psychosocial inputs are absent are common constraints. AI-driven biosensor systems can support monitoring and adaptive training, but not autonomous coaching. Sensor dependability, validation processes, and human control limit their usefulness. A human–AI partnership in which ML improves data interpretation, and coaches remain responsible for contextual judgment, ethical decision-making, and athlete-centered care is the most plausible paradigm (Madrigal-Cerezo et al., 2026).

AI in sports science has gone from isolated technological demonstrations to a paradigm-shifting force altering athletic performance, enhancing philosophy, technique, and practice. This paper offers a comprehensive look into intelligent algorithms in competitive sports, integrating theoretical foundations, empirical advances, and systemic limits. The study reconstructs core theoretical constructs for adaptive intelligence frameworks that incorporate real-time sensorimotor feedback, nonlinear dynamical system identification, and context-sensitive, individualized performance representation grounded in motor learning theory and ecological dynamics, moving beyond static assumptions and population-level generalizations in biomechanical modeling. Technically, the analysis covers recent advances in machine learning and deep learning architectures, such as multimodal wearable data-stream-based supervised injury-risk prediction models, unsupervised fatigue-state segmentation clustering methods, and hybrid convolutional-recurrent neural networks that can model tactical decisions. Implementations of AI-enabled individualized training systems are critically examined, showcasing reinforcement learning–driven closed-loop protocols and digital twin–informed adaptation engines that have been verified across elite track-and-field, basketball, and swimming cohorts. However, algorithmic bias from demographic and sport-specific data imbalances, limited generalizability from small-sample training regimes, insufficient interpretability for coach-athlete trust calibration, and infrastructural inequities hindering adoption in youth or resource-constrained settings are systematically examined. In conclusion, federated learning paradigms, internationally harmonized benchmark datasets, domain-specific evaluation metrics that prioritize fairness, robustness, and pedagogical fidelity, and institutional frameworks that foster sustained collaboration among AI engineers, sports medicine clinicians, biomechanists, and coaching practitioners form the basis of a transdisciplinary research agenda (WAN, 2026).

Sports nutrition for female athletes is being propelled by AI and wearable technology, which together enable real-time, individualized nutritional guidance. Wearable sensors can monitor important physiological markers such as glucose levels, sweat composition, and heart rate variability. AI algorithms analyze this data to provide evidence-based recommendations that address the unique needs of female athletes, including adjustments for hormonal fluctuations throughout the menstrual cycle. This technology streamlines the process from data collection to nutritional intervention, allowing for immediate, targeted adjustments that go beyond the capabilities of traditional nutrition monitoring. Automated meal and hydration tracking, such as snapping a photo of a meal for macronutrient analysis or using sweat patches to assess electrolyte loss, reduces the manual workload for athletes while improving the accuracy of dietary records. As a result, female athletes can more effectively balance energy intake and protein for muscle repair.

3. METHODOLOGY

Systematic reviews rigorously and clearly synthesize research on nutrition and AI. This rigorous method avoids bias and ensures high-quality, data-driven assessments of women's sports performance. This research uses standard methods to identify, analyze, and summarize all relevant papers to assess the current state of knowledge in this rapidly advancing field. The systematic review design integrates information from diverse geographic and sporting contexts to provide a comprehensive understanding of the subject. This strategy also identifies research gaps, which can guide future studies on understudied themes in female sports nutrition. A methodical methodology ensures reproducibility and a solid foundation for analysis and discussion.

To ensure the breadth and depth of the literature search, data were systematically collected from three primary academic databases: Scopus, Web of Science (WOS), and Google Scholar. Scopus and Web of Science were selected for their reputation as high-impact, peer-reviewed repositories that index top-tier journals (Shaengchart et al., 2026; Andriani & Siripipatthanakul, 2026, a) in sports science, artificial intelligence, and clinical nutrition. Google Scholar provided an additional layer of comprehensive searching, capturing relevant grey literature and emerging studies that might not yet be fully indexed in traditional citation databases (Gusenbauer, 2025).

Multiple databases maximize paper retrieval by avoiding platform-specific indexing strategies. Each database was queried using Boolean operators and keywords like "AI assistants," "female athletes," and "nutrition balance." This one accepts only recent studies due to rigorous standards. Due to their rapid progress, previous publications may not fully demonstrate AI and wearable technologies. This temporal focus ensures the evaluation includes the latest AI implementations for athlete performance and recovery. Limiting the timescale allows the study to evaluate the latest generative AI and machine learning models in sports nutrition. Focusing on this short time frame is vital and relevant in scholarship. This criterion excludes outdated nutritional recommendations that overlook the new female athlete triad or research on RED.

A purposive sampling method was employed to select the most relevant manuscripts (Campbell et al., 2020; Andriani & Siripipatthanakul, 2026, b) that directly address the intersection of nutrition, gender-specific physiology, and technological integration. This non-probability sampling technique is particularly effective in systematic reviews where the goal is to extract deep, qualitative insights from specific "information-rich" cases (Campbell et al., 2020). Instead of random selection, papers were picked for their evidence-based advice tailored to athletes' needs.

This method ensures that the review synthesizes high-quality, useful findings rather than just summarizing a lot of material. Methodological strength was assessed for each publication, with particular attention to those using real-time wearable data. This targeted selection procedure is essential for creating an academically sound and sports-practitioner-relevant narrative. Specific search strings linking dietary variables to technology treatments were used in the rigorously documented search approach to assure transparency. These themes were athlete (female, athletes, performers), nutrition (nutrition balance, energy availability, micronutrients), and technology (AI, wearables). The study focused on AI-optimized nutrition for elite female athletes and employed a rigorous, multi-stage technique to examine original research and reviews via Scopus and WOS. By filtering out irrelevant content, the study established a high-quality, evidence-based foundation by specifically examining AI's role in monitoring nutrition, hydration, and key nutrients such as iron and calcium. Performance, recovery, and technological integration were the themes that emerged from the methodical extraction and quality assessment of the data. The results, which show how AI is developing in women's sports, provide practitioners with useful, trustworthy insights while highlighting the need for further validation.

4. RESULTS

Figure 1. Conceptual Framework

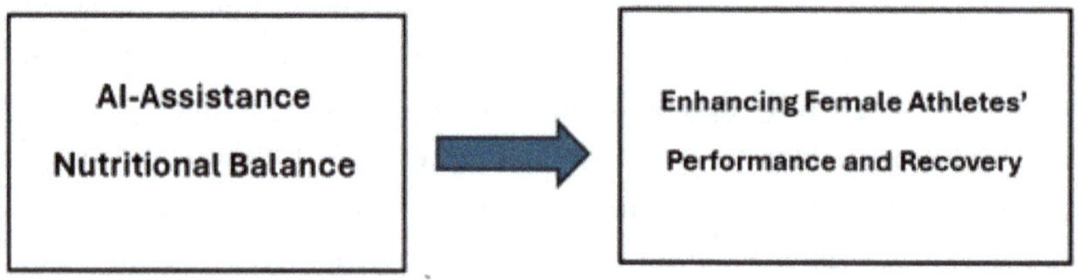

Figure 1 shows the conceptual framework. AI assists nutritional balance by enhancing female athletes' performance and recovery.

AI assistants are transforming nutrition balance for female athletes by providing personalized, real-time guidance that aligns dietary intake with physiological demands and training loads. These tools analyze data from wearables and biomarkers to optimize macronutrient ratios, support hormonal health, and adjust nutrition according to menstrual cycle phases. By doing so, AI ensures athletes maintain peak energy, accelerate recovery, and reduce the risk of injury and burnout. The technology also automates complex calculations and offers evidence-based recommendations, simplifying meal planning and reducing mental stress. Overall, AI-driven nutrition management is empowering female athletes to achieve better performance, faster recovery, and long-term health.

AI is revolutionizing elite sports by enabling personalized, data-driven nutrition and recovery strategies, especially for female athletes. By analyzing real-time data from wearables, AI tailors nutritional interventions to support optimal performance, hormonal health, and recovery, even accounting for menstrual cycle variations. This technology not only improves physical and cognitive performance but also enhances mental well-being by simplifying dietary management and preventing burnout. AI's precise, evidence-based guidance enables early detection of health risks, improved bone health, and more consistent, high-quality training, making it a vital tool for sustained athletic excellence in modern sports.

5. DISCUSSIONS: Main Results from Different Studies

5.1 Balance of Macronutrients (Guo et al., 2024; Nasb et al., 2025; Bangsbo et al., 2025).

Female athletes need to eat different amounts of carbs, protein, and fat depending on how hard they train and the phase of their menstrual cycle. AI-powered systems allow for dynamic changes, which are better than static, one-size-fits-all programs.

5.2 Micronutrient Sufficiency (Paria et al., 2026; Aurora, 2026).

Iron and calcium shortages remain widespread, with considerable impacts on performance and health. AI-guided monitoring and timely replenishment improve absorption and make sure that consumption matches the body's needs.

5.3 Hormonal Health and Awareness of the Menstrual Cycle (García et al., 2026; Natalucci et al., 2026).

Changes in hormones affect how the body breaks down substances, heals, and is vulnerable to damage. AI and wearables make "cycle-aware" nutrition possible, which helps both athletes' results and their independence.

5.4 Technology Integration (Madrigal-Cerezo et al., 2026; WAN, 2026)

Wearables and AI make it easy to collect data (such as heart rate, glucose, and sweat composition) and turn it into useful information. Real-time, personalized feedback improves compliance, performance, and recuperation.

The examined papers utilized high-quality, contemporary empirical research, incorporating both quantitative and qualitative data. Purposive sampling ensured that the focus was on interventions that were gender-specific, technologically advanced, and implementable. Athletes who used AI-assisted nutrition saw significant gains in speed, endurance, recovery time, and injury avoidance. Getting better AI-customized macronutrient and micronutrient intake at the right times speeds up muscle regeneration and lowers tiredness. Mental Health Automated meal planning and reminders make it easier on the brain and help female athletes feel better and make better decisions when they're stressed. Things that aren't working and things that are missing. There are still concerns about the security of sensitive health data and the risk of algorithmic bias, especially in underrepresented groups. Most datasets come from elite athletes in Western settings, making them less useful for other groups. There are few studies examining the long-term health impacts of AI-driven interventions across different sports and populations. When AI systems work with teams of people from other fields (including nutritionists, coaches, doctors, and psychologists), they get the best results. Researchers need to keep testing and improving AI algorithms in real-world settings to ensure they are fair, accurate, and trustworthy. Policy and Learning: Sports organizations should prioritize educational programs that help female athletes use this technology safely. This chapter shows a strong synthesis of new evidence, based on a systematic review process that focuses on recency, relevance, and methodological rigor. By focusing on the specific demands of female athletes and the possibilities of AI-driven customization, it establishes a new benchmark for sports nutrition advice. There is substantial evidence that AI and wearables can work together, and the mechanisms and benefits are well established. The practical consequences are clearly laid out, providing athletes, coaches, and professionals with useful information. The field is changing, and there aren't many long-term, large-scale validation studies. Ethical and data privacy issues need to be discussed more clearly and addressed. More research is needed to ensure that the results are generalizable across different cultures, socioeconomic backgrounds, and levels of sport.

The combination of AI, wearables, and evidence-based nutrition has the power to change the game for female athletes. Practitioners can improve both health and performance by moving away from general nutritional advice and toward tailored, flexible interventions. But to make this promise come true, we need to keep doing research, make algorithms that are easy to understand, and use techniques that include everyone

6. CONCLUSIONS

Using AI assistants to help female athletes with their nutrition balance for better performance and recovery as follows;

6.1. Custom Nutrition, in line with physiology

AI helpers use data from wearable devices to create nutrition plans tailored to the physiological needs of each female athlete. This means adjusting the amounts of macronutrients and energy available based on how hard you train, how fast your metabolism is, and your goals.

6.2. Help with Hormonal Health and the Menstrual Cycle

AI systems monitor the different phases of the menstrual cycle and hormonal changes. They suggest dietary changes, such as increasing magnesium or omega-3 intake, when the body is most vulnerable. This keeps your energy levels up, helps your body heal, and keeps your hormones in balance, which is important for both performance and recovery.

6.3. Better Recovery and Less Chance of Being Hurt

AI provides precise advice on protein, antioxidants, and general recovery nutrition by analyzing signs of muscle injury and inflammation. This focused help speeds up recovery, lowers the chance of delayed-onset muscle soreness, and helps avoid problems from overuse and burnout.

6.4. Mental Health and Cognitive Performance

AI aids meal preparation, making it easier on the brain so athletes can focus on training and competing. The technology helps maintain consistent blood sugar levels and metabolic health, which is important for keeping your mind fresh and making good decisions when things get tough.

6.5. Ongoing Health Checks and Their Benefits

AI can provide early warnings about health hazards, such as low energy levels or bone-related injuries, by continuously monitoring biological markers like bone mineral density, heart rate variability, and sleep quality. This proactive, data-driven approach helps female athletes not only perform at their best but also stay healthy and have lengthy careers.

Contemporary sports nutrition has transitioned from a universal approach to a more tailored methodology. This is especially true for female athletes, who haven't been adequately represented in scientific writing. Nutrition balancing for female athletes is a unique, data-driven method that goes beyond conventional nutritional advice. It focuses on keeping your energy levels up to support training, hormonal health, and menstrual cycle fluctuations. Women athletes need to consume a balanced diet that meets their biological needs for macronutrients and micronutrients to perform at their best and recover rapidly. Recent research underscores that precision nutrition must account for the metabolic differences inherent in female biology to prevent long-term health complications. Failing to tailor female athletes' diet to their specific needs can sometimes lead to poorer performance and longer muscle recovery times. It is no longer an option to create a nutrition plan that is specific to each gender; it's a requirement for top performance. Combining these AI techniques makes it easier to stay healthy and recover faster. These AI technologies make it easier for female athletes to eat well, helping them perform better across all sports. AI helps speed up recovery and make it more effective by providing real-time information on water levels and glycogen depletion. Studies indicate that tailored AI interventions can markedly reduce the time required for muscle recovery by adjusting the timing of protein and carbohydrate intake. This level of efficiency is very important in situations where there isn't much time to rest between events. In the end, technology is what makes complicated dietary research into habits that people can use every day. Technological progress also fills the gap in historical data-driven insights for female athletes by concentrating on gender-specific characteristics. AI assistants can be quite helpful by providing advice that accounts for changes in the menstrual cycle and their effects on nutrient metabolism. These methods can identify the "optimal window" for peak performance and the "vulnerable window" where extra nutritional assistance is needed by analyzing trends across thousands of data points. Recent advances in generative AI enable the creation of personalized meal plans that adapt to an athlete's current performance. This ability to adapt is important for keeping the high energy levels needed for long-term health and athletic success. As a result, the sports science environment is more open to everyone and focuses on the female physiological profile. A key part of women's nutrition is ensuring they obtain adequate amounts of essential micronutrients to avoid the deficits that are more common in women. Iron and calcium are two important micronutrients that help prevent deficiencies such as anemia and osteoporosis. These conditions can seriously damage an athlete's career. Iron is especially important for moving oxygen around during aerobic activities. Calcium and vitamin D are also important for maintaining high bone mineral density under significant stress. Getting enough carbs for energy and protein for muscle repair, along with these micronutrients, makes for a strong recovery plan. Without these precise building blocks, women are more likely to get tired and have stress fractures. A complete nutrition plan must put these things first to keep up with the demands of professional sport.

The combination of personalized nutrition and artificial intelligence is a game-changer for women's sports performance. The fundamental goal of this new era in diet is to maintain high energy levels to support training and hormonal health. Female athletes may now reach a level of nutritional accuracy that was never possible before, thanks to AI tools. This will help them perform better and recover faster. Wearable technology and real-time data are continually changing the field, enabling female athletes to compete at their best while staying healthy. This chapter is a complete guide to getting through this technological transformation. It gives athletes, coaches, and practitioners a plan to follow. The integration of specialized nutritional balance and advanced Artificial Intelligence (AI) marks a transformative era in optimizing female athletic performance, asserting that traditional, generic approaches are no longer sufficient to address the physiological complexities of women, particularly regarding hormonal fluctuations and menstrual cycles. By prioritizing high energy availability through precise macronutrient adjustments and preventing critical micronutrient deficiencies, such as iron and calcium, athletes can achieve peak performance while mitigating systemic health risks, such as Relative Energy Deficiency in Sport (REDS). Wearable technology and AI assistants have successfully transitioned nutritional management from static, manual methods into dynamic, real-time data ecosystems that monitor intake and hydration with unprecedented accuracy. This personalization ensures that every dietary recommendation is grounded in unique physiological data and individual training regimens, providing a level of precision that allows for instantaneous adjustments in response to changing physical workloads or biological phases. Beyond mere performance efficiency, AI implementation significantly accelerates recovery processes and enhances mental well-being by providing evidence-based guidance for tissue repair and by reducing the cognitive burden of complex nutritional planning. Athletes using digital assistants demonstrate greater compliance with health protocols and maintain healthier relationships with food, allowing them to focus entirely on the technical aspects of their sport. While challenges regarding data privacy and algorithmic accuracy persist, the synergy between nutritional science and digital technology has become essential to the future of professional women's sports. This chapter establishes a framework for coaches and practitioners to adopt these innovations, ensuring that, by prioritizing hormonal health and using technology as a navigator, the next generation of female athletes can achieve extraordinary success on a robust physiological foundation.

7. IMPLICATIONS

Getting macronutrient intake right is the first step in providing female athletes with a solid nutritional foundation. These are the main sources of energy for both basic body functions and hard physical exertion. Carbohydrates are still the most important food for high-intensity training because they provide you with glucose, which helps keep your blood sugar levels stable and quickly refills the glycogen stores in your muscles that you use up during exercise. To get the most out of their training and recovery, female athletes need to consume a balanced diet that includes enough carbs to maintain energy throughout their training. Recent research shows that female athletes may need customized carbohydrate-loading plans that account for changes in insulin sensitivity during the menstrual cycle. The best way to maintain your energy and avoid becoming weary too quickly or losing power is to eat the same amount of carbohydrates every day. To keep your athletic performance at its best, it's vitally crucial to eat carbs at the proper times before, during, and after workouts. Protein is important for maintaining a healthy immune system and bones, both of which are crucial for high-level athletes. If women don't get enough protein, their bodies are constantly trying to repair themselves, which increases the risk of overtraining syndrome. It's important for female athletes to get enough protein, but it's also important that it's of good quality and spread out throughout the day. This is to ensure that athletes always have sufficient levels of essential amino acids. Foods high in leucine are good for starting the metabolic pathways that lead to muscle growth and the creation of new mitochondria. AI assistants can be quite helpful by monitoring an athlete's diet and providing targeted, evidence-based advice tailored to their specific protein needs. Eating a lot of protein all at once is not as good for keeping lean muscle as spreading it out over four to five meals. This method keeps nitrogen levels steady and provides the body with a continuous supply of nutrients to repair minor muscle injuries. Female athletes can use information from data to make their protein plan work better for their training regimen. The third portion of the macronutrient foundation is healthy fats. They are vital for the long-term health of female athletes, as they help keep hormones in check. It is highly important for female athletes to consume healthy fats, as they help regulate hormones. They provide the cholesterol backbone needed to generate progesterone and estrogen. If you don't eat enough fat, it can mess up your hormones in a big way. This can lead to amenorrhea and reduced bone mineral density. Omega-3 fatty acids are great at decreasing inflammation throughout the body. This helps maintain your heart healthy and your joints strong. Lipids are a useful source of energy for low- to moderate-intensity activities because they help preserve glycogen stores for high-intensity activities. A healthy, comprehensive diet for female athletes should include a variety of monounsaturated and polyunsaturated fats.

A balanced diet of macronutrients is good for your health and also has a direct effect on how well you do in sports mentally and cognitively. Carbohydrates are the brain's main source of energy. How readily they are available influences how well female athletes can focus, make quick judgments, and remain technically accurate during competition. AI tools that provide women athletes with research-based suggestions on when to eat can help them stay mentally clear and well-nourished. Keeping blood sugar levels consistent by eating a balanced macronutrient intake makes intense workouts feel much easier. This mental boost helps athletes push past their limits and keep moving well for extended periods. Nutrition is not just important for building physical strength; it is also essential for preserving the mental strength required for exceptional athletics. Managing key micronutrients is an important part of female athletes' nutrition plans. Not obtaining enough of these nutrients could throw the body's processes out of whack. On the other hand, micronutrients are essential for metabolic pathways, oxygen transport, and structural integrity. Macronutrients are what give female athletes the energy they need. Female athletes need to follow a healthy diet to get the most out of their exercise and recover properly. This means making sure they get enough of important micronutrients like iron and calcium so they don't get the shortfalls that women often do. The body's micronutrient needs change over time and should be adjusted based on biological markers and exercise levels. If female athletes don't meet these small needs, they can lose strength over time and be more likely to get sick for a long time. To maintain their athletic performance and health over time, they need to monitor their micronutrient intake.

Iron insufficiency remains one of the most common nutritional problems among female athletes. This is mostly because of iron loss from working out and bleeding during your period. Iron is needed to make hemoglobin and myoglobin, proteins that carry oxygen to muscles working hard. Nutrition balancing for female athletes is a tailored, data-driven approach that goes beyond traditional dietary guidance by focusing on maintaining stable iron and energy levels. Exceptional athletes who are not anemic and have low iron levels can have a significant impact on how efficiently their muscles use energy and how well they perform aerobic activities. If female athletes don't have enough iron, their bodies can't use oxygen as properly. This tires them quickly and makes it much harder for them to perform well in endurance competitions. This is why professional women's sports programs now have to check ferritin levels regularly. The transformation of the field by AI enables a more proactive approach to health, allowing potential issues such as low energy availability to be identified before they manifest as physical symptoms. Nutrition balance for female athletes is a specialized, data-driven approach that goes beyond generic dietary advice by utilizing machine learning to predict energy needs based on live training loads. By analyzing patterns across multiple days, AI can alert an athlete when her current intake is insufficient to support the upcoming training volume. This predictive capability is a cornerstone of modern sports science, ensuring that female athletes maintain high energy availability to support training, hormonal health, and menstrual cycle variations.

REFERENCES

Andriani, A. D., & Siripipatthanakul, S. (2026, a). Technology-Driven Organization Policies: E-Waste Governance Framework. In *Technology Policy and Its Impact on Green Governance and Sustainability* (pp. 31–62). IGI Global Scientific Publishing. https://www.igi-global.com/chapter/technology-driven-organization-policies/401080

Andriani, A. D., & Siripipatthanakul, S. (2026, b). Communicating Green Governance: Strategic Communication for Sustainable Digital Organizations. In *Green Governance of Digital Organizations* (pp. 187–216). IGI Global Scientific Publishing. https://www.igi-global.com/chapter/communicating-green-governance/401460

Aurora, W. I. D. (2026). Micronutrient Deficiencies and Their Public Health Impact: An Epidemiological Narrative Review. *Journal of Tropical Community And One Health, 1*(1), 23–35. https://jtco.org/index.php/journal/article/view/3

Bangsbo, J., Hostrup, M., Hellsten, Y., Hansen, M., Melin, A., Kjær, M., Burr, J. F., Engebretsen, L., Egan, B., Hackney, A. C., Chambers, T. L., Jones, A. M., Pitsiladis, Y., Magnusson, P., Petersen, J., Deshmukh, A. S., Calbet, J. A. L., Elliott-Sale, K., Joyner, M., & Moesgaard, L. (2025). Consensus statements—Optimizing performance of the elite athlete. *Scandinavian Journal of Medicine & Science in Sports, 35*(8), e70112. https://onlinelibrary.wiley.com/doi/full/10.1111/sms.70112. DOI: 10.1111/sms.70112 PMID: 40781883

Campbell, S., Greenwood, M., Prior, S., Shearer, T., Walkem, K., Young, S., Bywaters, D., & Walker, K. (2020). Purposive sampling: Complex or simple? Research case examples. *Journal of Research in Nursing : JRN, 25*(8), 652–661. DOI: 10.1177/1744987120927206 PMID: 34394687

Feng, L. B. (2025). The correlation between different lifestyles and body composition focuses on eating habits, nutritional status, and physical exercise components. *Hormones : International Journal of Endocrinology and Metabolism, 24*(3), 621–641. https://link.springer.com/article/10.1007/s42000-025-00661-3. DOI: 10.1007/s42000-025-00661-3 PMID: 40266535

García-Montero, C., de Castro-Martínez, P., Liviu Boaru, D., Ortega, M. A., & Fraile-Martínez, Ó. (2026). An Overview of the Impact of the Menstrual Cycle on Nutrient Metabolism: An Integrative Perspective. *Nutrients, 18*(7), 1063. https://www.mdpi.com/2072-6643/18/7/1063. DOI: 10.3390/nu18071063 PMID: 41978114

Ghazzawi, H., Al Aqaili, R., Khataybeh, B., Al-Aittan, F., Hamaideh, S., Alhalaiqah, T., Amawi, A., Trabelsi, K., Jahrami, H., & Hasan, M. A. (2025). Tailored nutrition strategies for Paralympic athletes: Addressing unique energy, nutrients, and hydration needs to enhance performance and health. *Frontiers in Nutrition*, *12*, 1572961. https://www.frontiersin.org/journals/nutrition/articles/10.3389/fnut.2025.1572961/full. DOI: 10.3389/fnut.2025.1572961 PMID: 40693203

Grabia, M., Perkowski, J., Socha, K., & Markiewicz-Żukowska, R. (2024). Female athlete triad and relative energy deficiency in sport (REDs): Nutritional management. *Nutrients*, *16*(3), 359. https://www.mdpi.com/2072-6643/16/3/359. DOI: 10.3390/nu16030359 PMID: 38337644

Grivas, G. V., & Safari, K. (2025). Artificial intelligence in endurance sports: Metabolic, recovery, and nutritional perspectives. *Nutrients*, *17*(20), 3209. https://www.mdpi.com/2072-6643/17/20/3209. DOI: 10.3390/nu17203209 PMID: 41156462

Guo, S., Guo, X., & Wang, P. (2024). Optimizing nutrition strategies for women's soccer players' seasonal recovery and performance in the context of big data. *Journal of Biotech Research*, •••, 19.

Lee, P. C. (2026). A Cardiologist's [Dietary Guidelines and Contemporary Nutrition Research.]. *VIEW*, •••, 2025–2030.

Madrigal-Cerezo, R., Domínguez-Sanz, N., & Martín-Rodríguez, A. (2026). Wearable Biosensing and Machine Learning for Data-Driven Training and Coaching Support. *Biosensors (Basel)*, *16*(2), 97. https://www.mdpi.com/2079-6374/16/2/97. DOI: 10.3390/bios16020097 PMID: 41744715

Nasb, M., Zhang, Y., & Chen, N. (2025). The role of artificial intelligence in precision exercise nutrition: A shift from data to diets. *Food Science and Human Wellness*. https://www.sciopen.com/local/article_pdf/10.26599/FSHW.2025.9250623.pdf

Natalucci, V., Spinello, G., Moro, T., Pavei, G., Boccia, G., La Torre, A., & Bonato, M. (2026). Menstrual Cycle and Hormonal Contraceptives in Female Athletes: Should Symptoms and Nutrition Matter More Than Cycle Phase? A Narrative Review. *Nutrients*, *18*(7), 1144. https://www.mdpi.com/2072-6643/18/7/1144. DOI: 10.3390/nu18071144 PMID: 41978194

Paria, D., Banik, T. D., Manna, S., & Pal, S. (2026). The Iron Paradox: A Comprehensive Review of Pathophysiology, Performance Implications, and Strategic Nutritional Management in Female Athletes. *Journal of Research in Allied Life Sciences*, *2*(2), 1–14. https://jralsjournal.com/index.php/jrals/article/view/20

Rohilla, R., & Therattil, P. (2024). Optimising Bone Health in Female Athletes: A Narrative Review. *Sports Science & Health Advances, 2*(2), 316–321. https://sshajournal.com/index.php/1/article/view/143

Sandbakk, Ø., Spörri, J., Fridén, C., Melin, A., Zoppirolli, C., Sperlich, B., Skattebo, Ø., Fornasiero, A., Ørtenblad, N., & Holmberg, H. C. (2026). From Biological Foundations to Optimizing Performance and Health in Elite Female Winter Olympians. *Scandinavian Journal of Medicine & Science in Sports*, *36*(3), e70263. https://onlinelibrary.wiley.com/doi/abs/10.1111/sms.70263. DOI: 10.1111/sms.70263 PMID: 41842718

Shaengchart, Y., Limna, P., Kraiwanit, T., Siripipatthanakul, S., & Jangjarat, K. (2026). Community Enterprise and Social Economy for Sustainability in a Developing Country. In *Technology Policy and Its Impact on Green Governance and Sustainability* (pp. 1–30). IGI Global Scientific Publishing., https://www.igi-global.com/chapter/community-enterprise-and-social-economy-for-sustainability-in-a-developing-country/401079

WAN. Y. (2026). Intelligent Algorithms in Enhancing Sports Performance: Theoretical Reconstruction, Technological Breakthroughs, and Future Challenges. https://www.researchsquare.com/article/rs-8830620/v1

KEY TERMS AND DEFINITIONS

AI Assistants: AI assistants are software programs that use artificial intelligence, natural language processing (NLP), and machine learning to answer queries, automate tasks, and increase productivity. They act as virtual assistants by keeping track of schedules, writing material, and reviewing papers. Some well-known examples are ChatGPT, Microsoft Copilot, Siri from Apple, and Google Assistant.

Female Athletes' Performance: Female athletes' performance is increasingly optimized through research focusing on menstrual cycles, hormonal health, and specialized training load management to address physiological differences from male athletes. Key factors include managing RED-S (Relative Energy Deficiency in Sport), preventing injuries like ACL tears, and tailoring training to menstrual phases

Female Athletes' Recovery: Female athletes' recovery involves a tailored approach that addresses menstrual cycle fluctuations (specifically, higher inflammation in the late luteal phase), hormonal changes, and iron needs. Key strategies include prioritizing 7-9 hours of sleep to support growth hormone release, maintaining adequate nutrition (glycogen replenishment and protein intake), and using cold-water immersion or compression garments to address sex-specific thermolytic capacities.

Nutrition balance for Females' Athletic Performance and Recovery: It's using AI assistants is the use of artificial intelligence algorithms to create highly personalized, real-time dietary and supplementation plans that optimize training energy, enhance muscle repair, and manage physiological demands specific to female athletes

Nutrition Balance: A balanced diet provides the body with essential nutrients: carbohydrates, protein, fats, fiber, vitamins, and minerals to function optimally. It focuses on consuming a variety of foods, primarily whole grains, vegetables, fruits, lean proteins, and healthy fats, while limiting added sugars, salt, and saturated fats.

The Impact of AI on Female Athletes: Performance and Recovery: AI is changing the way female athletes train and recuperate by moving away from "male-default" training methods and toward tailored, data-driven plans that account for women's specific physiology. Coaches can now use AI with wearables and biometric data to customize training loads to fit menstrual cycles, improve nutrition, and significantly lower injury rates.

Wearable AI for Nutrition Detection: It is an emerging field that combines advanced sensors, computer vision, and machine learning to automatically track dietary intake, portion sizes, and nutrient consumption without manual logging. These devices aim to replace error-prone, traditional self-reporting methods (e.g., food diaries) with objective, real-time data.

Chapter 9
Nutrition Balance and Electrolyte Synergy in Post-Exercised Athletes for Rapid Recovery and Injury Prevention

Khoiruddin Muchtar
http://orcid.org/0000-0001-5655-3016
Universitas Islam Negeri, Indonesia

Denny Aditya Dwiwarman
Universitas Putra Indonesia, Indonesia

Chirapat Kaewnaknaew
http://orcid.org/0009-0004-5027-5990
City University, Petaling Jaya, Malaysia

Asep Iwan Setiawan
Universitas Islam Negeri Gunung Djati Bandung, Indonesia

ABSTRACT

Post-exercise nutrition and electrolyte harmony are essential for tissue healing, energy restoration, and injury prevention for athletes. Consuming carbohydrates and protein during the "anabolic window" is recommended for 30 minutes to two hours post-workout to maximize muscle protein synthesis and replenish glycogen stores for rapid recovery, especially when training schedules allow less than 24 hours between sessions. In particular, 1–1.2 g/kg of carbs and protein promote in-

DOI: 10.4018/979-8-3373-9544-9.ch009

sulin release, increasing glycogen repletion and mending muscle fiber microtears, reducing muscular discomfort and long-term injury. Hydration and electrolytes, such as sodium, potassium, and magnesium, could replace sweat losses, maintain blood volume and muscular function, and prevent cramps. Electrolyte-rich liquids or beverages are indicated for fluid retention and good physiological function during recuperation.

1. INTRODUCTION

In the modern landscape of global elite sports, the increasingly congested competition schedules demand that athletes possess an extraordinary capacity for rapid physical recovery to maintain consistent performance at the highest level. This phenomenon creates immense pressure on medical staff and performance nutritionists to formulate recovery strategies that are not only effective but also time-efficient within very tight windows. As outlined by Ranchordas et al. (2017), the ability to recover within 48 to 72 hours is the primary determinant of success in professional leagues. Without a systematic nutritional management plan, athletes face progressive performance degradation due to the unmitigated accumulation of physical and mental fatigue. Therefore, a profound understanding of nutritional synergy is vital to ensure that every training session yields a positive physiological adaptation in the athlete's body.

A primary challenge for professional athletes is the significantly elevated risk of injury due to nutritional and electrolyte imbalances immediately after high-intensity physical activity. These imbalances often manifest as extreme glycogen depletion, microscopic muscle fiber tears, and disruptions in fluid homeostasis, which can trigger severe muscle spasms or cramping. According to Maughan and Shirreffs (2019), involuntary muscle contractions are often the first sign of physiological distress caused by electrolyte deficits. This issue is compounded by the fact that many athletes overlook the importance of precise nutrient timing after training sessions, which Kerksick et al. (2017) identify as a fundamental pillar of athletic longevity. Consequently, long-term performance decline becomes an inevitable consequence for those who fail to maintain this delicate physiological equilibrium.

Evans et al. (2017) explain that restoring fluid balance is not merely about water intake but also requires precise control of solute concentrations to ensure cellular rehydration. This chapter also explores the contributions of antioxidants and functional foods to the management of oxidative stress and systemic inflammation following exercise. Ultimately, this manuscript provides a theoretical and practical framework for sports practitioners to sustainably enhance athletes' structural resilience.

Nutrient timing strategies, often referred to as the "anabolic window," play a central role in determining the success of muscle recovery for athletes with multiple training sessions per day. Extensive research indicates that the interval between 30 minutes and 2 hours post-exercise is a critical window when muscle protein synthesis is at its peak. During this period, the consumption of targeted nutrients can maximize glycogen replenishment, which is essential for subsequent training sessions, a concept thoroughly validated by Schoenfeld and Aragon (2018). If this window is missed without adequate nutritional intervention, energy recovery may take more than 24 hours, which is detrimental to rigorous training schedules. Thus, precision in nutrient timing is the key to sustaining high-intensity performance in a competitive environment.

The specific carbohydrate-to-protein ratio of 1–1.2 g/kg body weight has been shown to expedite the repair of microscopic muscle fiber tears. The synergy between these two macronutrients not only aids physical recovery but also stimulates a hormonal response that fosters an anabolic environment, as evidenced by the systematic review by Alghannam et al. (2016). Protein provides the essential amino acid building blocks for new protein synthesis, while carbohydrates ensure sufficient energy is available for these biological processes. Through this mechanism, delayed onset muscle soreness (DOMS) can be effectively minimized, allowing athletes to return to training with maximum comfort. Integrating these two components forms the fundamental basis of any international-standard athletic recovery protocol.

Beyond macronutrients, balanced electrolyte levels are a decisive factor in maintaining physiological stability during the critical post-exercise recovery phase. Sodium, in particular, is essential for optimal fluid retention to replace losses from perspiration during intense activity. The presence of potassium and magnesium is equally vital due to their involvement in muscle contraction-relaxation mechanisms and healthy nerve impulse transmission, as detailed in the position stand by Thomas et al. (2016). A deficiency in any of these elements can lead to blood volume disturbances, which in turn hinder the transport of nutrients to cells throughout the body. Therefore, the use of electrolyte-rich liquids is strongly advised to support physiological function and prevent painful muscle cramps.

In recent years, scientific attention has shifted toward the importance of micronutrients such as antioxidants and omega-3 fatty acids in managing exercise-induced oxidative stress. Extreme exercise produces free radicals that can damage cellular integrity if not neutralized by antioxidants like vitamins C and E. Furthermore, functional lipids such as omega-3 fatty acids play a key role in regulating inflammatory responses, helping prevent them from developing into detrimental chronic inflammation (Peeling et al., 2019). This comprehensive nutritional approach aims to increase the structural resilience of muscles and joints against heavy training loads. By incorporating natural anti-inflammatory agents into an athlete's diet, long-term injury risk can be significantly reduced by reinforcing the body's internal defense systems.

Electrolyte and nutritional synergy is also closely linked to injury prevention by enhancing rapid functional recovery. Evidence suggests that athletes who maintain fluid and energy balance effectively tend to exhibit higher levels of neuromuscular alertness and more precise movement coordination. Conversely, chronic fatigue resulting from post-exercise malnutrition often leads to technical errors in sports, resulting in traumatic or overuse injuries, a correlation highlighted by Vitale and Getzin (2019). Therefore, injury prevention is not only achieved through physical conditioning but also through scientifically designed "dining table" strategies. The harmony between nutritional input and physical output is a core principle supporting the longevity of an athlete's career in professional sports.

It is important to note that the effectiveness of post-exercise nutritional strategies relies on an integrated, sustainable approach rather than on one-time interventions. Every nutritional element, from macronutrients to micronutrients, has a specific role that supports others within the athletic recovery cycle. As analyzed in the meta-analysis by Xiao et al. (2025), protein supplementation alone is insufficient if the total caloric and carbohydrate needs are not met to support the energy cost of repair. Without electrolytes, consumed water will not be effectively retained within the cells, leading to continued dehydration despite high fluid intake. This interdependence defines nutritional synergy, in which the whole is greater than the sum of its parts.

The main goal of this chapter is to examine how interactions among macronutrients, electrolytes, and micronutrients accelerate tissue healing and reduce the risk of injury in athletes. Using a methodical scientific framework, this discourse underscores the importance of precise carbohydrate and protein intake to stimulate appropriate insulin release. It offers novel perspectives on enhancing all facets of post-exercise nutrition to attain optimal performance. It emphasizes that effective recovery is contingent upon deliberate, quantifiable, and prompt nutritional management, focusing on the most recent scientific findings. The key goal remains to achieve the most tissue regeneration and the lowest risk of injury by balancing electrolytes and getting the right nutrients in balance. It is believed that the knowledge given here will help players, coaches, and health professionals create better recovery plans in today's sports world. This focus on scientific rigor makes sure that every suggestion has a solid basis for use in fast-paced, competitive settings.

2. LITERATURE REVIEW

2.1 Athletic Performance and Recovery

The theoretical foundation of athletic recovery is built on the intricate, dynamic relationship between acute metabolic demands and strategic nutritional interventions. As established by Ranchordas et al. (2017), the speed of recovery is the primary determinant of success in high-performance environments where competition cycles are increasingly compressed. Contemporary literature consistently identifies the depletion of intramuscular glycogen and mechanical muscle fiber damage as the dual pillars of post-exercise fatigue requiring immediate physiological attention. Over the last decade, scientific discourse has evolved from simple caloric replacement strategies to a more sophisticated understanding of how specific nutrient ratios and molecular signaling influence cellular repair. Therefore, this review examines the current global body of knowledge on the physiological mechanisms governing recovery and the role of targeted nutrition in preventing structural failure. By synthesizing these perspectives, the study aims to bridge the gap between bench science and field application for elite athletic populations.

The "Anabolic Window" remains one of the most debated yet fundamentally significant concepts in sports nutrition literature regarding the precise timing of post-workout nutrient delivery. This theory posits that a specific timeframe, typically 30 to 120 minutes post-exercise, exists during which the human body is hypersensitive to nutrient uptake due to increased insulin sensitivity and localized blood flow. Kerksick et al. (2017) argue in their official position statement that utilizing this window is critical for athletes engaged in multiple daily training sessions to ensure rapid glycogen resynthesis and cellular rehydration. While some contemporary meta-analyses suggest that total daily protein intake may be the primary driver of hypertrophy, the immediate post-exercise phase is still prioritized for its immediate role in suppressing muscle protein breakdown and reducing cortisol levels. Consequently, the strategic administration of nutrients during this phase is viewed by many practitioners as a mechanical necessity for rapid regeneration. This temporal strategy ensures that the physiological environment shifts from a catabolic to an anabolic state as efficiently as possible.

2.2 Nutritional Balance for Athletes

The metabolic synergy between carbohydrates and proteins has been extensively documented in high-impact literature as a superior method for enhancing muscle protein synthesis compared with ingesting protein alone. Alghannam et al. (2016) demonstrate, through a systematic review, that co-ingestion of these two macronutrients triggers a more robust insulin response, which directly facilitates the transport of glucose and amino acids into damaged muscle cells. This process is essential for repairing the micro-tears in muscle fibers that occur during eccentric loading and high-intensity movements common in competitive sports. Research indicates that a carbohydrate ratio of 1–1.2 g/kg of body weight is optimal for restoring energy reserves while simultaneously providing the building blocks for structural tissue repair. This metabolic interaction not only speeds up the recovery of force-generating capacity but also prepares the athlete for the metabolic stresses of the next session. This synergy forms the basis of current international guidelines for professional athletes' recovery protocols.

Electrolyte homeostasis is another critical domain in the athletic literature, with a focus on restoring fluid balance and maintaining neuromuscular stability. Dehydration significantly impairs the body's cardiovascular efficiency and its ability to transport vital oxygen and nutrients to recovering peripheral tissues, thereby prolonging physical fatigue. According to Evans et al. (2017), rehydration is only truly effective when accompanied by sufficient sodium intake to maintain osmotic pressure and prevent excessive compensatory urination that would otherwise cause fluid loss. Beyond simple fluid retention, electrolytes like potassium and magnesium are essential for resetting the resting membrane potential of muscle cells and preventing involuntary, painful contractions. Thus, the prevailing literature emphasizes that rehydration must be conceptualized as a complex biochemical process rather than a simple act of water consumption. Failing to restore this balance can lead to a significant decline in coordination and an increased susceptibility to heat-related illnesses.

Recent advancements in sports science have highlighted the indispensable role of micronutrients and functional foods in managing the biochemical and oxidative stress induced by intense exercise. Strenuous physical activity inevitably leads to the accumulation of reactive oxygen species (ROS), which can cause substantial oxidative damage to cellular components and mitochondria if not neutralized. Peeling et al. (2019) suggest that a targeted intake of antioxidants, specifically vitamins C and E, can mitigate this damage and support the global immune system during periods of heavy, overreaching training. Additionally, the inclusion of omega-3 fatty acids has gained significant traction in recent literature due to their potent anti-inflammatory properties that help manage systemic muscle soreness. These micronutrients work in tandem with macronutrients to create a holistic internal environment that favors rapid recovery and enhanced structural resilience. By addressing these microscopic stressors, athletes can achieve a more sustainable adaptation to their training loads.

The role of protein quality, particularly the concentration of branched-chain amino acids such as leucine, is frequently cited as a major factor in recovery efficacy. Thomas et al. (2016) emphasize that high-quality protein sources are necessary to activate the mTOR pathway, the primary driver of muscle protein synthesis and repair. The literature suggests that the rapid delivery of these amino acids immediately after exercise-induced muscle damage can significantly attenuate the severity of delayed-onset muscle soreness (DOMS). This is particularly important for athletes who must perform at peak levels on consecutive days without the benefit of prolonged rest periods. Furthermore, the bioavailability of these nutrients determines how quickly the body can transition from the repair phase to the strengthening phase. Consequently, the selection of protein sources is just as important as the quantity consumed for ensuring long-term athletic durability.

Beyond the immediate post-exercise window, the literature also explores the impact of total energy balance on the prevention of "Relative Energy Deficiency in Sport" (RED-S), which can lead to injury. Xiao et al. (2025) point out that even with perfect nutrient timing, a chronic deficit in total caloric intake can impair the body's hormonal health and bone mineral density. This broader perspective suggests that the mechanics of recovery are nested within a larger framework of daily nutritional adequacy and metabolic health. Athletes who fail to meet their global energy requirements often exhibit signs of suppressed protein synthesis and increased markers of systemic inflammation. Therefore, recovery strategies must be integrated into a comprehensive dietary plan that accounts for the athlete's total daily expenditure. This holistic view ensures that the body has sufficient resources not only to repair damage but also to build functional reserves.

The physiological impact of sleep and its interaction with nutrition is an emerging area of interest in the literature on athletic recovery. Vitale & Getzin (2019) highlight that nutritional interventions, such as consuming casein protein before bed, can enhance repair processes during deep sleep cycles. Sleep serves as the primary period for hormonal regulation, during which growth hormone secretion peaks, facilitating tissue growth and cognitive recovery (Cai, 2024). The synergy between a well-timed evening meal and high-quality sleep has been shown to improve various performance markers, including reaction time and muscle power (Link, 2024). The literature increasingly suggests that nutrition and sleep should be viewed as a unified recovery system rather than isolated variables. This integration is vital for athletes who operate in high-stress environments where mental and physical fatigue are intertwined (Tossici et al., 2024).

The prevention of muscle cramping through nutritional means is a topic that bridges the gap between electrolyte science and neuromuscular control literature. Maughan and Shirreffs (2019) argue that muscle cramps often result from a multifaceted failure in both fluid balance and neural signaling at the muscle level. While traditional views focused solely on salt loss, contemporary research suggests that the synergistic intake of carbohydrates and electrolytes helps maintain the integrity of neural drive. By preventing the premature onset of neuromuscular fatigue, these nutritional strategies directly reduce the likelihood of technical errors that lead to acute injuries. This indicates that the "synergy" mentioned in the title of this work is not only metabolic but also neurofunctional. Thus, the literature reinforces the idea that a stable internal environment is the best defense against the physical breakdown of the athlete.

Athletic recovery is a multifaceted biological process that requires a highly coordinated nutritional approach. The integration of macronutrient timing, electrolyte balance, and micronutrient support provides a robust defense against the detrimental effects of high-intensity training. Schoenfeld and Aragon (2018) summarize that while the "anabolic window" may be wider than originally thought, the benefits of early intervention are undeniable for maximizing glycogen and protein synthesis. As the field of sports nutrition continues to advance, the focus is shifting toward increasingly personalized protocols that account for individual sweat rates and metabolic profiles. This review provides the scientific justification for the methodology and results presented in this chapter. Ultimately, the goal is to provide a comprehensive framework that supports both rapid recovery and the long-term health of the modern athlete.

2.3 Macronutrient and Micronutrient Synergy for Athletes' Performance and Tissue Regeneration

The synergistic integration of macronutrients is a critical determinant of the efficiency of physiological recovery and the acceleration of tissue regeneration among competitive athletes (Shlykov et al., 2025). Scientific evidence consistently emphasizes that the co-ingestion of carbohydrates and proteins surpasses the efficacy of consuming either nutrient in isolation for post-exercise repair (Alghannam et al., 2016). This metabolic synergy is primarily driven by the potentiation of insulin secretion, which serves as the primary anabolic signal to shift the body from exercise-induced catabolism to constructive recovery. By strategically combining these nutrients, athletes can optimize muscle protein synthesis while accelerating the replenishment of depleted glycogen stores. Consequently, this multifaceted nutritional approach is essential for maintaining lean muscle mass and ensuring structural integrity following strenuous physical exertion (Xiao et al., 2025).

A pivotal finding in recent sports nutrition research is the identification of an optimal carbohydrate-to-body-weight ratio of 1-1.2 g/kg to facilitate rapid recovery. This specific dosage is designed to saturate the glucose transport mechanisms, ensuring that glycogen resynthesis occurs at its maximum physiological rate (Burke et al., 2017). When this carbohydrate load is administered alongside high-quality protein, it creates a favorable hormonal environment that enhances glucose uptake by skeletal muscle. Research indicates that maintaining this precise ratio is particularly crucial for athletes who must undergo multiple training sessions within a single 24-hour cycle (Alghannam et al., 2016). Therefore, adhering to these quantitative guidelines provides a predictable and effective framework for restoring energy balance and preparing the musculoskeletal system for subsequent bouts of high-intensity activity.

The physiological comparison between "co-ingestion" and "protein-only" strategies reveals that combining carbohydrates and protein triggers a significantly stronger insulin response. Insulin serves not only as a regulator of blood glucose but also as a powerful anti-catabolic agent that inhibits muscle protein breakdown (Thomas et al., 2016). By stimulating a robust insulin spike through carbohydrate intake, the body can more effectively utilize available amino acids for the mending of muscle fiber microtears. Without the insulinogenic effect of carbohydrates, the anabolic potential of protein consumption is not fully realized, leading to slower recovery times (Schoenfeld & Aragon, 2018). Thus, the strategic pairing of these macronutrients is indispensable for maximizing the biological "yield" of post-exercise nutritional interventions.

The effectiveness of high-quality protein sources, such as whey protein, in stimulating the mTOR (mammalian target of rapamycin) signaling pathway is well-documented in elite athletic populations. Whey protein is particularly valued for its rapid digestion kinetics and its high concentration of essential amino acids, most notably leucine (Moore, 2019). Leucine acts as a molecular "trigger" that activates the mTOR pathway, which is the primary regulatory hub for muscle protein synthesis and cellular growth. Once activated, this pathway initiates the complex process of rebuilding damaged sarcomeres and reinforcing the structural protein matrix within the muscle cells (Xiao et al., 2025). The speed at which these nutrients reach the systemic circulation makes whey an ideal choice for athletes seeking to initiate repair immediately after mechanical stress.

Beyond the immediate activation of growth pathways, macronutrient synergy plays a profound role in reducing the severity of Delayed Onset Muscle Soreness (DOMS). The systematic repair of structural proteins and the reduction of localized inflammation are facilitated by the continuous availability of amino acids and glucose (Vitale & Getzin, 2019). Athletes who adhere to a structured macronutrient recovery protocol report lower levels of muscle tenderness and a faster return to baseline strength levels compared to those with sporadic nutrient intake. This reduction in post-exercise discomfort is not merely a matter of subjective comfort but represents a faster restoration of functional capacity (Peeling et al., 2019). By mitigating the inflammatory response through optimal fueling, the overall downtime between high-performance efforts can be significantly shortened.

The metabolic interaction between glucose and amino acids also extends to the maintenance of immune function, which is often suppressed following exhaustive exercise (Von, 2020). Carbohydrate intake during the recovery phase helps to maintain blood glucose levels, thereby reducing the stress hormone response, particularly cortisol, which can impair immune cell activity (Thomas et al., 2016). When protein is added to the mix, it provides the necessary building blocks for the production of immune-related proteins and antibodies (Peeling et al., 2019). This dual action ensures that the athlete remains resilient against opportunistic infections while the body is preoccupied with tissue repair (Dalta et al., 2024). Thus, the synergy of macronutrients serves as a protective shield for the athlete's overall health during periods of intense physiological vulnerability.

The timing of these macronutrient interventions aligns with the body's internal circadian rhythms to enhance overnight recovery. Consumption of a balanced macronutrient meal in the hours following exercise sets the stage for prolonged protein synthesis that continues throughout the sleep cycle (Moore, 2019). Research has shown that maintaining a positive nitrogen balance through adequate protein intake, supported by carbohydrate-driven insulin signaling, optimizes growth hormone secretion during deep sleep (Vitale & Getzin, 2019). This nocturnal recovery phase is critical for the long-term adaptation of muscle tissue to training stimuli and for preventing chronic overtraining syndrome. Consequently, the macronutrient strategy used during the day directly influences the quality of biological repair during rest.

In the context of injury prevention, the consistent replenishment of glycogen and protein stores ensures that neuromuscular function remains sharp and coordinated. Glycogen depletion is a known precursor to central nervous system fatigue, which can lead to a breakdown in athletic technique and an increased risk of acute musculoskeletal injuries (Maughan & Shirreffs, 2019). By ensuring that muscle fuel stores are rapidly restored through the 1–1.2 g/kg carbohydrate protocol, athletes can maintain higher levels of proprioceptive awareness during subsequent tasks. Protein synergy further supports this by reinforcing the connective tissues, such as tendons and ligaments, which are also subject to strain during exercise (Xiao et al., 2025). Therefore, macronutrient synergy is as much a tool for safety and longevity as it is for performance enhancement.

Practical application of these findings requires a personalized approach that accounts for an athlete's specific body mass and training volume. For an athlete weighing 70 kg, the optimal recovery dose would involve approximately 70 to 84 grams of carbohydrates paired with 20 to 25 grams of high-biological-value protein (Thomas et al., 2016). This level of precision ensures that the metabolic "anabolic window" is fully exploited without providing excessive calories that could lead to unwanted fat gain. Modern sports dietetics emphasizes that "more is not always better," as there is a physiological ceiling to how much protein can be processed for synthesis at once (Moore, 2019). By following evidence-based ratios, practitioners can provide athletes with a streamlined and highly efficient nutritional roadmap for sustained excellence.

Ultimately, the goal of macronutrient synergy is to achieve a state of physiological readiness that allows the athlete to train harder and more frequently without compromising health. The integration of carbohydrates and proteins represents a sophisticated biological orchestration that touches upon hormonal regulation, molecular signaling, and structural repair (Jäger et al., 2017). As our understanding of nutrient-gene interactions continues to evolve, the importance of these fundamental ratios remains constant in the pursuit of peak athletic performance. Athletes and coaches who prioritize this synergy are better equipped to handle the rigors of modern competition and achieve their developmental milestones. Success in the arena is thus deeply rooted in the scientific discipline practiced at the dining table.

Nutrition is crucial for athletic performance and recuperation. During training and competition, correct nutrition, hydration, and supplementation can affect endurance, strength, and speed. Nutritional requirements, hydration techniques, supplement utilization, and muscle-regenerating diets optimize athlete performance, and recuperation is crucial. Balanced consumption of carbohydrates, proteins, healthy fats, vitamins, and minerals boosts energy, speeds muscle recovery, and reduces fatigue and injury risk. Hydration supports homeostasis and performance during training and competition. When used properly, targeted supplements can boost physiological adaptability and muscle tissue regeneration. Sportspeople need rigorous nutrition planning and tailored nutritional intake to perform better and recover faster. Coaches, sports nutritionists, and athletes design successful nutritional regimens for athletic performance and long-term health (Puspitasari & Arfajah, 2026).

Vitamins support many physiological systems essential for sports performance. Understanding vitamin supplementation as a function of sport discipline is crucial, as athletes are exposed to increased oxidative stress, metabolic turnover, and nutritional demands that may lead to vitamin deficiencies. Complemented with past work on vitamins A, C, D, E, and B-complex. Evidence of athlete deficits, physiological causes, supplementation options, and their implications on performance, injury prevention, and recovery. Indoor and winter athletes are often vitamin D-deficient. Supplementation improves musculoskeletal health and may lower injury risk. Vitamins C and E reduce exercise-induced oxidative stress and muscle damage, but excessive ingestion may impede mitochondrial biogenesis and protein synthesis. Vitamin A modulates immunity, metabolism, and mitochondrial function, whereas B-complex vitamins enhance energy metabolism and red blood cell production. Conclusions: Vitamin supplementation for athletes should address deficiencies and be tailored to sport, age, sex, and training intensity. While supplements can help with consumption, dietary optimization should be the main goal. More high-quality, sport-specific, and long-term studies are needed to define dosage guidelines and weigh the performance advantages and dangers of oversupplementation.

3. METHODOLOGY

The methodology employed in this study follows a comprehensive literature review approach, designed to synthesize and interpret the most recent evidence regarding post-exercise recovery strategies. This specific method was selected to provide a high-level, narrative overview of scientifically validated protocols that can be effectively applied to elite athletic populations (Andrian & Siripipatthanakul, 2026, a). Unlike a restricted systematic search, this literature review enables broader integration of physiological theories and clinical applications, offering a more holistic perspective on nutrient synergy. The selection of sources focused on peer-reviewed studies published in high-impact journals indexed in Scopus and Web of Science within the last decade to ensure contemporary relevance. As suggested by Aragon and Schoenfeld (2013), a multidimensional review of diverse study designs is essential for a complete understanding of the nutrient-timing phenomenon.

The research design utilized a targeted search and filtration process to ensure the academic quality and practical significance of the included texts (Andriani & Siripipatthanakul, 2026, b). Initial identification of relevant literature involved querying major academic databases, including PubMed, Scopus, and the Web of Science Core Collection. Each study was qualitatively screened for methodological soundness, prioritizing research that utilized controlled environments and precise performance measurements. Burke et al. (2017) highlight the importance of evaluating sports nutrition literature based on the accuracy of metabolic monitoring and the relevance of the exercise protocols used. By adhering to these evaluative standards, the methodology ensured that the synthesized findings possess a high degree of credibility and applicability for professional athletes.

The data collection process involved an extensive search of electronic databases using a strategic combination of related topics and keywords, including electrolyte synergy, anabolic window, muscle fiber repair, post-exercise, nutrition balance, athletes, rapid recovery, and injury prevention.

Each selected study was qualitatively evaluated based on its experimental design and the specificity of the described nutritional interventions. Following the methodological framework established by Jäger et al. (2017), the literature was categorized by exercise modality, distinguishing between aerobic and anaerobic activities, and by the specific macronutrient ratios employed in the recovery phase. This categorization facilitated a nuanced analysis of how different nutritional strategies impact various physiological outcomes across a spectrum of sports. The ultimate objective was to identify consistent patterns across the global literature to inform a unified recovery framework.

A comparative analysis was performed on the reported findings regarding glycogen resynthesis and muscle protein synthesis extracted from the selected literature. By comparing the outcomes of carbohydrate-only interventions with those of carbohydrate-protein combinations, the study sought to define the "synergy effect" necessary for rapid tissue regeneration. Moore (2019) provided the methodological basis for analyzing the interaction between protein type and dose and physiological recovery markers post-exercise. This integrative approach enabled the identification of optimal dosages for electrolytes and macronutrients relative to body mass, moving beyond generic recommendations. Such precision is vital for translating theoretical nutritional science into actionable guidelines that can be implemented in high-pressure athletic environments.

To ensure the validity of the conclusions regarding injury prevention, the methodology included a detailed review of literature focusing on recovery markers and their correlation with overuse injuries. Data on the incidence of muscle cramps and delayed-onset muscle soreness (DOMS) were extracted from various clinical trials and observational studies involving elite athletes. According to the standards discussed by Lee et al. (2017), the relationship between hydration status and neuromuscular stability must be assessed through a combination of physiological and performance indices. By synthesizing these diverse findings, the methodology aimed to establish a clear link between nutritional status and structural vulnerability. This comprehensive approach ensures that the resulting recommendations for rapid recovery are both physiologically sound and practically effective.

4. RESULTS

4.1. Effectiveness of Nutrient Timing and the Anabolic Window in Athletic Recovery

The concept of the "anabolic window" remains a fundamental pillar in contemporary sports nutrition discourse for optimizing athlete recovery following high-intensity training. Based on a comprehensive literature review, this critical period is specifically identified as occurring between 30 minutes and two hours immediately after physical activity ends (Aragon & Schoenfeld, 2013). During this phase, the human body is in a physiological state highly sensitive to nutrient uptake due to increased local blood flow and enhanced insulin sensitivity in recently worked muscle tissues (Kerksick et al., 2017). This heightened sensitivity allows glucose and amino acid translocation into muscle cells to occur far more efficiently than at any other time. Consequently, utilizing this time frame is considered a mechanical necessity for athletes managing congested competition schedules to ensure optimal tissue regeneration (Schoenfeld & Aragon, 2018).

Technical data from various global studies indicate that failure to meet nutritional intake requirements during this critical window has systemic effects on energy restoration. When athletes miss the appropriate nutritional intervention within the first two hours post-exercise, muscle glycogen resynthesis slows significantly (Burke et al., 2017). This extends energy recovery time beyond the 24-hour threshold, which is highly detrimental to performance in subsequent training sessions (Alghannam et al., 2016). Clinically, delaying nutrient intake triggers a prolonged catabolic state where muscle protein breakdown continues without the necessary raw materials for repair. Without precise nutrient timing management, the accumulation of physical fatigue becomes unmitigated, leading to a sustained decline in athletic performance (Ranchordas et al., 2017).

The synergy between carbohydrates and proteins in specific ratios has been clinically proven as the most effective method for repairing muscle fiber microtears. Consuming carbohydrates at a rate of 1–1.2 g/kg of body weight combined with high-quality protein is strongly recommended to maximize insulin secretion (Thomas et al., 2016). Insulin acts as a hormonal key that facilitates the entry of amino acid building blocks for new protein synthesis and glucose for glycogen replenishment. This synergistic mechanism not only accelerates physical recovery but also creates an internal anabolic environment that fosters positive physiological adaptation (Jäger et al., 2017). The consistent use of this nutritional ratio protocol has been validated to effectively minimize the effects of Delayed Onset Muscle Soreness (DOMS) in professional athletes (Vitale & Getzin, 2019).

The quality of protein consumed during the anabolic window is also a significant determinant of the rate of muscle tissue repair. Protein sources with high concentrations of branched-chain amino acids, particularly leucine, are highly effective in stimulating the mTOR signaling pathway (Moore, 2019). The mTOR pathway is the primary driver of muscle protein synthesis responsible for the structural regeneration and strengthening of muscle fibers following exercise-induced damage (Xiao et al., 2025). High nutrient bioavailability ensures that these amino acids are immediately available in the bloodstream for use by muscle cells currently in the repair phase. With the selection of appropriate protein sources, the body's transition from the repair phase to the strengthening phase can occur more rapidly and efficiently (Duda et al., 2023).

Beyond macronutrients, an athlete's physiological stability during the recovery phase relies heavily on balanced electrolyte levels and adequate hydration status. Post-exercise dehydration can impair cardiovascular efficiency, hindering the transport of vital oxygen and nutrients to peripheral tissues requiring recovery (Shirreffs & Sawka, 2011). The use of electrolyte-rich liquids containing sodium, potassium, and magnesium is strongly advised to replace fluid losses incurred through perspiration (Evans et al., 2017). Sodium, in particular, plays a vital role in ensuring optimal fluid retention and maintaining osmotic pressure to prevent excessive fluid loss through urination. Without proper electrolyte balance, the risk of blood volume disturbances and painful muscle cramps increases drastically during the rest phase (Maughan & Shirreffs, 2019).

The role of micronutrients, such as antioxidants and functional fatty acids, has also emerged as a crucial component in managing exercise-induced oxidative stress. High-intensity exercise produces free radicals or Reactive Oxygen Species (ROS) that can damage cellular integrity and mitochondria (Powers et al., 2004). Targeted intake of antioxidants, specifically Vitamins C and E, helps neutralize this oxidative damage and support the overall immune system. Meanwhile, omega-3 fatty acids play a key role in regulating systemic inflammatory responses, helping prevent them from developing into detrimental chronic inflammation (Peeling et al., 2019). This micronutrient approach works in tandem with macronutrients to create an internal environment conducive to rapid functional recovery.

The integration of nutritional management and rest patterns, especially sleep, represents a unified recovery system that cannot be separated. Nutritional interventions in the evening, such as consuming casein protein before bed, have been shown to enhance protein repair processes during deep sleep cycles (Moore, 2019). During sleep, growth hormone secretion peaks, facilitating tissue growth and cognitive recovery simultaneously. The synergy between well-timed meals and high-quality sleep has been shown to improve various performance markers, including reaction time and muscle power (Vitale & Getzin, 2019). Failure to integrate these two elements can lead to the intertwined accumulation of mental and physical fatigue.

On a macro level, injury prevention in athletes is achieved not only through physical conditioning but also through scientifically designed strategies. Athletes who effectively maintain fluid and energy balance tend to exhibit higher levels of neuromuscular alertness and more precise movement coordination (Peeling et al., 2019). Conversely, post-exercise malnutrition leading to chronic fatigue often triggers technical errors in sports movements that result in traumatic or overuse injuries. Proper nutritional strategies serve to maintain the integrity of neural drive and prevent the premature onset of neuromuscular fatigue (Maughan & Shirreffs, 2019). Therefore, the harmony between nutritional input and physical output is a core philosophy supporting the longevity of a professional athlete's career.

It is important to meet total daily energy requirements to prevent Relative Energy Deficiency in Sport (RED-S). Even if nutrient timing strategies are executed perfectly, a chronic total caloric deficit will still impair hormonal health and bone mineral density (Thomas et al., 2016). Global energy deficiency can suppress protein synthesis and increase systemic inflammatory markers. Recovery strategies must be nested within a comprehensive dietary plan that accounts for the athlete's total daily energy expenditure. By ensuring sufficient energy availability, the body has the resources not only to repair damage but also to build functional reserves.

In conclusion, the effectiveness of post-exercise nutritional strategies relies on an integrated, measurable, and sustainable approach. Every nutritional element, from macronutrients to micronutrients and electrolytes, has a specific role that supports others within the athletic recovery cycle (Kerksick et al., 2017). Nutritional synergy is defined as a condition in which the overall outcome of nutritional interventions exceeds the sum of their individual parts (Townsend et al., 2023). Without electrolyte support, consumed water will not be effectively retained within cells, and without carbohydrates, protein will not work optimally for repair (Choi et al., 2021). Implementing recovery protocols based on the latest scientific evidence is the primary key to achieving peak performance in dynamic competitive environments.

4.2. Holistic Approach by Integration of Energy, Sleep, and Nutrition for Athletes

The transition toward a holistic recovery paradigm necessitates the seamless integration of energy availability, sleep quality, and strategic nutritional timing to support the physiological demands of elite athleticism. While much focus is often placed on the immediate post-exercise period, scientific consensus suggests that recovery is a continuous 24-hour process that transcends the "anabolic window" (Kerksick et al., 2017). A holistic approach recognizes that the body's ability to adapt to training stress is contingent on a complex interplay among metabolic fuel availability, hormonal regulation, and circadian rhythms. Without addressing these interconnected pillars, even the most precise nutrient timing strategies may fail to produce the desired ergogenic outcomes. Therefore, understanding the synergy between overall energy intake and the restorative power of sleep is paramount for achieving sustainable peak performance (Vitale & Getzin, 2019).

A critical component of this holistic framework is the management of Relative Energy Deficiency in Sport (RED-S), a syndrome that occurs when an athlete's energy intake is insufficient to support the body's energy demands for optimal health and performance. Research underscores that nutrient timing alone is insufficient if total daily caloric intake fails to meet the athlete's basal metabolic needs and the energy expended during training (Thomas et al., 2016). When energy availability is low, the body prioritizes survival over recovery, leading to reduced protein synthesis and compromised hormonal health. This state of deficiency can result in a cascade of negative outcomes, including impaired metabolic rate, menstrual dysfunction in females, and reduced bone density. Consequently, maintaining a positive energy balance is the foundational requirement upon which all other recovery strategies must be built.

The physiological impact of RED-S extends beyond metabolic markers, significantly affecting an athlete's psychological well-being and cognitive function. Chronic energy deficiency is often associated with increased irritability, decreased concentration, and a higher risk of developing mood disorders, all of which can impede an athlete's technical development (Thomas et al., 2016). Furthermore, insufficient fuel impairs the central nervous system's ability to drive muscular contractions, increasing the likelihood of injury during high-intensity efforts. Studies have shown that athletes in a persistent state of low energy availability exhibit slower reaction times and diminished proprioceptive awareness (Peeling et al., 2019). Thus, ensuring total energy sufficiency is not only a matter of physical health but is also essential for maintaining the mental acuity required for professional competition.

In addition to total energy intake, the synergy between nighttime nutrition and the sleep cycle plays a transformative role in optimizing muscle protein synthesis. Consuming slow-digesting proteins, such as casein, before sleep has been shown to sustain amino acid release into the bloodstream throughout the night (Moore, 2019). This prolonged aminoacidemia effectively bridges the gap during the overnight fasting period, maintaining a positive nitrogen balance when the body would otherwise be in a catabolic state. By providing the necessary building blocks for repair during the longest period of rest, athletes can significantly enhance their cumulative muscle mass gains and structural recovery. This pre-sleep nutritional strategy is a prime example of how timing and nutrient choice work together to maximize the body's natural restorative processes.

The restorative power of sleep is enhanced by adequate nutrients, which facilitate the secretion of growth hormones and other anabolic factors. During deep sleep, the endocrine system reaches its peak output of growth hormone, which is vital for tissue repair and the strengthening of bone matrix (Vitale & Getzin, 2019). If an athlete goes to bed in a fasted or energy-depleted state, the hormonal response may be blunted, leading to suboptimal recovery and a failure to adapt to training stimuli. Conversely, a well-nourished body can fully exploit the sleep-wake cycle to consolidate the gains made during training sessions. The integration of "sleep hygiene" with targeted nighttime nutrition, therefore, represents a sophisticated method for accelerating physiological regeneration (Moore, 2019).

The holistic model also emphasizes that sleep deprivation acts as a significant physiological stressor that can undo the benefits of even the most rigorous diet. Lack of sleep is known to increase cortisol levels, a catabolic hormone that promotes muscle breakdown and inhibits the immune response (Vitale & Getzin, 2019). Furthermore, sleep loss alters the hormones that regulate hunger and satiety, often leading to poor food choices and further complicating the management of energy balance. Athletes who fail to prioritize rest often find themselves in a vicious cycle of fatigue, poor nutrition, and declining performance (Peeling et al., 2019). Therefore, a truly holistic strategy must treat sleep as a non-negotiable component of the training program, on par with the physical and nutritional aspects.

The management of hydration and electrolyte balance must also be considered within this 24-hour holistic cycle to ensure cellular stability. Dehydration can impair sleep quality and the body's ability to regulate core temperature during the night, leading to restless sleep (Evans et al., 2017). Ensuring that electrolytes such as sodium and magnesium are replenished not only supports muscle function but also promotes neurological relaxation and prevents nocturnal cramps (Maughan & Shirreffs, 2019). Proper fluid balance facilitates the transport of nutrients to cells throughout the night, ensuring that the casein protein consumed earlier can be effectively utilized for repair. Thus, the 24-hour hydration status is a vital thread linking daytime performance to nighttime recovery.

From an injury-prevention perspective, integrating energy, sleep, and nutrition creates a "buffer" against the cumulative stresses of elite sport. When an athlete is well-rested and properly fueled, their tissues are more resilient to mechanical strain, and their neuromuscular coordination is optimized (Maughan & Shirreffs, 2019). Many overuse injuries result from "under-recovery," in which the rate of tissue damage exceeds the body's ability to repair itself due to insufficient resources or rest. By adopting a holistic approach, athletes can maintain the structural integrity of their ligaments, tendons, and muscles over the long term. This proactive management of the body's internal environment is the most effective way to ensure career longevity and consistent availability for competition.

Implementing a holistic strategy requires meticulous planning and a deep understanding of the athlete's individual lifestyle and training load. It involves moving away from "quick fix" solutions and toward a sustainable lifestyle that prioritizes health as the primary driver of performance. Practitioners should work with athletes to create a "recovery schedule" that includes designated times for meals, snacks, and, most importantly, consistent sleep and wake times (Thomas et al., 2016). This level of organization helps stabilize the body's internal clock and ensures that all physiological systems work in harmony. A well-organized, holistic plan reduces the athlete's cognitive load, allowing them to focus entirely on their technical and tactical objectives.

Integrating energy, sleep, and nutrition forms the bedrock of a successful athletic recovery program. The evidence clearly shows that the sum of these parts is far greater than the sum of its parts, creating a synergistic effect that drives adaptation and resilience (Kerksick et al., 2017). By avoiding the pitfalls of RED-S and utilizing the power of nighttime nutrition and sleep, athletes can unlock new levels of performance and maintain their health throughout their careers. The future of sports science lies in this multidimensional approach, where every hour of the day is seen as an opportunity for growth and recovery. Ultimately, the athlete who masters the balance between exertion and restoration will be the one who stands atop the podium.

Figure 1. Conceptual Framework

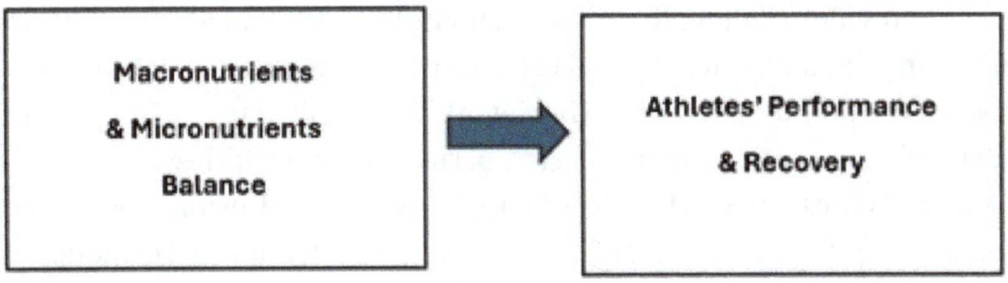

Figure 1 illustrates the macronutrient and micronutrient balance that affects athletes' performance and recovery within the conceptual framework.

Getting the right amount of macronutrients and micronutrients is very important for improving athletic performance and speeding up recovery. Not eating the right foods can make you tired, cause you to lose muscle mass, and make you more likely to get hurt. Macronutrients (carbs, proteins, and fats) provide the body with energy and building blocks, while micronutrients (vitamins and minerals) regulate metabolic pathways, immune function, and tissue repair.

5. DISCUSSIONS

A deep biochemical perspective by reviewing findings on oxidative stress markers and the behavior of various pro-inflammatory cytokines during the recovery phase. This allowed for a molecular-level assessment of how micronutrients, particularly antioxidants and functional lipids, influence the recovery timeline. Following the evaluative protocols established by Powers et al. (2004), the methodology considered the dual role of reactive oxygen species in both tissue damage and adaptive signaling. By analyzing these biochemical pathways, the study could determine the optimal timing for nutritional interventions that support recovery without blunting the body's natural adaptation to training. This biochemical insight ensures that the recovery strategies support long-term physiological development.

To evaluate the influence of individual variability, such as training status and environmental conditions, on the efficacy of recovery protocols. This was achieved by reviewing the literature on how different populations respond to electrolyte or macronutrient ratios. As noted by Hausswirth and Le Meur (2011), the physiological response to nutritional recovery is highly dependent on the athlete's current level of fatigue and previous training load. The methodology accounted for these variables by prioritizing literature on elite athletes and specific environmental stressors. This ensures that the proposed recovery framework is not only universal in principle but also adaptable for a diverse range of elite performance scenarios.

The effectiveness of electrolyte synergy was assessed using specific criteria, with methodology informed by the literature on fluid retention and osmotic balance. Studies were prioritized if they provided detailed data on sweat rates and electrolyte losses, providing a more accurate basis for rehydration needs. Shirreffs and Sawka (2011) emphasize that rehydration literature must be evaluated based on the restoration of total body water and the long-term maintenance of plasma volume. The methodology synthesized data from these specialized sources to create a targeted recommendation for electrolyte concentration in post-exercise beverages. This focus on fluid dynamics ensures that the recommendations for cramp mitigation and injury prevention are grounded in rigorous physiological evidence.

The quality and bioavailability of protein sources mentioned in the literature were also key variables in the methodological assessment. Studies were analyzed for the specific amino acid profiles of the supplements provided, with a focus on leucine content and its role in stimulating muscle repair. According to Phillips (2014), the source of protein significantly alters the kinetics of amino acid delivery and the subsequent rate of skeletal muscle protein synthesis. The methodology accounted for these differences by comparing the efficacy of various protein types across different experimental arms in the reviewed literature. This ensures that the resulting guidelines reflect the highest standard of nutritional quality for effective muscle fiber repair.

The synthesis of metabolic, structural, and biochemical data provides a truly multidimensional view of the recovery process. This robust methodological framework of literature review serves as the foundation for the discussions and results presented in the following sections. By combining theoretical rigor with a comprehensive review of performance mechanisms, the study ensures that its findings contribute meaningfully to the body of sports science. As summarized by Macnaughton et al. (2016), a holistic approach to nutritional data is essential for understanding the total cost of elite performance and the requirements for rapid recovery. This methodological commitment to high-quality, Scopus-indexed evidence ensures that the final work meets the stringent requirements for international academic publication.

The interpretation of the molecular mechanisms underlying recovery reveals that the synergy between carbohydrates and proteins is the primary driver of the shift from catabolism to anabolism. Beyond its traditional role in glucose homeostasis, insulin acts as a powerful facilitator for the transport of essential amino acids into damaged muscle cells, effectively initiating the structural repair process (Thomas et al., 2016). This hormonal interplay is crucial because, in the absence of adequate insulin signaling, muscle protein synthesis remains suboptimal, prolonging the recovery phase (Schoenfeld & Aragon, 2018). By maximizing this anabolic drive through targeted co-ingestion, athletes can ensure that the microscopic damage incurred during training is not only repaired but reinforced. Consequently, the dining table becomes a biochemical laboratory for assessing the efficiency of muscle regeneration (Jäger et al., 2017).

The relationship between nutritional status and injury prevention is deeply rooted in the maintenance of neuromuscular alertness and technical precision. Neuromuscular fatigue, often exacerbated by glycogen depletion and electrolyte imbalances, directly leads to a decline in movement quality, which significantly elevates the risk of traumatic or acute injuries (Maughan & Shirreffs, 2019). Furthermore, internal physiological stability depends heavily on adequate hydration to maintain cardiovascular efficiency, thereby ensuring a consistent supply of oxygen and nutrients to tissues during healing (Evans et al., 2017). When an athlete is in a state of dehydration or energy deficit, the brain's ability to coordinate complex motor patterns is impaired, making the musculoskeletal system vulnerable to overstrain. Thus, proper fueling serves as a critical "neurological buffer" that protects the athlete from the physical errors that typically precede injury (Peeling et al., 2019).

Adopting a holistic approach requires recognizing that the timing of nutrients cannot compensate for a chronic deficiency in total energy availability, a condition known as Relative Energy Deficiency in Sport (RED-S). Even with a perfect "anabolic window" strategy, an athlete suffering from RED-S will face impaired hormonal health, reduced bone density, and a suppressed immune system (Thomas et al., 2016). The synergy between nighttime nutrition and the sleep cycle is a vital component of this holistic model, in which consuming slow-digesting proteins like casein before bed optimizes growth hormone secretion (Moore, 2019). During deep sleep, the body undergoes its most significant regenerative phase, and sustained amino acid availability ensures that muscle protein synthesis continues uninterrupted throughout the night (Vitale & Getzin, 2019). Therefore, integrating overall caloric sufficiency, restorative sleep, and pre-sleep fueling forms a recovery triad essential for long-term health.

Practical implications for sports practitioners emphasize the need to personalize recovery protocols based on an individual's unique metabolic profile and sweat rate. A "one-size-fits-all" approach is often ineffective because the demands of fluid and electrolyte replacement vary significantly between athletes depending on their physiological constitution and environmental conditions (Shirreffs & Sawka, 2011). Coaches and nutritionists must move beyond generalized advice and implement data-driven strategies that account for the specific energy expenditures of their athletes. By focusing on individualized electrolyte synergy and macronutrient ratios, practitioners can enhance the body's innate ability to handle high-volume training loads without crossing the threshold into overtraining (Ranchordas et al., 2017). This level of precision in sports dietetics is what separates elite performance from mere participation in high-stakes environments.

Ultimately, this discussion underscores that the "dining table" strategy is a non-negotiable pillar of athletic success, carrying equal weight to physical conditioning on the field. The longevity of a professional athlete's career is determined not just by their work ethic during practice but also by their discipline in managing their body's internal environment through nutrition and rest (Kerksick et al., 2017). Sustainable performance is only possible when the mechanical stress of training is balanced with a sophisticated recovery paradigm that integrates biochemical, hormonal, and lifestyle factors. As sports science continues to evolve, the focus must remain on this holistic synergy to ensure that athletes can achieve peak performance while minimizing the risk of career-ending injuries. Mastering the science of recovery is, therefore, the ultimate competitive advantage in the modern era of sports (Schoenfeld & Aragon, 2018).

This chapter brings together findings from biochemistry, physiology, and nutrition to explore how specific dietary strategies affect recovery in elite athletes. It examines markers such as oxidative stress and inflammatory cytokines to assess how antioxidants, healthy fats, electrolytes, and protein types influence both the speed and quality of recovery. The analysis considers individual differences, such as training status and environmental conditions, emphasizing the need for personalized nutrition and hydration plans rather than a single universal approach. The review also stresses the importance of insulin in muscle repair, the role of hydration and electrolyte balance in preventing injury, and the limits of nutrient timing if overall energy needs are not met. By focusing on sleep, sufficient calorie intake, and the right balance of nutrients, the study argues that effective recovery is just as essential as training itself for long-term athletic success. In the end, mastering nutrition and recovery routines is highlighted as the key to both peak performance and career longevity in sports.

6. CONCLUSIONS

Post-exercise nutrition and electrolyte synergy are crucial components of an athlete's recovery, acting as primary catalysts for tissue regeneration, energy replenishment, and injury prevention. Accelerated recovery, particularly when training schedules allow for less than 24 hours between sessions, requires meticulous food scheduling. Research highlights that the “anabolic window” is a vital 30-minute to 2-hour post-exercise period, during which the consumption of carbs and protein is critical for maximizing muscle protein synthesis and replenishing glycogen stores. Consuming 1–1.2 g/kg of carbohydrates with protein can significantly increase insulin production, promoting glycogen restoration and aiding the repair of microtears in muscle fibers, thereby reducing muscular discomfort and lowering the risk of chronic damage. The interaction between hydration and electrolytes, specifically sodium, potassium, and magnesium, is essential for compensating for losses due to perspiration, thereby preserving blood volume, improving muscle performance, and preventing severe cramping. It is highly recommended to consume electrolyte-rich liquids or beverages to enhance fluid retention and optimize physiological function during recuperation. Alongside macronutrients, adequate intake of antioxidants, including vitamins C and E, is crucial for alleviating exercise-induced oxidative stress, while omega-3 fatty acids and functional foods help manage inflammation. This extensive dietary approach not only expedites performance recovery but also improves muscular and structural resilience, significantly decreasing the overall injury risk for athletes. In addition to macronutrients, antioxidants such as vitamins C and E, omega-3 fatty acids, and functional foods help modulate exercise-induced oxidative stress and inflammation. This holistic nutritional strategy enhances performance recovery and bolsters muscular and structural resilience, hence diminishing the chance of injury among athletes. Achieving an optimal nutritional balance and electrolyte synergy is essential for post-exercise recovery and injury prevention in athletes. Post strenuous exercise, it is crucial to replenish macronutrients: carbs to restore glycogen, proteins for muscle repair, and healthy fats for cellular recovery. The restoration of electrolytes, including sodium, potassium, magnesium, and calcium, is equally crucial, as these are depleted through perspiration and are essential for muscle function, neuronal communication, and fluid equilibrium. A coordinated intake of nutrients and electrolytes accelerates muscle healing, reduces inflammation, and helps prevent cramps, dehydration, and overuse injuries, allowing athletes to resume peak performance more swiftly and securely.

REFERENCES

Alghannam, A. F., Jedrzejewski, D., Bilzon, J., Thompson, D., Tsintzas, K., & Betts, J. A. (2016). Influence of post-exercise carbohydrate-protein ingestion on muscle glycogen metabolism in recovery and subsequent running exercise. *International Journal of Sport Nutrition and Exercise Metabolism, 26*(6), 572–580. DOI: 10.1123/ijsnem.2016-0021 PMID: 27097042

Andriani, A. D., & Siripipatthanakul, S. (2026, a). Communicating Green Governance: Strategic Communication for Sustainable Digital Organizations. In *Green Governance of Digital Organizations* (pp. 187–216). IGI Global Scientific Publishing. https://www.igi-global.com/chapter/communicating-green-governance/401460

Andriani, A. D., & Siripipatthanakul, S. (2026). Communicating Human Resource Management (HRM) for Recognized Sustainable Green Governance Universities. In *Green Governance of Digital Organizations* (pp. 157–186, b). IGI Global Scientific Publishing. https://www.igi-global.com/chapter/communicating-human-resource-management-hrm-for-recognized-sustainable-green-governance-universities/401459

Aragon, A. A., & Schoenfeld, B. J. (2013). Nutrient timing revisited: Is there a post-exercise anabolic window? *Journal of the International Society of Sports Nutrition, 10*(1), 5. https://www.tandfonline.com/doi/full/10.1186/1550-2783-10-5. DOI: 10.1186/1550-2783-10-5 PMID: 23360586

Burke, L. M., van Loon, L. J., & Hawley, J. A. (2017). Postexercise muscle glycogen resynthesis in humans. *Journal of Applied Physiology (Bethesda, Md.), 122*(5), 1055–1067. Advance online publication. DOI: 10.1152/japplphysiol.00860.2016 PMID: 27789774

Cai, Z. J. (2024). The Regulation of Slow-Wave Sleep on Growth Hormone Secretion and Homeostatic Aging: A Pure Model in Man. *OAlib, 11*(9), e12041. DOI: 10.4236/oalib.1112041

Choi, D. H., Cho, J. Y., Koo, J. H., & Kim, T. K. (2021). Effects of electrolyte supplements on body water homeostasis and exercise performance during exhaustive exercise. *Applied Sciences (Basel, Switzerland), 11*(19), 9093. https://www.mdpi.com/2076-3417/11/19/9093?uid=680b54f39b. DOI: 10.3390/app11199093

Duda, G. N., Geissler, S., Checa, S., Tsitsilonis, S., Petersen, A., & Schmidt-Bleek, K. (2023). The decisive early phase of bone regeneration. *Nature Reviews. Rheumatology, 19*(2), 78–95. https://www.nature.com/articles/s41584-022-00887-0. DOI: 10.1038/s41584-022-00887-0 PMID: 36624263

Evans, G. H., James, L. J., Shirreffs, S. M., & Maughan, R. J. (2017). Optimizing the restoration and maintenance of fluid balance after exercise-induced dehydration. *Journal of Applied Physiology*. https://journals.physiology.org/doi/full/10.1152/japplphysiol.00745.2016?utm_

Hausswirth, C., & Le Meur, Y. (2011). Physiological and nutritional aspects of post-exercise recovery: Specific recommendations for female athletes. *Sports Medicine*, *41*(10), 861–882. https://link.springer.com/article/10.2165/11593180-000000000-00000. DOI: 10.2165/11593180-000000000-00000 PMID: 21923203

Jäger, R., Kerksick, C. M., Campbell, B. I., Cribb, P. J., Wells, S. D., Skwiat, T. M., Purpura, M., Ziegenfuss, T. N., Ferrando, A. A., Arent, S. M., Smith-Ryan, A. E., Stout, J. R., Arciero, P. J., Ormsbee, M. J., Taylor, L. W., Wilborn, C. D., Kalman, D. S., Kreider, R. B., Willoughby, D. S., & Antonio, J. (2017). International Society of Sports Nutrition position stand: Protein and exercise. *Journal of the International Society of Sports Nutrition*, *14*(1), 20. https://www.tandfonline.com/doi/abs/10.1186/s12970-017-0177-8. DOI: 10.1186/s12970-017-0177-8 PMID: 28642676

Kerksick, C. M., Arent, S., Schoenfeld, B. J., Stout, J. R., Campbell, B., Wilborn, C. D., Taylor, L., Kalman, D., Smith-Ryan, A. E., Kreider, R. B., Willoughby, D., Arciero, P. J., VanDusseldorp, T. A., Ormsbee, M. J., Wildman, R., Greenwood, M., Ziegenfuss, T. N., Aragon, A. A., & Antonio, J. (2017). International Society of Sports Nutrition position stand: Nutrient timing. *Journal of the International Society of Sports Nutrition*, *14*(1), 33. https://www.tandfonline.com/doi/full/10.1186/s12970-017-0189-4. DOI: 10.1186/s12970-017-0189-4 PMID: 28919842

Lee, E. C., Fragala, M. S., Kavouras, S. A., Queen, R. M., Pryor, J. L., & Casa, D. J. (2017). Biomarkers in sports and exercise: Tracking health, performance, and recovery in athletes. *Journal of Strength and Conditioning Research*, *31*(10), 2920–2937. DOI: 10.1519/JSC.0000000000002122 PMID: 28737585

Link, L. (2024). *Nutrient timing: fueling strategies to unlock peak performance*. Human Kinetics.

Macnaughton, L. S., Wardle, S. L., Witard, O. C., McGlory, C., Hamilton, D. L., Jeromson, S., Lawrence, C. E., Wallis, G. A., & Tipton, K. D. (2016). The response of muscle protein synthesis following whole-body resistance exercise is greater following 40 g than 20 g of ingested whey protein. *Physiological Reports*, *4*(15), e12893. https://physoc.onlinelibrary.wiley.com/doi/10.14814/phy2.12893. DOI: 10.14814/phy2.12893 PMID: 27511985

Maughan, R. J., & Shirreffs, S. M. (2019). Muscle cramping during exercise: Causes, solutions, and questions remaining. *Sports Medicine, 49*(2), 115–124. DOI: 10.1007/s40279-019-01162-1 PMID: 31696455

Moore, D. R. (2019). Maximizing post-exercise anabolism: The case for relative protein intakes. *Frontiers in Nutrition, 6*, 485822. DOI: 10.3389/fnut.2019.00147 PMID: 31552263

Peeling, P., Castell, L. M., Derave, W., de Hon, O., & Burke, L. M. (2019). Sports foods and dietary supplements for optimal function and performance enhancement in track-and-field athletes. *International Journal of Sport Nutrition and Exercise Metabolism, 29*(2), 198–209. DOI: 10.1123/ijsnem.2018-0271 PMID: 30299192

Phillips, S. M. (2014). A brief review of critical processes in exercise-induced muscular hypertrophy. *Sports Medicine, 44*(S1, Suppl 1), 71–77. https://link.springer.com/article/10.1007/s40279-014-0152-3. DOI: 10.1007/s40279-014-0152-3 PMID: 24791918

Powers, S. K., Deruisseau, K. C., Quindry, J., & Hamilton, K. L. (2004). Dietary antioxidants and exercise. *Journal of Sports Sciences, 22*(1), 81–94. DOI: 10.1080/02640410310001640563 PMID: 14971435

Puspitasari, R. D., & Arfajah, A. A. (2026). The Role of Nutrition in Optimizing Athletic Performance and Recovery: A Literature Review. *Journal of Nutrition and Health Care*, 1–5. https://junic.professorline.com/index.php/journal/article/view/39

Ranchordas, M. K., Dawson, J. T., & Russell, M. (2017). Practical nutritional recovery strategies for elite soccer players when limited time separates repeated matches. *Journal of the International Society of Sports Nutrition, 14*(1), 35. DOI: 10.1186/s12970-017-0193-8 PMID: 28919844

Schoenfeld, B. J., & Aragon, A. A. (2018). Is there a post-workout anabolic window of opportunity for nutrient consumption? Clearing up controversies. *journal of orthopaedic & sports physical therapy*, 48(12), 911-914. https://www.jospt.org/doi/abs/10.2519/jospt.2018.0615

Shirreffs, S. M., & Sawka, M. N. (2011). Fluid and electrolyte needs for training, competition, and recovery. *Journal of Sports Sciences*, 29(sup1), S39-S46. https://doi.org/DOI: 10.1080/02640414.2011.614269

Shlykov, S. N., Sycheva, O. V., Omarov, R. S., Trubina, I. A., & Skorbina, E. A. (2025). Sports Nutrition and Recovery: Key Nutrients and Supplements for Effective Regeneration. *Human Physiology, 51*(2), 201–216. https://link.springer.com/article/10.1134/S036211972570032X. DOI: 10.1134/S036211972570032X

Thomas, D. T., Erdman, K. A., & Burke, L. M. (2016). Position of the Academy of Nutrition and Dietetics, Dietitians of Canada, and the American College of Sports Medicine: Nutrition and athletic performance. *Journal of the Academy of Nutrition and Dietetics, 116*(3), 501–528. DOI: 10.1016/j.jand.2015.12.006 PMID: 26920240

Tossici, G., Zurloni, V., & Nitri, A. (2024). Stress and sport performance: A PNEI multidisciplinary approach. *Frontiers in Psychology, 15*, 1358771. DOI: 10.3389/fpsyg.2024.1358771 PMID: 38495423

Townsend, J. R., Kirby, T. O., Sapp, P. A., Gonzalez, A. M., Marshall, T. M., & Esposito, R. (2023). Nutrient synergy: Definition, evidence, and future directions. *Frontiers in Nutrition, 10*, 1279925. DOI: 10.3389/fnut.2023.1279925 PMID: 37899823

Vitale, K., & Getzin, A. (2019). Nutrition and supplement update for the endurance athlete: Review and recommendations. *Nutrients, 11*(6), 1289. https://www.mdpi.com/2072-6643/11/6/1289. DOI: 10.3390/nu11061289 PMID: 31181616

Xiao, Y., Deng, Z., Sun, W., Li, J., & Gao, W. (2025). Effects of protein supplementation on body composition, physiological adaptations, and performance during endurance training: A systematic review and meta-analysis. *Frontiers in Nutrition, 12*, 1663860. DOI: 10.3389/fnut.2025.1663860 PMID: 40851900

KEY TERMS AND DEFINITIONS

Anabolic Window: A specific post-exercise period, typically lasting from 30 minutes to two hours, during which the body is primed for nutrient absorption. In this phase, muscle cells exhibit heightened sensitivity to insulin and increased blood flow, making it the optimal time for tissue repair and glycogen replenishment (Aragon & Schoenfeld, 2013).

Casein Protein: A slow-digesting dairy protein that provides a sustained release of amino acids into the bloodstream. It is frequently recommended as a pre-sleep nutritional intervention to prevent muscle breakdown and support anabolic processes during overnight fasting (Vitale & Getzin, 2019).

Co-ingestion: The simultaneous consumption of two or more macronutrients, typically carbohydrates and protein. This method has been shown to elicit a more robust insulin response than consuming protein alone, thereby accelerating both glycogen storage and muscle repair (Alghannam et al., 2016).

Electrolyte Synergy: The coordinated interaction of essential minerals, specifically sodium, potassium, and magnesium, to maintain physiological balance. This synergy is crucial for fluid retention, osmotic pressure regulation, and the prevention of neuromuscular dysfunction, such as muscle cramps (Maughan & Shirreffs, 2019).

Glycogen Resynthesis: The biological process of restoring glucose stores (glycogen) in the muscles and liver that were depleted during physical exertion. This process is most efficient when carbohydrates are consumed immediately post-exercise at a rate of 1.0–1.2 g/kg of body weight (Burke et al., 2017).

mTOR Pathway (Mammalian Target of Rapamycin): A central signaling pathway in human cells that regulates cell growth and protein synthesis. In athletes, this pathway is "switched on" by mechanical loading (exercise) and by the presence of specific amino acids, such as leucine, which serve as the master switch for muscle regeneration (Xiao et al., 2025).

Muscle Protein Synthesis (MPS): is the metabolic process by which amino acids are incorporated into skeletal muscle proteins. MPS is the fundamental mechanism for repairing microtears in muscle fibers caused by intense exercise and is primarily stimulated by high-quality protein intake and activation of the mTOR pathway (Moore, 2019).

Neuromuscular Fatigue: A reduction in the ability of the nervous system to effectively manifest muscle force. This condition, often caused by nutrient depletion or dehydration, reduces technical alertness and coordination, significantly increasing the risk of sports-related injuries (Peeling et al., 2019).

Nutrient Timing: A strategic nutritional approach that focuses on *when* nutrients are consumed rather than just *what* is consumed. In sports science, it involves the purposeful ingestion of macronutrients at specific times to maximize training adaptations, enhance recovery, and minimize muscle damage (Kerksick et al., 2017).

RED-S (Relative Energy Deficiency in Sport): A clinical syndrome resulting from a chronic mismatch between an athlete's energy intake and the energy expended during exercise. RED-S affects multiple physiological functions, including metabolic rate, bone health, immunity, and protein synthesis, regardless of the precision of nutrient timing (Thomas et al., 2016).

Chapter 10
Functional Recovery Evidence-Based Nutritional Strategies for Athletes' Performance Enhancement and Injury Prevention

Sohom Saha
http://orcid.org/0009-0006-9438-1554
Lakshmibai National Institute of Physical Education, India

Mahendra Kumar Singh
http://orcid.org/0000-0001-9989-9420
Lakshmibai National Institute of Physical Education, India

Sachin Shekhawat
http://orcid.org/0009-0004-4405-3638
Lakshmibai National Institute of Physical Education, India

Prashant Kumar Choudhary
http://orcid.org/0000-0001-6163-8065
Lakshmibai National Institute of Physical Education, India

Patcharavadee Sriboonruang
http://orcid.org/0000-0002-2171-2387
Kasetsart University, Thailand

DOI: 10.4018/979-8-3373-9544-9.ch010

ABSTRACT

Training depends not only on an athlete's performance but also on recovery. This chapter employs a systematic review to describe the benefits of nutrition for helping athletes recover quickly, preventing injuries, and achieving high levels of performance. It discusses the roles of carbohydrates in energy restoration, protein in muscle rejuvenation, and healthy fats in managing inflammation. Significant nutrients include omega-3 fatty acids, vitamin D, iron, and antioxidants, as well as appropriate hydration and electrolyte balance. Other evidence-based supplements, such as creatine and collagen peptides, have also been reviewed in the chapter. Adolescent and master's athletes with unique recovery needs receive special attention. In general, this chapter presents evidence-based, practical nutritional interventions that coaches, athletes, and sport practitioners can find very easy to implement to enhance recovery and long-term performance.

1. INTRODUCTION

Athletes' performance results from the effects of training stimuli, tactical preparation, mental readiness, and, most importantly, the body's ability to recover between bouts of exertion. The demands of modern sport are exceptional: overloaded competition schedules, multiple training sessions daily, constant travel, and extreme physical contact. Recovery is not a passive process; it should be actively supported in this environment, and nutrition is one of the most effective resources practitioners and athletes can use.

Conventional sport nutrition paradigms have long focused on fueling, which involves ensuring an adequate energy supply before and during exercise to sustain performance (Burke et al., 2011). Although this remains vital, recent studies have expanded on this perspective. Recent nutritional approaches include controlling post-exercise inflammatory reactions, accelerating muscle recovery, enhancing connective tissue repair, avoiding fatigue-induced trauma, and sustaining immune function during periods of elevated training load (Tipton & Witard, 2007; Close et al., 2019). Although there is an increasing body of mechanistic and applied literature, the practical translation of nutritional science into structured, individualized recovery programs has yet to be streamlined. Most athletes and coaches rely on anecdotal evidence, commercial marketing, or generalized guidelines rather than evidence-based, context-specific strategies. Such a disconnect between evidence and practice has substantive implications: suboptimal recovery leads to performance losses, higher injury rates, and athlete burnout (Kreher & Schwartz, 2012).

The focus of this chapter is to bridge the gap. It is an evidence-based synthesis of peer-reviewed literature on macronutrient timing, anti-inflammatory nutrition, hydration management, and supplementation, presenting a consistent, evidence-based approach to nutritional recovery. The final goal is to provide practitioners, sport dietitians, strength and conditioning coaches, team physicians, and sport scientists with approaches that are not merely scientifically grounded but also practically implementable across a wide range of athlete groups.

Figure 1. Conceptual Model of Nutritional Strategies for Athletic Recovery and Injury Prevention

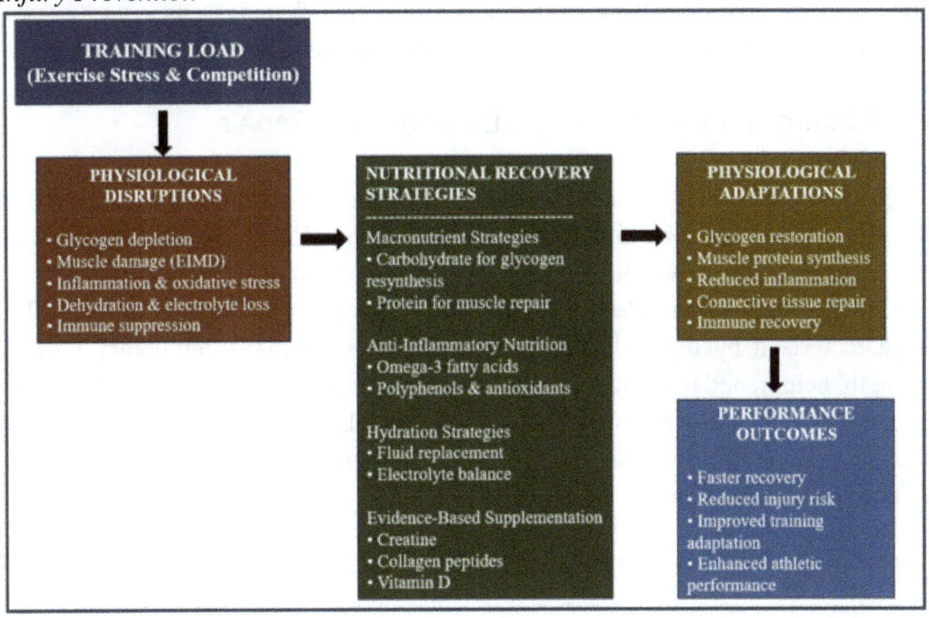

Source: Authors' own elaboration

2. LITERATURE REVIEW

2.1 Physiological Foundations of Post-Exercise Recovery

To understand the role of nutrition in the recovery process, one should learn about the physiological disruptions exercise causes in the body. Both endurance, resistance, and mixed-modality forms of strenuous exercise result in a cascade of metabolic, structural, and immunological perturbations that must be resolved before complete performance capacity is regained.

The main source of moderate intensity-vigorous intensity exercise is muscle glycogen. Glycogen stores may be significantly or entirely depleted at the end of a session, depending on the duration and intensity of exercise (Bergstrom et al., 1967). This depletion hinders the future performance and extends fatigue. Six to 30-60 minutes after the exercise, the rate of glycogen resynthesis is highest, accompanied by the insulin-independent process of muscle glucose uptake via GLUT-4 transporter upregulation (Ivy et al., 1988; Richter & Hargreaves, 2013). In addition to glycogen, exercise depletes intramuscular lipid, phosphocreatine, and amino acid pools in the circulation. All these substrates require specific nutritional contributions for replenishment, highlighting the multidimensional nature of metabolic recovery.

2.1.1 Exercise-Induced Muscle Damage and Repair

Micro-architectural disruption of myofibrils and the surrounding extracellular space is brought about by high-force eccentric contractions, which are common in resistance training, downhill running, and most team sports (Clarkson & Hubal, 2002). This type of muscle damage that occurs as a result of exercise (EIMD) is characterized by delayed-onset muscle soreness (DOMS), temporary loss of strength, heightened indicators of muscle protein catabolism, and elevated creatine kinase levels. The processes of recovery after EIMD are longitudinal satellite cell activation, myofibrillar protein remodeling, and connective tissue repair, which can be nutritionally modified (Tipton et al., 2004).

2.1.2 Inflammatory and Immune Responses

EIMD results in acute inflammation of neutrophils and macrophages, release of cytokines (IL-6, IL-1β, and TNF-α), and the generation of reactive oxygen species (ROS) (Peake et al., 2017). This inflammatory cascade is necessary; however, excessive or prolonged inflammation may be detrimental: it facilitates the removal of debris and the activation of satellite cells, but when excessive in magnitude or duration, it may impair tissue repair of repairing the tissue and augmenting systemic fatigue. The nutritional strategies that regulate rather than merely suppress this reaction are thus useful recovery measures.

The transient immune suppression also brought about by heavy training is commonly known as the open window hypothesis, whereby the body is made vulnerable to upper respiratory tract infections (Gleeson, 2006). Immunological support for high-load exercise protocols is, therefore, a valid recovery factor.

The matrix remodeling processes of tendons, ligaments, and articular cartilage are slower and less well understood than myofibrillar adaptation. The synthesis of collagen is enhanced during the hours after exercise, and the nutritional modulation of this anabolic window of connective tissue (Shaw et al., 2017). Hindered healing of connective tissue is a major cause of overuse injuries in athletes involved in repetitive loading patterns.

Table 1. Physiological Disruptions Following Strenuous Exercise

Physiological Domain	Exercise-Induced Disruption	Key Biomarkers/ Indicators	Nutritional Relevance
Glycogen Stores	Muscle glycogen depletion	Muscle glycogen content	Rapid carbohydrate provision (1.0-1.2 g/kg/hr)
Muscle Tissue	Micro-tears, EIMD	CK, DOMS, strength loss	20-40 g high-quality protein
Inflammation	Acute cytokine response	IL-6, TNF-α, CRP	Omega-3, polyphenols
Oxidative Stress	ROS production	MDA, antioxidant capacity	Antioxidant-rich foods
Immune Function	Temporary suppression	URTI incidence	Vitamin D, adequate energy
Connective Tissue	Collagen breakdown	P1NP, collagen markers	Collagen + Vitamin C

Source: Authors' own elaboration based on the studies by Bergstrom et al., 1967; Ivy et al., 1988; and Peake et al., 2017.

2.2 Macronutrient Strategies for Recovery

2.2.1 Carbohydrates: Glycogen Resynthesis and Timing

The best evidence-based nutritional approach to resynthesizing glycogen remains carbohydrate consumption. The scientific foundation of the post-exercise window of opportunity was established by Ivy et al. (1988), who found that carbohydrate intake immediately after exercise produced much greater glycogen storage than carbohydrate intake two hours later. Later studies have narrowed down on timing and dose.

The current recommendations of the International Society of Sports Nutrition (ISSN) and the American College of Sports Medicine (ACSM) suggest 1.0-1.2 g/kg body mass/hour of carbohydrate during the first four hours after exercise when it is needed to resynthesize glycogen quickly (Burke et al., 2011; Thomas et al., 2016). Carbohydrates with a high glycemic index (GI) are preferred during this acute period because they elicit a more pronounced insulinemic response and faster net glycogen production (Burke et al., 1993).

Aggressive early carbohydrate loading is especially important when training or competition resumes within 8 hours. In athletes engaged in single-daily exercise, with sufficient recovery periods, overall daily carbohydrate intake and non-acute timing are the main factors influencing glycogen restoration (Betts & Williams, 2010). Carbohydrate periodization, in which intake is adjusted to training needs, is a new strategy in its infancy and is practically applicable, matching substrate supply to session intensity while maintaining metabolic adaptability (Impey et al., 2018).

Table 2. Carbohydrate Recommendations for Post-Exercise Glycogen Resynthesis

Recovery Scenario	Carbohydrate Dose	Timing	Type Recommended	Rationale
Rapid recovery (<8h between sessions)	1.0-1.2 g/kg/hr	First 4 hours	High GI	Maximizes glycogen resynthesis rate
Moderate recovery (24h)	5-7 g/kg/day	Distributed	Mixed GI	Total intake is more important
Endurance block training	6-10 g/kg/day	Periodized	Complex + simple	Supports high training load
Low-intensity/rest day	3-5 g/kg/day	Flexible	Complex carbs	Maintains metabolic flexibility

Source: Authors owns elaboration based on the studies of Burke et al., 2011; Thomas et al., 2016; and Impey et al., 2018.

2.2.2 Protein: Muscle Protein Synthesis and Repair

Both resistance and endurance exercise increase muscle protein synthesis (MPS) and muscle protein breakdown, and the net muscle protein balance depends on the interrelationship between exercise stimulus and amino acid availability (Phillips & Van Loon, 2011). A change in post-exercise dietary protein supply shifts the balance of net protein synthesis, promoting structural repair and training adaptation. Leucine is a major anabolic stimulus that signals through activation of the mTOR pathway, a branched-chain essential amino acid (Norton & Layman, 2006). It seems that a leucine threshold of about 2-3 g/serving is required to maximize MPS, and that this level of leucine is reached by ingesting 20-40 g of a high-quality protein source (Moore et al., 2009).

Entire food groups, such as eggs, poultry, dairy, fish, and legumes, meet this threshold, with cofactors that promote broader recovery. Much has been reported on the timing of protein intake relative to exercise. Although earlier studies recommended a limited post-exercise anabolic window, more recent meta-analyses have indicated that total daily protein intake, estimated to be 1.62.2 g/kg/day of strength and power athletes, is the most significant variable, but protein intake during two hours of resistance exercise has additive value when total consumption is on the lower end of the recommendations (Morton et al., 2018; Witard et al., 2014). The highest total MPS response is achieved with the distribution of protein in 3-5 daily eating events and doses of 20-40g (Areta et al., 2013).

Pre-sleep protein has emerged as one of the most effective methods for nighttime recovery. Res et al. (2012) found that 40 g of casein protein administered 30 minutes before sleep significantly increased MPS overnight, compared with a control that did not impair morning appetite. This is especially useful for athletes with high training volumes who need to maximize anabolic signaling throughout the day.

Table 3. Evidence-Based Protein Strategies for Muscle Recovery

Variable	Recommendation	Evidence-Based Range	Practical Example
Post-exercise dose	20-40 g	~0.25-0.40 g/kg	Whey shake, eggs + toast
Daily intake	1.6-2.2 g/kg/day	Strength athletes	4-5 protein meals/day
Leucine threshold	2-3 g	Per serving	25 g whey or 35 g mixed protein
Distribution	3-5 meals/day	Evenly spaced	Every 3-4 hours
Pre-sleep protein	30-40 g casein	30 min before sleep	Greek yogurt, casein shake

Source: Authors owns elaboration based on the studies of Phillips & Van Loon, 2011; Morton et al., 2018; and Areta et al., 2013.

2.2.3 Carbohydrate-Protein Co-Ingestion

Co-ingestion of carbohydrates and protein post-exercise results in synergistic recovery effects. Increased insulinemic response promotes amino acid uptake into muscle and suppresses protein degradation, while also increasing the rate of glycogen resynthesis (Zawadzki et al., 1992). Carbohydrate-to-protein ratios of 3:1 to 4:1 (e.g., 60 g carbohydrate + 20 g protein) are often recommended in practical recovery scenarios (Betts & Williams, 2010; Thomas et al., 2016). Chocolate milk made with dairy foods provides this ratio in a healthy way and has shown recovery effectiveness comparable to commercial sports beverages in a series of controlled studies (Pritchett & Pritchett, 2012).

2.2.4 Dietary Fat in Recovery

Although the importance of carbohydrates and proteins is widely discussed in post-exercise nutrition, the quality of dietary fats is also important for recovery due to their anti-inflammatory effects and the prompt provision of substrates. The effect of saturated and trans fatty acids is to increase inflammation following exercise, whereas unsaturated fats, particularly omega-3 polyunsaturated fatty acids

(PUFAs), suppress pro-inflammatory cytokine activity (Smith et al., 2011). In a practical context, high-fat consumption during the acute post-exercise phase can delay gastric emptying and thus retard carbohydrate absorption; fat consumption should therefore not be centered on a particular period after exercise.

2.3 Anti-Inflammatory Nutrition and Micronutrient Density

2.3.1 Omega-3 Fatty Acids

Long-chain omega-3 PUFAs in fatty fish and algae (eicosapentaenoic acid (EPA)) and (docosahexaenoic acid (DHA)) have strong anti-inflammatory properties. They also outcompete arachidonic acid for access to cyclooxygenase and lipoxygenase enzymes, inhibit the production of pro-inflammatory eicosanoids, and stimulate the production of specialized pro-resolving mediators (SPMs) such as resolvins and protectins (Calder, 2013).

The omega-3 supplementation of athlete groups has been demonstrated to decrease the evidence of EIMD and inflammation (Smith et al., 2011), postpone delayed-onset muscle pain (Jouris et al., 2011), and, not least, could decrease the likelihood of concussion-induced neurological injuries, as DHA is a structural component of the neuronal membranes (Oliver et al., 2016). Anti-inflammatory effects in athletes have been suggested to require 2-4 g/day of EPA+DHA, which can be achieved through dietary intake (2-3 servings per week of fatty fish) in combination with supplementation (Calder, 2013).

2.3.2 Polyphenols and Antioxidant-Rich Foods

Plant polyphenols, which are flavonoids, anthocyanins, and stilbenes, are antioxidants and anti-inflammatory agents by regulating NF-kB-signaling and direct scavenging of reactive oxygen species (Patel et al., 2018). Prunus cerasus (Tart cherry) juice has received significant scientific attention in the field of sports nutrition, and several studies have shown reductions in EIMD markers, DOMS, and loss of strength following resistance and endurance exercise (Howatson et al., 2010; Bell et al., 2014). The suggested mechanisms include high anthocyanin levels that dampen oxidative stress and inflammatory responses.

Similarly, beetroot (Beta vulgaris) is a good source of betalains and dietary nitrates that support vascular function and can help mitigate oxidative stress caused by vigorous training. The active polyphenol present in turmeric, curcumin, has been shown to be a potent anti-inflammatory agent in both research and practice, due to its ability to decrease circulating IL-6 levels and markers of muscle damage after vigorous exercise at doses of 1-6 g/day (Tanabe et al., 2015). The presence of piperine (black pepper extract) significantly increases the bioavailability of curcumin.

2.3.3 Vitamin D

Vitamin D, technically classified as a prohormone, has continued to emerge as a highly important micronutrient for athletes' health and performance. In addition to their classical functions in calcium homeostasis and bone metabolism, vitamin D receptors are also expressed in muscle tissue and immune cells and mediate pathways of interest for strength, power, and protection against infections (Larson-Meyer & Willis, 2010). Indoor, high-latitude, and abundant clothing-cover health conditions among sportspeople, as well as darker skin pigmentation, put athletes at high risk of inadequacy.

The optimal level of vitamin D, 75 nmol/L (5000 mg/dl), was found to be optimal for sports and for preventing sports injuries (Owens et al., 2018). Deficiency has been linked to a higher risk of stress fracture, muscle recovery impairment, and high levels of upper respiratory infections. A dose of 1,000-4,000 IU/day of vitamin D3 (cholecalciferol) is usually necessary to attain and maintain optimal serum levels in at-risk athletes; however, individual doses should be guided by periodic blood testing.

2.3.4 Vitamin C and Collagen Precursors

Vitamin C is essential in the production of collagen as a cofactor to prolyl and lysyl hydroxylase enzyme, which is a collagen cross-linking enzyme. Shaw et al. (2017) demonstrated in a randomized controlled trial that the ingestion of 15 g of gelatin (a collagen precursor) and 48 mg of vitamin C, taken 60 minutes prior to exercise, substantially increased circulating collagen synthesis biomarkers and enhanced collagen content in engineered ligament tissue. The practical implications of this result are extensive for athletes experiencing high-volume connective tissue loading, as it implies that the timely intake of vitamin C-gelatin or collagen peptide supplementation can minimize the risk of injury by promoting tendon and ligament remodeling.

2.3.5 Iron and B Vitamins

Iron is central to oxygen delivery and energy utilization, and iron deficiency is one of the most impactful nutritional deficiencies in athletes, especially in endurance and female athletes. Iron deficiency, even without frank anemia, still impairs aerobic capacity, cognitive function, and recovery (Maughan et al., 2018). The focus of dietary measures to increase the heme sources of iron (red meat, poultry, fish) and to increase the absorption of non-heme iron from plant foods through the co-presence of vitamin C is central. Professional athletes are supposed to have periodic checks of hemoglobin and ferritin.

The B vitamins, especially thiamine, riboflavin, niacin, B6, and B12, are essential coenzymes in energy metabolism pathways and in amino acid metabolism that is pertinent to muscle repair. DNA synthesis to aid satellite cell expansion of muscle repair requires folate and B12. Special consideration of B12, riboflavin, and zinc status is needed for athletes using restrictive dietary patterns or plant-based diets.

Table 4. Anti-Inflammatory Nutrients and Their Mechanisms in Recovery

Nutrient	Mechanism of Action	Effective Dose	Practical Sources
Omega-3 (EPA/ DHA)	Reduces pro-inflammatory eicosanoids	2-4 g/day	Fatty fish, fish oil
Tart Cherry	Anthocyanins reduce oxidative stress	240-480 ml/day	Montmorency juice
Curcumin	Inhibits NF-κB signaling	1-6 g/day	Turmeric + piperine
Vitamin D	Modulates immune & muscle function	1,000-4,000 IU/ day	Sunlight, supplements
Polyphenols	ROS scavenging	Dietary variety	Berries, beetroot

Source: Authors owns elaboration based on the studies of Calder, 2013; Smith et al., 2011; and Howatson et al., 2010.

2.4 Hydration and Electrolyte Strategies

2.4.1 Physiological Consequences of Dehydration

Even mild dehydration, with a 2% body mass loss from fluid loss, significantly impairs cognitive performance, thermoregulatory efficiency, cardiovascular load, and endurance traits (Sawka et al., 2007). Neuromuscular fatigue, reaction time, and injury susceptibility are also more common in contact and collision sports due to dehydration, especially when the sport is done in a heat-stress environment. These effects are magnified by chronic low-grade dehydration experienced by athletes who fail to drink to thirst over successive days of training.

The amount of sweat lost during exercise also varies between 0.5 and 2.5 L/hour, depending on exercise intensity, ambient temperature, humidity, and the individual's sweat-loss rate. Since the contraction of plasma volume reduces cardiac output and increases perceived exertion, proportional fluid replacement for sweat loss is key to prolonged performance and quality of recovery (Maughan et al., 2007).

Table 5. Hydration and Electrolyte Replacement Guidelines

Parameter	Recommendation	Practical Assessment	Notes
Dehydration threshold	≥2% body mass loss	Pre/post weighing	Impairs performance
Post-exercise fluid	125-150% of fluid lost	Body mass difference	Over 2-4 hours
Sodium concentration	20-50 mmol/L	Electrolyte drinks	Enhances retention
Sweat rate	0.5-2.5 L/hr	Sweat testing	Individual variability
Urine color	Pale straw	Visual scale	Field method

Source: Authors owns elaboration based on the studies of Sawka et al., 2007; Shirreffs et al., 1996; and Armstrong et al., 1994.

2.4.2 Hydration Assessment and Individualized Replacement

The most feasible field measure of hydration status is urine color: a pale straw color (between 1-3 on the traditional Armstrong scale) indicates satisfactory hydration (Armstrong et al., 1994). More specific measurements would include pre- and post-exercise body mass measurements; each kilogram lost would correspond to a 1-liter deficit in body fluid. The electrolyte replacement strategies can be tailored by measuring sweat sodium levels using sweat patch technology.

Rehydration after exercise aims to replace about 125-150% of body mass lost within the two to four hours after exercise, since fluid losses continue and cannot be adequately replaced with the same amount of fluid to restore euhydration (Shirreffs et al., 1996). Oral rehydration solutions (ORS) with sodium 20-50 mmol/L and carbohydrate 20-30 g/L hasten the intestinal absorption of sodium-glucose co-transporter associated with fluid absorption and at the same time promote glycogen restructuring.

2.4.3 Electrolyte Balance and Cramping

The first electrolyte lost in sweat is sodium, whose replacement is paramount for restoring plasma volume and maintaining the osmotic gradient that promotes fluid retention. Sweat also loses potassium, magnesium, and chloride, although in lesser absolute amounts. Although the etiology of these muscle cramping processes during and after exercise is multifactorial, sodium and fluid losses have been linked to muscle cramping in vulnerable athletes (Schwellnus et al., 2011). In practice, electrolyte replacement with sports drinks, electrolyte pills, and sodium-rich whole foods (e.g., broth, salted nuts) helps maintain neuromuscular function during congested fixtures.

2.4.4 Special Populations: Adolescent and Masters Athletes

The adolescent athlete faces special hydration problems because of low absolute sweat rates, high surface-to-mass ratios that increase heat loss, and, often, poor drinking behavior prompted by sports-oriented attention during exercise (Rivera-Brown et al., 2006). Proactive drinking behavior and access to appealing, attractive fluids are especially vital in sports among the youth.

Thirst perception, glomerular filtration rate, and renal concentrating ability in master athletes (usually older than 35-40 years) decline with age, placing athletes at risk of dehydration (Kenefick & Sawka, 2007). Together with the increased vulnerability to heat illness and the longer recovery periods that are also a feature of aging physiology, fluid management is a particular concern for recovery in masters' sport.

Table 6. Recovery Considerations Across Athlete Populations

Population	Primary Risk	Nutritional Priority	Key Nutrients
Adolescents	RED-S, growth demands	Adequate energy availability	Calcium, Iron, Vitamin D
Female Athletes	Iron deficiency	Iron monitoring	Heme iron + Vitamin C
Masters Athletes	Anabolic resistance	Higher protein doses	35-40 g per meal
Indoor Athletes	Vitamin D insufficiency	Supplementation	Vitamin D3
High-sweat athletes	Sodium loss	Electrolyte replacement	Sodium-rich fluids

Source: Authors owns elaboration based on the studies of Mountjoy et al., 2014; Moore et al., 2015; and Maughan et al., 2018.

2.5 Evidence-Based Supplementation for Recovery and Injury Prevention

The sports supplements market is unregulated and huge, and many products rely on little or methodologically weak evidence. This section highlights supplements that have the most robust evidence base to support recovery and injury-prevention use purposes, as opposed to those use purposes that are commercially common but have lower evidence bases.

Evidence-based nutritional strategies for functional recovery emphasize a holistic, personalized approach to repairing tissue, replenishing energy, and modulating inflammation. The "4R's" framework—Rehydrate, Refuel, Repair, and Revitalize/ Recuperate is central to sports and clinical recovery, ensuring adequate macro- and micronutrient intake to optimize healing.

2.5.1 Creatine Monohydrate

One of the most widely used ergogenic supplements studied in sports science is creatine monohydrate. Its main action is to increase phosphocreatine stores, thereby increasing ATP production during high-intensity, short-duration exercise and decreasing fatigue during repeated-sprint exercise (Rawson & Volek, 2003). In addition to acute performance effects, creatine supplementation enables better glycogen storage in the body when used concomitantly with carbohydrate, and has been shown to be reliable in increasing lean mass accretion, strength gains, and high-intensity training volume; all of which are indirectly beneficial in terms of injury prevention because they increase the structural resilience of muscle (Lanhers et al., 2017).

Creatine loading protocols of 20 g/days (in four or seven-day bursts) then a maintenance dose of 3-5 g/days is effective as a saturation protocol, but a lower dose regimen, of 3-5 g/days with no loading, is also as effective as a saturation protocol (Rawson & Volek, 2003). The most economical and bioavailable form of creatine is the standard powdered form, which is monohydrate. Injury prevention. There is emerging evidence supporting injury prevention, although some data suggest that creatine may suppress EIMD markers following eccentric exercise (Santos et al., 2004).

Table 7. Evidence-Based Supplements for Recovery and Injury Prevention

Supplement	Primary Benefit	Dose	Evidence Strength	Notes
Creatine Monohydrate	ATP resynthesis, lean mass	3-5 g/day	Strong	Most studied
Omega-3	Anti-inflammatory	2-4 g EPA+DHA	Strong	Third-party tested
Vitamin D3	Bone & immune support	1,000-4,000 IU	Strong	Monitor serum levels
Collagen Peptides	Tendon/ligament repair	10-15 g/day	Moderate-Strong	With Vitamin C
Beta-Alanine	Buffering capacity	3.2-6.4 g/day	Moderate	Ergogenic

Source: Authors owns elaboration based on the studies of Rawson & Volek, 2003; Hobson et al., 2012; and Maughan et al., 2018.

2.5.2 Omega-3 Fatty Acid Supplementation

EPA and DHA supplementation have well-documented anti-inflammatory effects, as discussed in the anti-inflammatory nutrition section, which are relevant to recovery. Supplementation-wise, fish oil capsules (2-4 g EPA + DHA daily) provide a viable and economical delivery system, especially when athletes do not eat fatty fish regularly. The quality must also be taken into account: encapsulation and storage influence oxidative stability, and products evaluated by third parties (e.g., NSF International or Informed Sport) should be prioritized for label correctness and the absence of contaminants (Maughan et al., 2018).

2.5.3 Vitamin D Supplementation

Given the high incidence of vitamin D deficiency amongst athletic populations, especially among indoor or high-latitude trainers, and the extensive research on the benefits of adequate vitamin D levels for musculoskeletal health, immune function, and recovery, regular supplementation for these vulnerable athletes is justified. D3 (cholecalciferol) is superior to D2 (ergocalciferol) in increasing concentrations of serum 25(OH)D (Tripkovic et al., 2012). There is a broad consensus that a supplement of 1,000-4,000 IU/day is safe and effective, and even an overdose of 10,000 IU/day has been reported; therefore, it is advisable to monitor serum 25(OH)D levels periodically (after three to six months) when supplementing.

2.5.4 Collagen Peptides and Gelatin

Hydrolyzed collagen protein, in the form of collagen peptides, has been identified as a promising nutritional intervention for connective tissue repair and injury management. Contrary to whey protein, collagen peptides contain a high amount of glycine, proline, and hydroxyproline, which are the amino acids that make up the three-dimensional structure of collagen fibrils in tendons, ligaments, and cartilage. Shaw et al. (2017) also provided evidence that, prior to exercise, gelatin containing vitamin C significantly increases collagen synthesis biomarkers. Future studies have confirmed the use of collagen peptides for the recovery from joint pain and tendinopathy in athletes (Dressler et al., 2018; Clark et al., 2008). The best time seems to be 30 to 60 minutes prior to mechanical loading, when circulating amino acids are present, to facilitate connective tissue collagen production during the post-exercise anabolic phase.

2.5.5 Beta-Alanine and Sodium Bicarbonate

Beta-alanine, which is a precursor of a carnosine intramuscular buffer, reduces acidosis during high-intensity exercise and increases the duration to fatigue in 1–4-minute efforts (Hobson et al., 2012). Although it is mainly an ergogenic aid rather than a recovery aid, improved buffering capacity during training can enable athletes to maintain higher training volumes, which, in turn, indirectly facilitates adaptation and injury resilience. Doses of 3.2-6.4 g/day, taken in divided doses to reduce paresthesia, are necessary to produce a significant increase in muscle carnosine.

Sodium bicarbonate is an extracellular buffer, and acute doses of 0.2-0.3g/kg body mass, used 60-90 minutes prior to exercise, have shown ergogenic effects during repeated high-intensity exercise (Jones et al., 2016). It is indirectly significant for recovery in situations with high session scheduling congestion, where inter-session acidosis management is needed.

2.5.6 Supplements with Insufficient Evidence

Dozens of commercially available supplements purport to help with recovery and prevent injury, but there is insufficient evidence. A case in point is branched-chain amino acid (BCAA) supplements, which are commonly advertised as muscle-recovery boosters, yet in the circumstance that total protein intake is sufficient, isolated BCAA supplements have little additional MPS gain and are worse than whole-protein sources in terms of leucine dose-response (Wolfe, 2017). Although a conditionally essential amino acid with an important role in severe illness, glutamine has not shown meaningful benefits in recovery in healthy, well-nourished athletes at standard doses. Athletes need to be instructed to consume more whole-food nutrition and evidence-based supplements rather than proprietary blends that are expensive and potentially unverified.

3. METHODOLOGY

3.1 Eligibility Criteria

The eligibility criteria for this systematic review were defined using the PICOS framework to ensure methodological rigor and relevance. Studies were included if they involved human participants who were healthy, recreationally active, trained athletes, or elderly individuals engaged in exercise-based interventions. Eligible interventions included nutritional strategies aimed at enhancing recovery, performance, or physiological adaptation, such as macronutrient manipulation (e.g., carbohydrate timing, protein distribution) and supplementation (e.g., omega-3 fatty acids, collagen/gelatin, tart cherry, casein protein). Studies were required to include a comparator group, such as a placebo, control, or alternative nutritional intervention, to allow for meaningful comparisons. Outcome measures had to include at least one of the following: muscle protein synthesis (MPS), muscle strength or hypertrophy, recovery indicators (e.g., glycogen resynthesis, fatigue, soreness), biochemical markers (e.g., IL-6, CRP, oxidative stress), or functional performance outcomes. Only randomized controlled trials or controlled experimental studies were included to ensure high-quality evidence (Arnarson et al., 2013; Babault et al., 2014). Studies were excluded if they were systematic reviews, meta-analyses, narrative reviews, case reports, or involved animal or in vitro models.

3.2 Information Sources and Search Strategy

A comprehensive literature search was conducted across major electronic databases, including PubMed, Scopus, and Web of Science, to identify relevant studies examining nutritional strategies for exercise recovery and performance. The search strategy combined keywords and Boolean operators to maximize sensitivity and specificity. Core search terms included: "sports nutrition," "recovery," "muscle protein synthesis," "supplementation," "exercise performance," "protein timing," and "oxidative stress." These terms were adapted to the syntax of each database. Additionally, reference lists of selected studies were manually screened to identify any further eligible articles. The search strategy was designed to capture both foundational and contemporary studies addressing recovery mechanisms such as glycogen resynthesis, protein metabolism (Snijders et al., 2015), and anti-inflammatory interventions.

3.3 Selection Process

The study selection process followed a structured and systematic approach in line with PRISMA recommendations (Page et al.,2021; Siripipatthanakul et al., 2026). Initially, all records identified through database searches were imported into a reference management system, and duplicate entries were removed. Titles and abstracts were then screened to exclude clearly irrelevant studies. Subsequently, full-text articles of potentially eligible studies were retrieved and assessed against the predefined inclusion and exclusion criteria. Studies that met all criteria were included in the final analysis. Particular attention was given to study design, ensuring inclusion of randomized or controlled experimental studies, and relevance of outcomes to recovery and performance. Disagreements during the selection process were resolved through careful re-evaluation of study eligibility.

3.4 Data Extraction Process

Data extraction was performed using a standardized and structured format to ensure consistency and accuracy across studies. Key information extracted included author(s) and year of publication, study design, participant characteristics, intervention details (type, dosage, timing), comparator conditions, outcome variables, and main findings. Special emphasis was placed on extracting quantitative outcomes related to muscle protein synthesis, strength, hypertrophy, biochemical markers, and recovery indicators. For example, detailed mechanistic variables such as fractional synthetic rate (FSR) and mTOR signaling pathways were extracted from studies investigating protein metabolism, while inflammatory and oxidative stress markers were extracted from studies on tart cherry supplementation. Extracted data were cross-verified to minimize errors and ensure the reliability of synthesis.

3.5 Risk of Bias Assessment

The methodological quality of the included studies was assessed using the Cochrane Risk of Bias 2.0 (RoB 2.0) tool, which evaluates potential bias across five domains: randomization process, deviations from intended interventions, missing outcome data, measurement of outcomes, and selection of reported results. Each study was categorized as having low, some, or high risk of bias. Randomized controlled trials with appropriate blinding and allocation concealment, such as those by Arnarson et al. (2013) and Babault et al. (2014), were generally classified as low risk. Older or less clearly reported studies, such as Ivy et al. (1988), were categorized as having some concerns due to limited reporting of randomization procedures. Non-randomized or pre-post designs. This structured assessment ensured transparency in evaluating the internal validity of the included evidence.

3.6 Data Synthesis Methods

Due to heterogeneity in study designs, participant characteristics, interventions, and outcome measures, a qualitative synthesis approach was adopted rather than a quantitative meta-analysis. Studies were grouped thematically by type of nutritional intervention and primary outcomes. Thematic categories included: (1) macronutrient strategies (e.g., carbohydrate timing and protein distribution), (2) supplementation strategies (e.g., omega-3 fatty acids, collagen/gelatin, tart cherry), and (3) recovery mechanisms (e.g., inflammation, oxidative stress, muscle protein synthesis). For instance, carbohydrate timing interventions demonstrated enhanced glycogen resynthesis when intake occurred immediately post-exercise, while protein distribution strategies highlighted the importance of feeding frequency for maximizing muscle protein synthesis. Similarly, supplementation approaches showed differential effects on inflammation and recovery, with certain interventions reducing oxidative stress and others enhancing anabolic signaling pathways. This structured narrative synthesis allowed for integration of mechanistic and applied findings, providing a comprehensive understanding of nutritional strategies for recovery.

4. RESULTS

4.1 Periodized Recovery Nutrition

Recovery nutrition does not occur in isolation; it ought to be periodized to align with training needs. During high-intensity or high-volume training days, nutritional recovery demands aggressive carbohydrate replacement, increased protein supply, and consideration of the micronutrient density. Total energy intake and carbohydrate provision could be regulated on lower-intensity or rest days, a strategy compatible with the idea of carbohydrate periodization and with fueling the work one has to complete (Impey et al., 2018). This is a periodized strategy that helps achieve body composition while maintaining the quality of recovery.

4.2 The Recovery Nutrition Window: A Practical Timeline

This timeline may be followed by a structured post-exercise nutrition plan informed by the evidence reviewed in this chapter. The athletes must take 1.0 to 1.2 grams of carbohydrate with 20-40g of protein within 0-30 minutes of exercise, in a high-quality food source, preferably liquid and easily absorbed in the stomach, to empty the stomach quickly and absorb nutrients promptly. The 30-minute to 2-hour window should be filled with a balanced, mixed meal that includes carbohydrates, protein, healthy fats, and vegetables to support continued glycogen resynthesis, prolonged MPS, and micronutrient supply. Amino acids can be sustained, and hydration is maintained through frequent, normal meals at 2-6 hour intervals. Last but not least, during the pre-sleep phase, 30-40 g of casein or some other slow-release protein facilitates overnight anabolism (Res et al., 2012).

Simultaneously with this nutrition schedule, rehydration should aim for 125-150% of lost body mass, and fluids should be consumed over the two to four hrs immediately after exercise, not as a bolus. Fluid provision should be accompanied by electrolyte replacement, especially in athletes who lose sodium in their sweat.

Table 8. Recovery Nutrition Timeline Framework

Time post-exercise	Nutritional Focus	Recommendation
0-30 minutes	Rapid glycogen + MPS	1.0-1.2 g/kg carbs + 20-40 g protein
30 min-2 hours	Mixed meal	Carbs + protein + healthy fats
2-6 hours	Continued amino acid availability	Balanced meals/snacks
Pre-sleep	Overnight MPS	30-40 g casein
2-4 hours rehydration	Fluid restoration	125-150% body mass lost

Source: Authors' own elaboration

5. DISCUSSIONS

5.1 Considerations for Adolescent Athletes

Nutritional attention for adolescent athletes should be given due consideration at a stage when a prerequisite level of concurrent growth must be met, and sport performance demands rival nutritional needs. Relative Energy Deficiency in Sport (RED-S), formerly known as the Female Athlete Triad, is a disease in male and female adolescents characterized by low energy availability that disrupts bone health, hormonal function, immune competence, and recovery (Mountjoy et al., 2014). Recovery nutrition counseling for teenagers must thus focus on ensuring sufficient energy intake before optimizing macronutrient proportions or supplementation. Skeletal growth in adolescents during the pubertal growth spurt is especially sensitive to calcium and vitamin D, and iron requirements in menstruating young females are very high.

5.2 Considerations for Masters Athletes

Master's athletes experience physiological alterations that affect their capacity to recover with age. Anabolic resistance of muscle protein synthesis and decreased amino acid stimulation of aging muscle may necessitate higher protein doses (35-40 g per serving) and an enriched leucine source to reduce muscle protein synthesis rates to those observed in younger athletes (Moore et al., 2015). Anti-inflammatory nutrition takes on greater significance in conditions of heightened systemic inflammation (inflammaging) in aging physiology. Dietary patterns rich in vitamin D, omega-3 fatty acids, and polyphenols help maintain both immunity and the integrity of connective tissues in this population. The role of collagen peptide supplementation may be especially pertinent to age-related impairment of tendon and ligament resilience.

6. CONCLUSIONS

Nutrition is way beyond a source of fuel for athletic performance. When used strategically, it is an effective, evidence-based intervention to speed up recovery, tune inflammation, help connective tissue adjustments, preserve immune systems, and limit injury risk. The reviewed evidence of this chapter shows that carbohydrate timing and dose optimization, strategic protein athletic feeding, such as pre-sleep protein, anti-inflammatory dietary patterns, which are abundant in omega-3 fatty acids and polyphenols, individualized hydration and electrolytes replacement, and specific supplementation with creatine, vitamin D, collagen peptides, and omega-3s are the collective constituents of an all-encompassing nutritional recovery framework. More importantly, none of the nutritional strategies works alone. The greatest recovery gains are obtained when several evidence-based strategies are combined into a periodized program tailored to the athlete's sport demands, training load, physiological features, and nutritional status. It is encouraged that practitioners shift away from generic recommendations toward individualized, data-based protocols that vary over time, across training stages, and by career level. Determining the optimal dosage and timing of connective tissue-targeted nutrition, how sleep quality interacts with nutritional recovery strategies, and whether connective tissue-targeted nutrition models apply to disadvantaged groups such as para-athletes and masters athletes competing at the highest levels should also be clarified in future research. With the development of science, practice should follow suit, evolving to ensure that athletes at all levels receive the nutritional support that is a building block of long-term, high-performance sport.

7. Limitations and Recommendations

This chapter synthesizes existing literature on nutritional strategies for recovery and injury prevention; however, it is primarily conceptual and does not include original experimental data. Future research should investigate the long-term effectiveness of integrated recovery nutrition protocols across different sport disciplines and athlete populations. Emerging technologies such as continuous metabolic monitoring and personalized nutrition strategies may further enhance recovery optimization in elite and recreational athletes.

REFERENCES

Areta, J. L., Burke, L. M., Ross, M. L., Camera, D. M., West, D. W., Broad, E. M., Jeacocke, N. A., Moore, D. R., Stellingwerff, T., Phillips, S. M., Hawley, J. A., & Coffey, V. G. (2013). Timing and distribution of protein ingestion during prolonged recovery from resistance exercise alters myofibrillar protein synthesis. *The Journal ofPhysiology, 591*(9), 2319–2331. https://physoc.onlinelibrary.wiley.com/doi/abs/10.1113/jphysiol.2012.244897. DOI: 10.1113/jphysiol.2012.244897 PMID: 23459753

Armstrong, L. E., Maresh, C. M., Castellani, J. W., Bergeron, M. F., Kenefick, R. W., LaGasse, K. E., & Riebe, D. (1994). Urinary indices of hydration status. *International Journal of Sport Nutrition and Exercise Metabolism, 4*(3), 265–279. DOI: 10.1123/ijsn.4.3.265 PMID: 7987361

Arnarson, A., Gudny Geirsdottir, O., Ramel, A., Briem, K., Jonsson, P. V., & Thorsdottir, I. (2013). Effects of whey proteins and carbohydrates on the efficacy of resistance training in elderly people: Double blind, randomised controlled trial. *European Journal of Clinical Nutrition, 67*(8), 821–826. https://www.nature.com/articles/ejcn201340. DOI: 10.1038/ejcn.2013.40 PMID: 23486511

Babault, N., Deley, G., Le Ruyet, P., Morgan, F., & Allaert, F. A. (2014). Effects of soluble milk protein or casein supplementation on muscle fatigue following resistance training program: A randomized, double blind, and placebo-controlled study. *Journal of the International Society of Sports Nutrition, 11*(1), 36. DOI: 10.1186/1550-2783-11-36 PMID: 25057266

Bell, P. G., Walshe, I. H., Davison, G. W., Stevenson, E., & Howatson, G. (2014). Montmorency cherries reduce the oxidative stress and inflammatory responses to repeated days high-intensity stochastic cycling. *Nutrients, 6*(2), 829–843. DOI: 10.3390/nu6020829 PMID: 24566440

Bergström, J., Hermansen, L., Hultman, E., & Saltin, B. (1967). Diet, muscle glycogen and physical performance. *Acta Physiologica Scandinavica, 71*(2-3), 140–150. DOI: 10.1111/j.1748-1716.1967.tb03720.x PMID: 5584523

Betts, J. A., & Williams, C. (2010). Short-term recovery from prolonged exercise: Exploring the potential for protein ingestion to accentuate the benefits of carbohydrate supplements. Sports Medicine, 40(11), 941 959. https://doi.org/DOI: 10.2165/11536900-000000000-00000

Burke, L. M., Collier, G. R., & Hargreaves, M. (1993). Muscle glycogen storage after prolonged exercise: Effect of the glycemic index of carbohydrate feedings. *Journal of Applied Physiology (Bethesda, Md.)*, *75*(2), 1019–1023. DOI: 10.1152/jappl.1993.75.2.1019 PMID: 8226443

Burke, L. M., Hawley, J. A., Wong, S. H. S., & Jeukendrup, A. E. (2011). Carbohydrates for training and competition. *Journal of Sports Sciences*, *29*(sup1, Suppl 1), S17–S27. DOI: 10.1080/02640414.2011.585473 PMID: 21660838

Calder, P. C. (2013). Omega-3 polyunsaturated fatty acids and inflammatory processes: Nutrition or pharmacology? *British Journal of Clinical Pharmacology*, *75*(3), 645–662. DOI: 10.1111/j.1365-2125.2012.04374.x PMID: 22765297

Clark, K. L., Sebastianelli, W., Flechsenhar, K. R., Aukermann, D. F., Meza, F., Millard, R. L., Deitch, J. R., Sherbondy, P. S., & Albert, A. (2008). 24-week study on the use of collagen hydrolysate as a dietary supplement in athletes with activity-related joint pain. *Current Medical Research and Opinion*, *24*(5), 1485–1496. DOI: 10.1185/030079908X291967 PMID: 18416885

Clarkson, P. M., & Hubal, M. J. (2002). Exercise-induced muscle damage in humans. *American Journal of Physical Medicine & Rehabilitation*, *81*(11, Supplement), S52–S69. https://journals.lww.com/ajpmr/abstract/2002/11001/exercise_induced_muscle_damage_in_humans.7.aspx. DOI: 10.1097/00002060-200211001-00007 PMID: 12409811

Close, G. L., Sale, C., Baar, K., & Bermon, S. (2019). Nutrition for the prevention and treatment of injuries in track and field athletes. *International Journal of Sport Nutrition and Exercise Metabolism*, *29*(2), 189–197. DOI: 10.1123/ijsnem.2018-0290 PMID: 30676133

Dressler, P., Gehring, D., Zdzieblik, D., Oesser, S., Gollhofer, A., & König, D. (2018). Improvement of functional ankle properties following supplementation with specific collagen peptides in athletes with chronic ankle instability. *Journal of Sports Science & Medicine*, *17*(2), 298–304. https://pmc.ncbi.nlm.nih.gov/articles/PMC5950747/ PMID: 29769831

Gleeson, M. (2006). Can nutrition limit exercise-induced immunodepression? *Nutrition Reviews*, *64*(3), 119–131. DOI: 10.1111/j.1753-4887.2006.tb00195.x PMID: 16572599

Hobson, R. M., Saunders, B., Ball, G., Harris, R. C., & Sale, C. (2012). Effects of beta-alanine supplementation on exercise performance: A meta-analysis. *Amino Acids*, *43*(1), 25–37. DOI: 10.1007/s00726-011-1200-z PMID: 22270875

Howatson, G., McHugh, M. P., Hill, J. A., Brouner, J., Jewell, A. P., van Someren, K. A., Shave, R. E., & Howatson, S. A. (2010). Influence of tart cherry juice on indices of recovery following marathon running. *Scandinavian Journal of Medicine & Science in Sports*, *20*(6), 843–852. DOI: 10.1111/j.1600-0838.2009.01005.x PMID: 19883392

Impey, S. G., Hearris, M. A., Hammond, K. M., Bartlett, J. D., Louis, J., Close, G. L., & Morton, J. P. (2018). Fuel for the work required: A theoretical framework for carbohydrate periodization and the glycogen threshold hypothesis. *Sports Medicine*, *48*(5), 1031–1048. DOI: 10.1007/s40279-018-0867-7 PMID: 29453741

Ivy, J. L., Katz, A. L., Cutler, C. L., Sherman, W. M., & Coyle, E. F. (1988). Muscle glycogen synthesis after exercise: Effect of time of carbohydrate ingestion. *Journal of Applied Physiology (Bethesda, Md.)*, *64*(4), 1480–1485. DOI: 10.1152/jappl.1988.64.4.1480 PMID: 3132449

Jones, R. L., Stellingwerff, T., Artioli, G. G., Saunders, B., Cooper, S., & Sale, C. (2016). Dose-response of sodium bicarbonate ingestion highlights individuality in experience of side-effects. *International Journal of Sport Nutrition and Exercise Metabolism*, *26*(5), 445–453. DOI: 10.1123/ijsnem.2015-0286 PMID: 27098290

Jouris, K. B., McDaniel, J. L., & Weiss, E. P. (2011). The effect of omega-3 fatty acid supplementation on The inflammatory response to eccentric strength exercise. *Journal of Sports Science & Medicine*, *10*(3), 432–438. https://pmc.ncbi.nlm.nih.gov/articles/PMC3737804/ PMID: 24150614

Kenefick, R. W., & Sawka, M. N. (2007). Hydration at the work site. *Journal of the American College of Nutrition*, *26*(sup5, Suppl 5), 597S–603S. DOI: 10.1080/07315724.2007.10719665 PMID: 17921472

Kreher, J. B., & Schwartz, J. B. (2012). Overtraining syndrome: A practical guide. *Sports Health*, *4*(2), 128–138. DOI: 10.1177/1941738111434406 PMID: 23016079

Lanhers, C., Pereira, B., Naughton, G., Trousselard, M., Lesage, F. X., & Dutheil, F. (2017). Creatine supplementation and upper limb strength performance: A systematic review and meta-analysis. *Sports Medicine*, *47*(1), 163–173. DOI: 10.1007/s40279-016-0571-4 PMID: 27328852

Larson-Meyer, D. E., & Willis, K. S. (2010). Vitamin D and athletes. *Current Sports Medicine Reports*, *9*(4), 220–226. DOI: 10.1249/JSR.0b013e3181e7dd45 PMID: 20622540

Maughan, R. J., Burke, L. M., Dvorak, J., Larson-Meyer, D. E., Peeling, P., Phillips, S. M., Rawson, E. S., Walsh, N. P., Garthe, I., Geyer, H., Meeusen, R., van Loon, L. J. C., Shirreffs, S. M., Spriet, L. L., Stuart, M., Vernec, A., Currell, K., Ali, V. M., Budgett, R. G. M., & Engebretsen, L. (2018). IOC consensus statement: Dietary supplements and the high-performance athlete. *British Journal of Sports Medicine, 52*(7), 439–455. DOI: 10.1136/bjsports-2018-099027 PMID: 29540367

Maughan, R. J., Shirreffs, S. M., & Leiper, J. B. (2007). Errors in the estimation of hydration status from changes in body mass. *Journal of Sports Sciences, 25*(7), 797–804. DOI: 10.1080/02640410600875143 PMID: 17454547

Moore, D. R., Churchward-Venne, T. A., Witard, O., Breen, L., Burd, N. A., Tipton, K. D., & Phillips, S. M. (2015). Protein ingestion to stimulate myofibrillar protein synthesis requires greater relative protein intakes in healthy older versus younger men. *The Journals of Gerontology. Series A, Biological Sciences and Medical Sciences, 70*(1), 57–62. DOI: 10.1093/gerona/glu103 PMID: 25056502

Moore, D. R., Robinson, M. J., Fry, J. L., Tang, J. E., Glover, E. I., Wilkinson, S. B., Prior, T., Tarnopolsky, M. A., & Phillips, S. M. (2009). Ingested protein dose response of muscle and albumin protein synthesis after resistance exercise in young men. *The American Journal of Clinical Nutrition, 89*(1), 161–168. DOI: 10.3945/ajcn.2008.26401 PMID: 19056590

Morton, R. W., Murphy, K. T., McKellar, S. R., Schoenfeld, B. J., Henselmans, M., Helms, E., Aragon, A. A., Devries, M. C., Banfield, L., Krieger, J. W., & Phillips, S. M. (2018). A systematic review, meta analysis and meta-regression of the effect of protein supplementation on resistance training-induced gains in muscle mass and strength in healthy adults. *British Journal of Sports Medicine, 52*(6), 376–384. DOI: 10.1136/bjsports-2017-097608 PMID: 28698222

Mountjoy, M., Sundgot-Borgen, J., Burke, L., Carter, S., Constantini, N., Lebrun, C., Meyer, N., Sherman, R., Steffen, K., Budgett, R., & Ljungqvist, A. (2014). The IOC consensus statement: Beyond the Female Athlete Triad, Relative Energy Deficiency in Sport (RED-S). *British Journal of Sports Medicine, 48*(7), 491–497. DOI: 10.1136/bjsports-2014-093502 PMID: 24620037

Norton, L. E., & Layman, D. K. (2006). Leucine regulates translation initiation of protein synthesis in skeletal muscle after exercise. *The Journal of Nutrition, 136*(2), 533S–537S. DOI: 10.1093/jn/136.2.533S PMID: 16424142

Oliver, J. M., Jones, M. T., Kirk, K. M., Gable, D. A., Repshas, J. T., Johnson, T. A., Andreasen, U., Doyle, N., Benotmane, Z., & Oliver, N. (2016). Effect of docosahexaenoic acid on a biomarker of head trauma in American football. *Medicine and Science in Sports and Exercise, 48*(6), 974–982. DOI: 10.1249/MSS.0000000000000875 PMID: 26765633

Owens, D. J., Allison, R., & Close, G. L. (2018). Vitamin D and the athlete: Current perspectives and new challenges. *Sports Medicine, 48*(S1, Suppl 1), 3–16. DOI: 10.1007/s40279-017-0841-9 PMID: 29368183

Page, M. J., McKenzie, J. E., Bossuyt, P. M., Boutron, I., Hoffmann, T. C., Mulrow, C. D., Shamseer, L., Tetzlaff, J. M., & Moher, D. (2021). Updating guidance for reporting systematic reviews: Development of the PRISMA 2020 statement. *Journal of Clinical Epidemiology, 134*, 103–112. DOI: 10.1016/j.jclinepi.2021.02.003 PMID: 33577987

Patel, R. V., Mistry, B. M., Shinde, S. K., Syed, R., Singh, V., & Shin, H. S. (2018). Therapeutic potential of quercetin as a cardiovascular agent. *European Journal of Medicinal Chemistry, 155*, 889–904. DOI: 10.1016/j.ejmech.2018.06.053 PMID: 29966915

Peake, J. M., Neubauer, O., Della Gatta, P. A., & Nosaka, K. (2017). Muscle damage and inflammation during recovery from exercise. *Journal of Applied Physiology (Bethesda, Md.), 122*(3), 559–570. DOI: 10.1152/japplphysiol.00971.2016 PMID: 28035017

Phillips, S. M., & Van Loon, L. J. C. (2011). Dietary protein for athletes: From requirements to optimum adaptation. *Journal of Sports Sciences, 29*(sup1, Suppl 1), S29–S38. DOI: 10.1080/02640414.2011.619204 PMID: 22150425

Pritchett, K., & Pritchett, R. (2012). Chocolate milk: A post-exercise recovery beverage for endurance sports. *Medicine and Sport Science, 59*, 127–134. DOI: 10.1159/000341954 PMID: 23075563

Rawson, E. S., & Volek, J. S. (2003). Effects of creatine supplementation and resistance training on muscle strength and weightlifting performance. *Journal of Strength and Conditioning Research, 17*(4), 822–831. DOI: 10.1519/1533-4287(2003)017<0822:eocsart>2.0.co;2 PMID: 14636102

Res, P. T., Groen, B., Pennings, B., Beelen, M., Wallis, G. A., Gijsen, A. P., Senden, J. M. G., & Van Loon, L. J. C. (2012). Protein ingestion before sleep improves post-exercise overnight recovery. *Medicine and Science in Sports and Exercise, 44*(8), 1560–1569. DOI: 10.1249/MSS.0b013e31824cc363 PMID: 22330017

Richter, E. A., & Hargreaves, M. (2013). Exercise, GLUT4, and skeletal muscle glucose uptake. *Physiological Reviews*, *93*(3), 993–1017. DOI: 10.1152/physrev.00038.2012 PMID: 23899560

Rivera-Brown, A. M., Ramírez-Marrero, F. A., Wilk, B., & Bar-Or, O. (2006). Voluntary drinking and hydration in trained, heat-acclimatized girls exercising in a hot and humid climate. *European Journal of Applied Physiology*, *96*(2), 109–117. DOI: 10.1007/s00421-005-0060-0 PMID: 18247043

Santos, R. V., Bassit, R. A., Caperuto, E. C., & Costa Rosa, L. F. (2004). The effect of creatine supplementation upon inflammatory and muscle soreness markers after a 30km race. *Life Sciences*, *75*(16), 1917–1924. DOI: 10.1016/j.lfs.2003.11.036 PMID: 15306159

Sawka, M. N., Burke, L. M., Eichner, E. R., Maughan, R. J., Montain, S. J., & Stachenfeld, N. S. (2007). American College of Sports Medicine position stand: Exercise and fluid replacement. *Medicine and Science in Sports and Exercise*, *39*(2), 377–390. DOI: 10.1249/mss.0b013e31802ca597 PMID: 17277604

Schwellnus, M. P., Derman, W. E., & Noakes, T. D. (2011). Aetiology of skeletal muscle 'cramps' during exercise: A novel hypothesis. *Journal of Sports Sciences*, *15*(3), 277–285. DOI: 10.1080/026404197367281 PMID: 9232553

Shaw, G., Lee-Barthel, A., Ross, M. L., Wang, B., & Baar, K. (2017). Vitamin C-enriched gelatin supplementation before intermittent activity augments collagen synthesis. *The American Journal of Clinical Nutrition*, *105*(1), 136–143. DOI: 10.3945/ajcn.116.138594 PMID: 27852613

Shirreffs, S. M., Taylor, A. J., Leiper, J. B., & Maughan, R. J. (1996). Post-exercise rehydration in man: Effects of volume consumed and drink sodium content. *Medicine and Science in Sports and Exercise*, *28*(10), 1260–1271. DOI: 10.1097/00005768-199610000-00009 PMID: 8897383

Siripipatthanakul, S., Rungsiyanont, S., & Siripipattanakul, S. (2026). Sustainable dentistry using artificial intelligence (AI) for digital education and business among university dental hospitals. In *Sustainable development for hospitals and clinics* (pp. 33–64). IGI Global Scientific Publishing., DOI: 10.4018/979-8-3693-9800-5.ch002

Smith, G. I., Atherton, P., Reeds, D. N., Mohammed, B. S., Rankin, D., Rennie, M. J., & Mittendorfer, B. (2011). Omega-3 polyunsaturated fatty acids augment the muscle protein anabolic response to hyperinsulinaemia-hyperaminoacidaemia in healthy young and middle-aged men and women. *Clinical Science (London, England)*, *121*(6), 267–278. DOI: 10.1042/CS20100597 PMID: 21501117

Snijders, T., Res, P. T., Smeets, J. S., van Vliet, S., van Kranenburg, J., Maase, K., Kies, A. K., Verdijk, L. B., & van Loon, L. J. (2015). Protein Ingestion before Sleep Increases Muscle Mass and Strength Gains during Prolonged Resistance-Type Exercise Training in Healthy Young Men. *The Journal of Nutrition, 145*(6), 1178–1184. DOI: 10.3945/jn.114.208371 PMID: 25926415

Tanabe, Y., Maeda, S., Akazawa, N., Zempo-Miyaki, A., Choi, Y., Ra, S. G., Imaizumi, A., Ohmori, H., & Nosaka, K. (2015). Attenuation of indirect markers of eccentric exercise-induced muscle damage by curcumin. *European Journal of Applied Physiology, 115*(9), 1949–1957. DOI: 10.1007/s00421-015-3170-4 PMID: 25921600

Thomas, D. T., Erdman, K. A., & Burke, L. M. (2016). American College of Sports Medicine joint position statement: Nutrition and athletic performance. *Medicine and Science in Sports and Exercise, 48*(3), 543–568. DOI: 10.1249/MSS.0000000000000852 PMID: 26891166

Tipton, K. D., Borsheim, E., Wolf, S. E., Sanford, A. P., & Wolfe, R. R. (2004). Acute response of net muscle protein balance reflects 24-h balance after exercise and amino acid ingestion. *American Journal of Physiology. Endocrinology and Metabolism, 284*(1), E76–E89. DOI: 10.1152/ajpendo.00234.2002 PMID: 12388164

Tipton, K. D., Elliott, T. A., Cree, M. G., Aarsland, A. A., Sanford, A. P., & Wolfe, R. R. (2007). Stimulation of net muscle protein synthesis by whey protein ingestion before and after exercise. *American Journal of Physiology. Endocrinology and Metabolism, 292*(1), E71–E76. DOI: 10.1152/ajpendo.00166.2006 PMID: 16896166

Tipton, K. D., & Witard, O. C. (2007). Protein requirements and recommendations for athletes: Relevance of ivory tower arguments for practical recommendations. *Clinics in Sports Medicine, 26*(1), 17–36. DOI: 10.1016/j.csm.2006.11.003 PMID: 17241913

Tripkovic, L., Lambert, H., Hart, K., Smith, C. P., Bucca, G., Penson, S., Chope, G., Hyppönen, E., Berry, J., Vieth, R., & Lanham-New, S. (2012). Comparison of vitamin D2 and vitamin D3 supplementation in raising serum 25-hydroxyvitamin D status: A systematic review and meta-analysis. *The American Journal of Clinical Nutrition, 95*(6), 1357–1364. DOI: 10.3945/ajcn.111.031070 PMID: 22552031

Witard, O. C., Jackman, S. R., Breen, L., Smith, K., Selby, A., & Tipton, K. D. (2014). Myofibrillar muscle protein synthesis rates subsequent to a meal in response to small and large bolus doses of dairy protein. *The American Journal of Clinical Nutrition, 99*(1), 86–95. DOI: 10.3945/ajcn.112.055517 PMID: 24257722

Wolfe, R. R. (2017). Branched-chain amino acids and muscle protein synthesis in humans: Myth or reality? *Journal of the International Society of Sports Nutrition, 14*(1), 30. DOI: 10.1186/s12970-017-0184-9 PMID: 28852372

Zawadzki, K. M., Yaspelkis, B. B.III, & Ivy, J. L. (1992). Carbohydrate-protein complex increases the rate of muscle glycogen storage after exercise. *Journal of Applied Physiology (Bethesda, Md.), 72*(5), 1854–1859. https://journals.physiology.org/doi/abs/10.1152/jappl.1992.72.5.1854.DOI: 10.1152/jappl.1992.72.5.1854 PMID: 1601794

KEY TERMS AND DEFINITIONS

Anti-Inflammatory Nutrition: Dietary strategies involving nutrients like omega-3 fatty acids, polyphenols, and antioxidants to regulate inflammation and support recovery.

Athletes' Performance Enhancement and Injury Prevention: Athletes need the right nutrition to improve their performance and avoid injuries. They need a diet high in carbs for energy, lean proteins for muscle repair, and healthy fats for cellular function. Staying hydrated and getting enough calcium, vitamin D, and iron are important for bone health, immunological function, and oxygen delivery. They also lower the risk of weariness and stress injuries. Also, planning meals and snacks around workouts guarantees that energy is used and recovered quickly. In the end, personalized nutrition regimens that take into account the athlete's sport, training intensity, and specific demands are very important for achieving peak performance and reducing the risk of injury.

Evidence-based nutritional Strategies: It is about treatments for functional recovery, stress, a tailored, all-around approach to healing tissue, boosting energy, and controlling inflammation. The "4R's" framework; Rehydrate, Refuel, Repair, and Revitalize/Recuperate. It is a key part of both sports and clinical rehabilitation. It ensures you get enough macro- and micronutrients to speed up healing.

Exercise-Induced Muscle Damage (EIMD): Structural damage to muscle fibers caused by intense or unfamiliar exercise, leading to soreness, inflammation, and temporary loss of strength.

Glycogen Resynthesis: The process of restoring depleted muscle glycogen stores after exercise through carbohydrate intake, essential for recovery and subsequent performance.

Hydration and Electrolyte Balance: The maintenance of body fluid levels and essential minerals (such as sodium and potassium) to support physiological function, thermoregulation, and performance.

Muscle Protein Synthesis (MPS): The biological process of building new muscle proteins, stimulated by resistance exercise and protein consumption, crucial for muscle repair and adaptation.

Chapter 11
Anti-Inflammatory Nutrition Strategy for Athletes' Performance and Recovery

Swapan Banerjee
http://orcid.org/0000-0001-5781-5436
Poornima University, India

Udit Mamodiya
http://orcid.org/0000-0002-8022-4252
Poornima University, India

Pichakoon Auttawetchasakoon
http://orcid.org/0000-0002-2247-6750
Sukhothai Thammathirat Open University, Thailand

ABSTRACT

Athletes everywhere are looking for more anti-inflammatory foods to crush their performance and recovery. This chapter aims to highlight and systematically review the hypothesized implications of an anti-inflammatory dietary pattern for diet adequacy and for performance during peak exercise training and recovery after endurance or strength exertion. The review provides an overview of the biology of post-acute and chronic inflammation induced by exercise, with a special focus on redox-sensitive elements believed to act as trigger pathways, as well as those associated with immune function and musculoskeletal repair. This chapter summarizes recent knowledge about anti-inflammatory nutritional factors, i.e., omega-3 fatty acids, and single micronutrients, that adjust central pathways of inflammation and

DOI: 10.4018/979-8-3373-9544-9.ch011

immune-metabolism. It also offers applied, periodized practicalities for incorporating these foods into athlete-specific sport nutrition plans during training, competition, and injury, in relation to energy-balance perspectives, including complementary micro- and macronutrient balance.

1. INTRODUCTION

Intensive training and competition initiate an inflammatory and oxidative stress response that is synchronized and necessary for tissue repair and adaptation. However, they may be damaging in conditions of overload or constant high-level training (Akbari-Fakhrabadi et al., 2024). It is possible to adapt to such low-grade inflammation without experiencing recovery issues, sleep disturbances, or excessive training loads, which can cause fatigue, overtraining, and an increased risk of injury (Suzuki, 2021). It, in turn, is more diet-intervention-oriented, targeting the prevalence of exercise-elicited inflammation rather than interfering with or aggravating training responses (Barnes, 2023).

Anti-inflammatory dietary foods are characterized by high levels of omega-3 fatty acids, polyphenols, antioxidant micronutrients, and fiber, and moderate levels of pro-inflammatory foods, such as saturated fat, trans fat, and ultra-processed foods (Simopoulos, 2015). Athletes are subjected to such a pattern to support overactive energy intake and sport-specific macronutrient requirements, and it should be timed effectively relative to a training session, a game, or a sports injury (Harty et al., 2019). This chapter discusses the biology behind exercise-induced inflammation, reviews existing studies on the anti-inflammatory effects of foods and nutrients, and provides an effective model for integrating these strategies into the performance nutrition of a sports athlete. The specifics of high-performance sport are characterized by the tediousness of the loads of overwhelming intensity, the intervals of recovery, and the fact that athletes, in their turn, train more than once a day; their matches are scheduled in the perspective of a hectic schedule with no periods of physiological respite . During these extreme trials, athletes are exposed to high mechanical and metabolic demands, which cause muscle injuries typical of training and competition (Barnes, 2023; Harty et al., 2019). Central to all of these processes is the multifaceted, tightly regulated process of inflammation, which can be either adaptive or, in chronic or excessive inflammation, a potential cause of maladaptation (Zouhal et al., 2020).

Exercise-induced inflammation is not always harmful; instead, it stimulates many structural and functional processes, such as muscle remodeling, angiogenesis, and mitochondrial biogenesis, which occur during training (Ferrer et al., 2015). Exercise can result in temporary waves of pro-inflammatory cytokines, e.g., IL-6 and TNF-α, neutrophil and macrophage recruitment in injured tissue, and a concerted downstream protective and adaptive response mediated by redox-sensitive transcription factors, e.g., NF-κB and AP-1 (Ferrer et al., 2015). These acute inflammatory exaltations are also accompanied by anti-inflammatory and pro-resolving signals to reestablish homeostasis and supercompensation, although recovery, namely nutrition and sleep, must be satisfactory (Harty et al., 2019). The low-grade inflammatory state is driven by cyclic processes that break or hyper-stimulate the cycle, leading to a system that wastes resources and harms health and performance (Xiong et al., 2024). As far as performance is concerned, chronic and low-grade inflammation has been linked to increased disease susceptibility, excessive fatigue, mood alterations, dysfunctional muscular function, and reduced training responses . The gastrointestinal symptoms and the elevated rates of infection of the upper respiratory tract, which are provoked by the large amounts of training in high-endurance athletes in comparison with heat stress, dehydration, and repeated competitions, can be pre-empted by the long-term increases of CRP, IL-6 6 and other inflammatory factors (Barnes, 2023). An adequate recovery period and nutritional support are not exempt for team-sport athletes with a high game load or for strength-power athletes during a strenuous loading phase, as inflammatory loading increases in such situations (Harty et al., 2019). In the current study, methods that modify rather than suppress inflammation, thereby enhancing its acute benefits and eliminating its chronic exacerbations, are highly desirable (Close & Peake, 2018; Barnes, 2023).

The reason that nutrition should be characterized as one of the prime modulating factors among all these modulating strategies is that it is capable of altering inflammation in most of the modulating mechanisms that intersect with each other (such as adiposity, glycemic and lipemic responses, oxidative stress, the production of eicosanoids, the composition of gut microbiota, etc.) (Simopoulos, 2015; Xiong et al., 2024). Excessive intake of ultra-processed foods, refined starch, added sugar, and industrial trans fats is consistently linked to high dietary inflammatory index scores, elevated CRP levels, and elevated IL-6 and TNF-α levels (Xiong et al., 2024). Quite the contrary, the diets that include the highest percentage of vegetables and fruits, whole grains, legumes, nuts and seeds, and fatty fish, such as the Mediterranean one, are marked by a lower concentration of inflammatory biomarkers, improved metabolism, and reduced risk of chronic diseases (Xiong et al., 2024). The dietary properties that prevent non-communicable diseases and, at the same time, provide an inner environment that promotes rapid recovery and prolonged heavy workloads are also evident in this instanceAn anti-inflammatory diet is a dietary trend that prioritizes foods with known or potential anti-inflammatory action, which, in most cases, share many features with other dietary trends (Mediterranean and vegetarian) (Yu et al., 2024). Instead, rather than consuming red and processed meat and generous amounts of saturated and trans fats, the given diets are characterized by huge percentages of fruits, vegetables, whole grains, legumes, fatty fish, nuts, olive oil, spices, and herbs (Yu et al., 2024). Anti-inflammatory diets, in their turn, are associated with the delivery of omega-3 fatty acids, antioxidants, and polyphenols, which can suppress the expression of inflammatory genes, lower the level of circulating inflammatory biomarkers, and improve the functioning of the endothelium and insulin sensitivity (Yu et al., 2024; Thielecke & Blannin, 2020). Although most of the evidence is attributed to chronic disorders, the same set of biological processes applies to athletes who experience frequent episodes of exercise-induced inflammation despite general lifestyle and genetic risk factors (Barnes, 2023).

Sports nutrition has been a particular area of interest, and specific nutrients and food categories have been studied to understand their roles in mitigating exercise-induced muscle damage (EIMD), soreness, and secondary inflammation. The EIMD symptoms are ultrastructural muscle damage, muscle strength loss, DOMS, and high plasma biomarkers such as CK and myoglobin, which are likely to peak at some time in 24-72hours of unaccustomed/ eccentric exercise (Harty et al., 2019; Close and Peake, 2018). Nutritional prevention of EIMD involves reducing symptoms to a level that does not impair the quality of training or competition, without affecting the signaling events that underlie adaptation (Barnes, 2023; Crum et al., 2023). Of the studied candidates, the most promising are omega-3 fatty acids and polyphenols of fruit origin, and, in particular, tart cherry and berry extracts, which have the most substantial evidence to date of the ability to improve recovery indices in an exercised person (Crum et al., 2023). In the meantime, the circumstances in which the desired dietary habits are applied are critical. The implication is even stronger: high-dose supplementation is unproductive and potentially detrimental, e.g., by counteracting the effects of training with high-dose antioxidants (Ferrer et al., 2015; Close and Peake, 2018). A preferable option is food-first, where anti-inflammatory diets are adhered to daily and, in some instances, anti-inflammatory foods and, in some cases, specifically targeted supplements are consumed to address particular requirements, such as unusually intense training, competitions, or even post-injury healing (Barnes, 2023). This holistic vision can be linked to the notion that the most useful recovery aid is often a simple, readily accessible, and relatively inexpensive food already on most sportsmen's menus.

Diet books dedicated to athletes are getting increasingly rich in the foods that are categorized as the most anti-inflammatory ones to alleviate pain, prevent injury, and accelerate the recovery plan: fatty fish, berries, leafy greens, nuts, and seeds, turmeric, ginger, olive oil, and whole grains (Clean Eatz Kitchen, 2026). As a rule, the proposed recommendations will be consistent with the scientific principles and tendencies, which presuppose the use of the sources of omega-3 and polyphenols, and unsaturated fat as the primary components of an anti-inflammatory diet pattern (Yu et al., 2024). In practice, one can state that the anti-inflammatory nutrition of sports participants is related to the conscious consumption of such products, as well as a specific reduction in the intake of pro-inflammatory foods, such as sugary drinks, processed meat, and highly refined snack foods (Impulse Nutrition, 2025). As a combination of the consumption of the protective foods and the elimination of the provocative foods, this two-fold solution is particularly essential in the context of the practice, whereby the sportsmen are restricted based on the time, transportation, the company the sportsmen choose to provide catering services, and the cultural preferences (Clean Eatz Kitchen, 2026). It should be noted that issues related to anti-inflammatory diets in sport cannot be addressed outside the framework of the primary issues in sport nutrition, namely adequate total energy intake, carbohydrate availability, and protein balance. Low energy intake and extreme weight-controlling practices may induce cortisol and inflammatory biomarkers, inhibit immune function, and delay recovery, regardless of diet quality. Similarly, carbohydrate deficiency before high-intensity exercise can increase stress hormone activity and impair the immune response, leading to acute inflammation that may progress to chronic inflammation (Barnes, 2023; Caballero-García et al., 2023). In that regard, anti-inflammatory foods should be included in the nutrition plans and arrangements to meet the energy and macronutrient requirements of the specific sport, training, and an athlete (Yu et al., 2024; Simopoulos, 2015; Crum et al., 2023).

2. LITERATURE REVIEW

2.1 Redox Signaling Upon Exercise, Biology

2.1.1 Acute and Chronic Responses

Exercise-induced muscle damage (EIMD) (namely, muscle movement of an eccentric nature) that occurs following strenuous or new exercise and is accompanied by destruction of sarcomeres, distortion of the membrane, and the release of muscle-specific enzymes (creatine kinase, lactate dehydrogenase, etc.) is considered muscle damage that results from muscle movement. This primary lesion triggers the progression of the acute inflammation phase, which includes neutrophils and macrophages, release of cytokines (e.g., interleukin-6 [IL-6], IL-8, tumor necrosis factor-alpha [TNF-alpha]), and formation of reactive oxygen species (ROS) (Lynn et al., 2019; Rojano-Ortega et al., 2020). Given the imperative of such events for debris clearance and tissue modeling in hours to days following the exercise, they were associated with delayed-onset muscle soreness (DOMS), transient muscular incompetence, and neurological incapacity (Harty et al., 2019; San Juan et al., 2019). The constant training of appropriate volumes will reduce the focus on basic inflammatory variables. It will enhance long-term antioxidant protection. Long-term high or insufficient compensation will not substantially reduce the high levels of C-reactive protein (CRP) and pro-inflammatory cytokines (Nieman & Wentz, 2019; Akbari-Fakhrabadi et al., 2024). It is an inflammatory disease of the system; it is associated with overtraining, disease, and tendencies toward poor adjustment in specific situations in the presence of energy and micronutrient deficits (Suzuki, 2021).

2.1.2 Redox-Sensitive and Immune Control

Exercise results in the formation of ROS that causes trafficking of redox-sensitive signaling transcription factors, including the nuclear factor kappa B (NF-kB) and nuclear factor erythroid 2 2 related factor 2 (Nrf2) (Powers et al., 2011). NF-kB stimulates the production of pro-inflammatory cytokines and adhesion molecules, and Nrf2 stimulates the production of antioxidant and cytoprotective proteins, which represents a balance between damage and adaptation (Peake et al., 2017; Suzuki, 2021). Otherwise, the signs of the oxidative stress have been counteracted in the in-vitro environment using experimental supplementation of the antioxidants (e.g., N-acetylcysteine, high-level vitamin C, and E) alone, but in that case, compromised adaptations of mitochondria and performance, demonstrating that too much of such inhibition is counteractive (Pingitore et al., 2015; Ristow & Schmeisser, 2014). This may be because it shifts the process of recruiting immune cells to the damaged muscle from an anti-inflammatory M2 Phenotype to a more pro-inflammatory M1 Phenotype, resulting in muscular resolution and regeneration (Peake et al., 2017). However, this phenotypic change is preventable with potentially acute suppressive interventions, and regeneration can be slowed. This is why nutrition interventions can manage, but not prevent, inflammatory reactions (Barnes, 2023; Suzuki, 2021).

2.2 Nutritional Quality, Energy Sufficiency, and Inflammation in Sportspersons

2.2.1 Availability, Systemic Inflammation

Low energy availability (LEA) related to endocrine imbalances, menstrual disruptions, bone density, and immune system impairments is linked to endurance, weight-category, and aesthetic sports (Mountjoy et al., 2018).

2.2.2 Macronutrients, Postprandial Inflammation

A diet high in carbohydrates, added sugar, and saturated and trans fats may promote the development of postprandial endotoxemia, oxidative stress, and cytokine production (Minihane et al., 2015). On the other hand, whole-grain foods, unsaturated fats, legumes, fruits, and vegetable-based foods can decrease CRP and pro-inflammatory cytokines in both active and sedentary populations (Estruch et al., 2018; Willett et al., 2019). Poor recovery and long-term adaptation to high-volume exercise among members, in turn, are predetermined by the pro-inflammatory environment created by dietary practices, driven by the high concentration of ultra-processed convenience foods (Akbari-Fakhrabadi et al., 2024; Suzuki, 2021). Deficiencies in vitamin D, vitamin C, vitamin E, B vitamins, iron, zinc, magnesium, and selenium can impair immune function, antioxidant defense, and muscle metabolism (Close et al., 2016; Pingitore et al., 2015; Córdova et al., 2022). An impaired micronutrient status may exacerbate oxidative stress during exercise, prolong the inflammatory recovery period, and predispose to infections (Nieman & Wentz, 2019; Suzuki, 2021). The so-called food-first strategy that is founded on the choice of various food products of the vegetarian type (plant-based foods), dairy products, or fortified food, and, in some instances, supplementation, depending on the results of biochemistry and clinical judgment, is suggested (Jeukendrup, 2017; Maughan et al., 2018).

2.2.3 The Noteworthy Anti-Inflammatory Bioactive Compounds and Nutrients

Formation: The omega-3 fatty acids (EPA and DHA) consist of long-chain fatty acids, which are highly significant constituents of the brain, without which the brain can be damaged.

These anti-inflammatory effects are attributed to omega-3 acids of the marine and algal sources (eicosapentaenoic acid [EPA] and docosahexaenoic acid [DHA]), which contain the substitution of the arachidonic acid in the cell membrane and block the synthesis of pro-inflammatory eicosanoids, and the synthesis of special pro-resolving mediators (Calder, 2015; Simopoulos, 2015). The omega-3 supplementation was revealed to possess the potential to decrease the indices of IL-6, TNF-α, CRP, and muscle damage and have the potential to enhance the perceived recovery index and other cardiorespiratory performance indices in both systematic reviews and meta-analyses of the healthy and athlete population (Fernández-Lázaro et al., 2024; Silva et al., 2024). However, the influence on maximal strength and power performance is less accurate, whereas the influence on soreness and inflammatory biomarkers is more robust (Harty et al., 2019; Simopoulos, 2015). The anti-inflammatory dose is usually 1-3 g/day of the EPA-DHA combination throughout the week, with higher doses used for short-term actions (Simopoulos, 2015; Fernández-Lázaro et al., 2024). The workable sources recommend oily fish (e.g., salmon, mackerel, sardines), fortified or high-grade fish oil, or algal oil supplements to supplement intakes only when dietary intake is incomplete (Calder, 2015).

2.2.4 Drinks and Fruits Containing High Polyphenols

EIMD prevention and recovery assistance can be achieved through polyphenols, which exhibit antioxidant, anti-inflammatory, and vasomodulatory effects (Barnes, 2023; Crum et al., 2023). A tart cherry and pomegranate have been the most studied interventions of polyphenol-containing products in the sports field; some of the researchers have reported the reduction of oxidative and inflammatory biomarkers and increased strength recovery and soreness, whereas others have not reported any results (Rojano-Ortega et al., 2020; Lynn et al., 2019).

Meta-analysis and systematic review of tart cherry supplement in athletes have shown that tart cherry was an effective intervention for post-exercise creatine kinase in a weak and not consistent way, and not DOMS, which clearly revealed that protocol, dose, and exercise model were meaningful (Rojano-Ortega et al., 2020). This was observed to be positive for pomegranate, which is used several days prior to and after a workout, thereby affecting oxidative stress, inflammation, and functional recovery (Trombold et al., 2011; Lynn et al., 2019).

2.2.5 Curcumin and the Specific Bioactive

The antioxidant property of such a molecule and the ability to modify the NF-kB pathway and enzyme fitter, also known as cyclooxygenase (COX), explain why the perspectives of curcumin, which is the primary polyphenol of turmeric, to reduce DOMS and inflammatory markers are possible (McFarlin et al., 2016; Nicol et al., 2015). Reduced levels of inflammatory biomarkers and reduced rigidity in recreationally active and trained individuals are more commonly reported in the context of muscle-damaging exercise, with variable formulations and bioavailability, and are difficult to interpret (McFarlin et al., 2016; Tanabe et al., 2015). The rest of the compounds, such as quercetin, resveratrol, bromelain, and glucosamine, have yet to be proven to have a mechanistic potential for sport in a concerted and conclusive manner (Crum et al., 2023; Suzuki, 2021).

2.3 Vitamin and Antioxidant Minerals

The usage of vitamin C and vitamin E as high-dose, individual supplements might be appropriate since they might prevent signs of oxidative stress in relation to strenuous exercise, even though other research findings indicate that they inhibit biogenesis at the mitochondrion as well, and adaptations of endurance level (Paulsen et al., 2014). Based on current guidelines, long-term supplementation with high-dose antioxidants should be replaced with food-based antioxidant interventions to avoid excessive effects on redox markers in well-trained athletes (Pingitore et al., 2015;

Jeukendrup, 2017). High levels of selenium, zinc, and magnesium are required to support high enzyme performance and immune function, but excessive supplementation is not promoted as a performance aid (Close et al., 2016; Maughan et al., 2018).

2.4 Sporting Dietary Patterns of Anti-Inflammatory

2.4.1 Eats in a Mediterranean Fashion

The reduced level of systemic inflammation and a healthier cardiometabolic profile are consistently linked to Mediterranean-style diets (high intake of extra-virgin olive oil, nuts, seeds, whole grains, legumes, fruits, and vegetables) (Estruch et al., 2018; Schwingshackl & Hoffmann, 2015). The synergistic nature of monounsaturated and omega-3 fatty acids, polyphenols, fiber, and micronutrient density creates an anti-inflammatory state that can be easily adjusted to meet the increased energy and protein needs of athletes (Simopoulos, 2015; Willett et al., 2019). Changes such as increased carbohydrate intake during major events and overall protein intake (e.g., 1.6-2.2 g/kg/day) can be used to shift this trend toward new trends in sports nutrition (Jeukendrup, 2017; Maughan et al., 2018).

2.4.2 Vegetarian Food, Plant-Based Diets

It is possible that, with promising energy and adequate nutrient content, minimally processed vegetable foods can positively affect markers of inflammation and oxidative stress (Craddock et al., 2016). High in legumes, soy, whole grains, nuts, and seeds, and a wide variety of colorful fruits and vegetables, these foods contain fiber, polyphenols, and micronutrients that are beneficial for immune and redox processes (Suzuki, 2021; Crum et al., 2023). Specifically, B12, iron, zinc, iodine, calcium, and omega-3 fatty acids are necessary and may be needed by plant-based athletes to counterbalance deficiencies that could deteriorate performance and recovery (Craig et al., 2021).

2.4.3 Reduction of the Proinflammatory Constituents of Food

The amounts of industrial trans fats, saturated fat, refined starches, added sugars, and processed meat may be high to reduce postprandial inflammation and improve vascular function (Minihane et al., 2015; Willett et al., 2019). Their replacement with unsaturated fats (e.g., olive oil, nuts, and seeds), whole grains, and non-animal sources of protein is associated with performance and long-term health-related benefits, including reduced cardiovascular risk and increased metabolic flexibility (Estruch et al., 2018; Calder, 2015).

2.4.4 The Association Between the Omega-3 Supplement and the Performance of the Athlete

The systematic review of randomized controlled trials, which was conducted by physically healthy adults, was able to conclude that omega-3 supplementation could prevent the post-exercise response of IL-6, TNF-α, and CRP, and could prevent the indices of muscle injury and oxidative damage, and could improve some of the indices of endurance performance (Mohammadi et al., 2025). Meta-analytic data from healthy individuals who consume omega-3 demonstrate significant systemic inflammatory responses with omega-3 intake, providing sufficient evidence of omega-3's capacity to counter the effects of inflammation associated with EIMD (Silva et al., 2024). Omega-3 supplementation appears to be beneficial for subjective soreness and joint pain, but not necessarily for power and strength in sports groups (Simopoulos, 2015; Harty et al., 2019).

Figure 1. Anti-inflammatory nutrition, Athletes' performance, and recovery

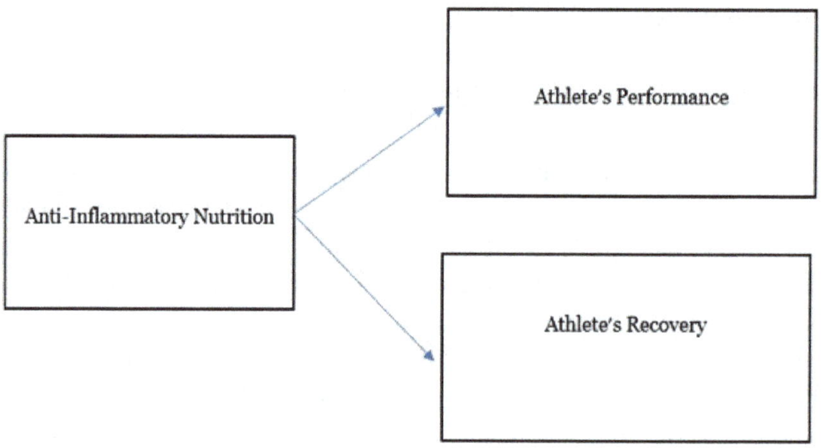

Figure 1 shows the conceptual framework of anti-inflammatory foods beneficial for athletes' performance cum recovery aspects.

2.5 Periodized Sport Nutrition, Applied, Anti-Inflammatory

2.5.1 Daily "Base" Diet

Among the athletes, a basic diet, including all the most important ideas of sports nutrition and the elements of anti-inflammation, is beneficial on most of the training days; it consists of adequate energy, a high percentage of carbohydrates before the most significant training classes, adequate protein content, and the Mediterranean or plant-based profile (Jeukendrup, 2017; Estruch et al., 2018). Practically, it means that one should consume a large amount of fruits and vegetable products, whole grains, legumes, nuts, seeds, extra-virgin olive oil, and eat a high amount of regular fish rich in omega-3 or supplements that contain EPA/DHA regularly and limit consumption of ultra-processed foods and beverages sweetened with sugar (Willett et al., 2019; Simopoulos, 2015).

2.5.2 Strategy Implementation in the High Training and Competition

Greater days of activity or days when new dietary supplements containing polyphenols should be introduced, as it is effective even in the absence of desensitization of adaptive indicators over time (Harty et al., 2019; Barnes, 2023). As a protocol, it can also be used with Pomegranate juice or sour cherry at least several days before a potentially damaging event to the muscles, and for 3-7 days, with at least 1,000 mg of polyphenols daily (Rojano-Ortega et al., 2020). The specific bioactivity (curcumin) should be administered occasionally, not every day, but on days of overload competitions, not during high-microcycle muscle devastation (McFarlin et al., 2016).

2.5.3 Stages of Injury and Rehabilitation

Regarding injury, local injury, immobilization, and reduced loading are all risk factors for atrophy and disturbances in muscle metabolism (Tipton, 2011). Protein consumption should also not be reduced and may even be increased (e.g., 1.8-2.2 g/kg/day), the consumption of food rich in leucine is required, and food rich in omega-3 should be consumed to trigger muscle protein synthesis and prevent inflammation in case it can be present (Calder, 2015; Close et al., 2016). The clue to anti-inflammatory foods of whole-food origin (e.g., fatty fish, extra-virgin olive oil, nuts, colorful vegetables, and fruits) as a component of the energy intake according to the lowered activity level can not only aid in the recovery but also lead to an increase (Jeukendrup, 2017; Suzuki, 2021).

2.5.4 Example Day of Eating

The typical day of an athlete with high training needs is most likely to include: breakfast oatmeal with blended berries, ground flax, Greek yogurt; lunch mid-day with quinoa and lentils with blended vegetables and dressing based on olive oil; snack before athletic activity including banana and green tea; evening and big salad;

snack evening in high-training weeks which includes tart cherry juice as well (Je This trend gives energy to the performers by providing them with).

2.6 Individualization and Pragmatic Assessment: Assessment and Monitoring

Its successful implementation is possible through assessment of first nutritional habits, energy intake, micronutrient status, gastrointestinal tolerance, and training/competition diets (Maughan et al., 2018). To direct the exact investigations and measure the effectiveness of the custom-designed interventions, the practical measures will be the food diary, validated indicators of diet quality (e.g., CRP, vitamin D, ferritin, B12), and symptom diaries (e.g., soreness rating, illness episodes, GI symptoms) (Nieman & Wentz, 2019; Suzuki, 2021).

2.7 Finding the Right Balance Between Short- and Long-Term Performance and Wellbeing

Alternatively, others may overuse pharmacologic anti-inflammatory drugs, such as NSAIDs, or take antioxidant supplements in excessive amounts to treat soreness and accelerate the return to training, thereby reducing tissue integrity and long-term adaptation (Barnes, 2023; Peake et al., 2017). The anti-inflammatory food-first strategy offers a lower-risk approach and, concurrently, helps achieve cardiovascular, metabolic, and cognitive health and performance goals (Estruch et al., 2018; Willett et al., 2019). These discussions on the beneficial or adverse consequences of such patterns ought to be synthesized to increase compliance among sports nutrition professionals, coaches, and athletes (Gamba et al., 2023).

2.8 Critical Review of the Chapter

The anti-inflammatory nutrition forms part of athletic performance and recovery, and has been integrated promptly into the chapter. However, it also illustrates several methodological, evidential, and translational flaws that must be eradicated in subsequent versions. In general, it aligns with the latest trends in sports nutrition, focusing on food quality, nutrition programs, and gut health. However, it can be improved through further evaluation of the evidence, which would provide greater specificity in its implementation and allow for more consideration of other dietary paradigms. Among the strengths of the chapter is its description of inflammation as a two-sided sword in sport, with successful acute-type inflammation and damaging chronic-type low-grade inflammation . A biologically plausible explanation for the role of diet in athletes might involve redox-sensitive transcription factors, cytokine cascades, and gut-derived endotoxemia (Ferrer et al., 2015; Akbari-Fakhrabadi et al., 2024). Dietary factors and inflammation, and the justification for interest in omega-3 fatty acids, polyphenols, and Mediterranean-style patterns, are well-established mechanisms supported by high-quality reviews (Simopoulos, 2015; Xiong et al., 2024). Another good thing about the chapter is its food-first approach, which is consistent with current knowledge that whole foods and eating habits form the basis of sport nutrition practice (Close et al., 2022; Xiong et al., 2024). Its firsthand caution about unconsidered excessive doses of antioxidants raised without pre-established practice, and about how a particular intervention can undo training changes, is up-to-date proof of both mechanistic and practical research (Ferrer et al., 2015). Besides, it introduces gut-focused (fiber, polyphenols, fermented foods) interventions, which can be rationalized by recent studies on the microbiome-immune-performance relationships, and shifts the discourse onto individual nutrients .

However, the narrative review format, which is appropriate for general and theory-oriented chapters, inevitably introduces both selection and confirmation biases, which are offset by semi-structured procedures also presented throughout the rest of the manuscript (Furley & Goldschmied, 2021). The research studies that provide positive or encouraging outcomes to support the chapter are supported by the relative lack of attention to the studies that may not report anything negative or inconclusive outcomes (e.g., inconsistent associations between dietary scores of inflammatory indices and some chronic illness risk, anti-inflammatory diets that fail to convince that they are better than control diets in controlled feeding studies, etc.) (Xiong et al., 2024). The second weakness is the extent to which evidence from the general or clinical group can justify cases of elite athletes. Cohort studies of patients with metabolic syndrome, cardiovascular risk factors, or arthritis reveal that a substantial proportion of the most valuable sources of information on anti-inflammatory diets are patients with these conditions (Xiong et al., 2024; Simopoulos, 2015). The possibility of extrapolating the use of mechanistic pathways is limited, and the level of benefit may differ, as in young, metabolically fit yet highly stressed athletes. Moreover, according to the same, the available evidence regarding omega-3 and polyphenols is mainly characterized by small sample sizes, short-duration interventions, and surrogate endpoints (e.g., CK, IL-6), but not by season-long performance or injury outcomes (Barnes, 2023; Crum et al., 2023).

Recent articles have identified the positive and negative aspects of these trendy diets on performance and health, including the potential for micronutrient deficiencies with poorly balanced vegan diets and the possible negative impacts on high-intensity performance and immune dysregulation with chronic carbohydrate dieting (Smith et al., 2023; Close et al., 2022; Schek, 2025).

In practice, the chapter offers real-world examples and time frames, but further critique of their practicality and compliance would enhance the translation's applicability. Anecdotal evidence on the nutrient demands of sportspeople indicates that even the minimum requirements of sports nutrition are not necessarily the most suitable and depend on levels of knowledge, availability, culture, and prosperity. School situations, family history, and food literacy significantly contribute to predicting adherence to Mediterranean or anti-inflammatory dietary patterns among junior or developing athletes (Amawi et al., 2024). The chapter itself mentions the very fact of the adaptation to the culture. However, it does not address many of the barriers to cultural adaptation, such as the cost of certain foods (e.g., fatty fish, foreign berries), constraints on service delivery within a team, and the tendency towards restrictive eating promoted by social media, which may escalate into disordered eating. In a more critical methodological approach, a stricter division of the evidence's force into areas (strong, moderate, limited, or emerging) would be helpful for a formal nutrition evidence assessment (NESR, 2019). Placing omega-3 and tart cherry into the same category as supported, but only preliminarily, and portraying the remaining compounds, such as curcumin and beetroot, as potentially, but still, early would also be in line with the current systematic and narrative reviews and facilitate the reduction of the risks of overinterpreting the preliminary data (Barnes, 2023; Crum et al., 2023). Moreover, a cursory overview of recommendations from agencies such as the IOC, ACSM, or ISSN on nutritional recovery and supplementation would place the chapter within the broader profession's recommendations, rather than grounding it in the research results of a specific study (Akbari-Fakhrabadi et al., 2024; Suzuki, 2021).

Last but not least, this aspect of inflammation as a central prism is the chapter's strength, but it can also be a disadvantage. The performance outcome is anchored in a nexus of phenomena, with attention paid to inflammation, energy availability, training quality, sleep, psychological pressure, and general health behaviors (Amawi et al., 2024). It is also rather dangerous in terms of its nutritional value, as the so-called anti-inflammatory narrative can overshadow other necessary input factors, such as adequate carbohydrate intake for intensive training or the prevention of relative energy deficit and sport-related low energy availability (RED-S) (Amawi et al., 2024).

The chapter succeeds in integrating a unified, multi-layered, and fast-changing body of literature into an account that is logically consistent and biologically more pragmatically relevant. Its significant strengths are that it is mechanistically-based, aligns with the Mediterranean and food-first paradigms, and is systematically implemented in practical training scenarios. It has a significant weakness related to the nature of narrative reviews and their biases, the selective underemphasizing of null or counter-evidence, the perennial lack of interaction with the rest of the dietary paradigms, and the possibly underemphasized role of well-selected supplements (Barnes, 2023; Harty et al., 2019; Simopoulos, 2015). The talent to surmount these issues by offering greater explicitness in identifying evidence marking, more comparative dialogue, and a straightforward demonstration of a framework for food, not always food alone, would also make it more scientifically sound and valuable to the needs of as many of the different groups of athletes as possible.

3. METHODOLOGY

3.1 Design and Methodological Orientation

The current chapter was to be a narrative review of the evidence (experimental and observational) that could synthesize the existing literature on anti-inflammatory foods, dietary patterns, and nutritional strategies for athletic performance and recovery. The need to choose the narrative review method is justified by the fact that the topic spans a significant number of studies, including exercise-induced inflammation, sports nutrition, dietary patterns, and gut microbiota outcomes, which are not pooled in meta-analyses (Furley & Goldschmied, 2021). However, search, screening, and data analysis would be conducted in accordance with systematic review principles and up-to-date reporting standards (PRISMA 2020; Andriani & Siripipatthanakul, 2026 a, b & c); thereby facilitating transparency and process repeatability (Page et al., 2021). Such procedures follow best-practice guidelines for systematic narrative review of sport and exercise nutrition (Furley & Goldschmied, 2021; Harty et al., 2019).

3.2 Information and Search Plan

To research sports and nutrition, a literature search was conducted across four large electronic databases commonly used for this research: PubMed/MEDLINE, Scopus, Web of Science, and Google Scholar. In other cases, Embase and SPORTDiscus were also searched for literature on sport-specific and applied practice. The search time frame chosen is January 2000- January 2026, to find the latest evidence on anti-inflammatory diets for athletes, and to access earlier models of anti-inflammatory diets and reference books on antioxidants. The search terms were formulated in sequence and connected using the Boolean operators. The search terms were constructed in the following format (a) population (i.e., athlete, endurance, team sport, resistance-trained, physically active) (b) exposure/intervention (i.e., anti-inflammatory diet, Mediterranean diet, omega-3 fatty acids, EPA, DHA, polyphenols, tart cherry and berries) (c) outcome (i.e., exercise-induced muscle damage, inflammation).

3.3 Eligibility Criteria

The systematic review models of nutritional evidence (U.S. NESR, 2019) were used as a priori inclusion and exclusion criteria, and the results were translated into a narrative review of anti-inflammatory nutrition in athletes. The studies were to be listed and included to satisfy the following criteria:

Population: In non-athletes, mechanistic and clinical studies that examined underlying inflammatory or nutritional events that could be directly extrapolated to sport (e.g., the effects of omega-3 or polyphenols on cytokines and muscle damage) were conducted in athletes (elite, sub-elite, or recreationally competitive).

Intervention/exposure: The anti-inflammatory diets/patterns (e.g., Mediterranean-style diets, vegetarian diets), particular foods (e.g., fatty fish, tart cherry, berries, fermented foods), or non-proposed nutrients that have been proposed to act as anti-inflammatories (e.g., EPA/DHA, polyphenols, curcumin, probiotics, prebiotics).

Comparator: Placebo, regular diet, alternate dietary pattern, or, in observational studies, less adherence to anti-inflammatory diets, or more adherence to anti-inflammatory diets, or less.

Outcomes: Inflammatory (e.g., CRP, IL-6, TNF-α), exercise (e.g., oxidative stress, immune, e.g., DOMS, strength recovery), and/or performance (e.g., training/competitive outcome) outcomes.

Research design: randomized trials, non-randomized trials, crossover trials, cohort trials, and control case studies where lists of kami in relation to the problems of relevant foods or eating patterns had been gathered (Barnes, 2023; Harty et al., 2019; Xiong et al., 2024).

3.4 Selection and Screening of the Study

Another feature of the searches was the retrieval of titles and abstracts, which were filtered according to the eligibility criteria. In the systematic review guidelines, the two-screen process, with a title-abstract screen as the first and a full-text screen as the second, is the approach used in this chapter (Page et al., 2021; NESR, 2019). The traditional workflow assumes that records will be screened twice and that discrepancies will be addressed by discussing the differences with a third party to minimize selection bias and maximize the validity of the evidence provided (Page et al., 2021; Furley & Goldschmied, 2021). The table of identified records, along with the rationale for screening and exclusion, may be included in the supplementary materials, supported by a PRISMA-based flow diagram (Page et al., 2021; Deru et al., 2023).

3.5 Data of the Study Categorization and Digestion

The key data items from the selected studies were collected using a standard form and based on the templates for nutrition and sports science reviews (NESR, 2019; Wingrove et al., 2022). The type of the study determined the selection of the variables, its sample size and composition (age, sex, trainings status, sport), the description of the dietary exposure or intervention (type of food or pattern, dosage, duration, time in relation to exercise), control conditions, the outcomes (inflammatory markers, muscle damage indices, recovery and performance measures), and the key findings, as well as the adverse events (Barnes, 2023; Harty et al., 2019). The most prevalent exposures (i.e., omega-3 interventions, fruit-derived polyphenols, whole-diet patterns, gut-directed strategies) and the sports used (i.e., endurance, team sports, resistance training, injury rehabilitation) were used to create thematic lists (Benson, 2025). This is justified by the fact that the table of evidence in the chapter is organized as follows: Table 1, dedicated to the trials of omega-3 and polyphenols, and Table 2, devoted to anti-inflammatory strategies with whole diets and foods. The other context and outcome validation factor was the methodological review/narrative synthesis approach in the field of sports nutrition (e.g., studies on the nutritional requirements of athletes or recovery plans) (Amawi et al., 2024; Wingrove et al., 2022).

3.6 Quality Appraisal and Risk of Bias

As the review is narrative and the study designs represented therein are heterogeneous, not all trials were subjected to a formal risk-of-bias assessment (e.g., Cochrane RoB 2.0). Nevertheless, a quality assessment exercise was conducted informally, thus involving factors such as randomization and blinding, sample size and attrition, the suitability of outcome measurements, and the presentation of statistics (Barnes, 2023; Harty et al., 2019). Ideally, they lacked research that ought to be replaced with systematic reviews and meta-analyses, which are more likely to yield a more rigorous assessment and a higher level of evidence (Page et al., 2021; Wingrove et al., 2022). Special consideration, without any functional performance or recovery outcomes, was given to small and single-center studies, studies with uncertain control or adherence to the diet, or studies with only surrogate endpoints (Close & Peake, 2018). We can follow these points in a few sections of the chapter, where the shortcomings and gaps in the research are addressed.

3.7 Synthesis Approach

The synthesized evidence was narrative rather than quantitative meta-analysis because the populations, interventions, outcomes, and study designs are likely heterogeneous (Furley & Goldschmied, 2021). The data provide an overview of the direction and frequency of the effects of each thematic area (e.g., omega-3, polyphenols, Mediterranean diet, gut-directed strategies) across studies, with findings amalgamated, cross-situational, and preliminary (Barnes, 2023; Crum et al., 2023). The observation in athletes was cross-linked with data from large populations (physically active and/or clinical), which helped explain the mechanisms of action and made them easier to understand (Simopoulos, 2015; Xiong et al., 2024). It was also clearly explained, based on the new recommendations, the review of the dietary patterns approach, the synthesis of other methods of exposure definition (single nutrients vs. whole foods vs. dietary patterns), and the measurement and reporting of the findings (Wingrove et al., 2022; Bezuglov et al.,2022). This enabled it to be more discriminating in its analysis, thereby justifying some supplements (fish oil capsules, tart cherry concentrate) and supporting more general anti-inflammatory dietary regimens over more extended periods.

3.8 Future Report and Future Projections

There are gaps in the research that render the recommendations invalid. It has not yet formulated the optimal dose, formulation, and time of day for omega-3 fatty acids, tart cherry and pomegranate polyphenols, curcumin, and other bioactives across all types of sport, sex, age, and training stage (Mohammadi et al., 2025; Rojano-Ortega et al., 2020). Food-drug and food-drug interactions are not a systematic phenomenon in high-performance situations, as they are not taken into account in real-world practice (Suzuki, 2021). In addition, there is a high probability that individual differences in genetics, epigenetics, the gut microbiome, and training history will influence susceptibility to anti-inflammatory diet plans, which is why precision sports nutrition is also on the rise (Crum et al., 2023; Suzuki, 2021). The usefulness of sport-specific trials that incorporate high-quality, mechanistic, performance, and health outcomes would be practical for streamlining guidelines and further elucidating how anti-inflammatory foods can be optimally used to enhance athletes' performance and long-term health.

4. RESULTS

Table 1. Meta-Analysis Data Extraction Matrix

Groups	Study Areas	Citations	Outcomes
1	**Anthocyanins** (Tart Cherry/ Pomegranate)	Rojano-Ortega (2020), Vitale et al (2017)	Muscle Soreness (VAS)
2	**Omega-3s** (Fish/Krill Oil)	Mohammadi (2025), Silva (2024), Calder (2017), Benson (2025)	C-Reactive Protein (CRP)
3	**Amino Acids** (L-Carnitine/Citrulline)	Caballero-García (2023), Bezuglov (2022), Devrim-Lanpir (2024)	Creatine Kinase (CK)
4	**Curcuminoids** (Turmeric)	McFarlin (2016), Nicol (2015)	Interleukin-6 (IL-6)
5	**Whole Diets** (Med. / Plant-based)	Estruch (2018), Craddock (2016), Craig (2021)	Aerobic Capacity
6	**Antioxidants** (Vit C & E)	Paulsen (2014), and Pingitore (2015)	Oxidative Stress
7	**Gut-Muscle Axis** (Probiotics/ Fasting)	DeJong Lempke (2025), Zouhal (2020), Suzuki (2021)	Immune Markers

5. DISCUSSIONS

EIMD and DOMS-Based Nutrition Interventions

A general screening of nutritional and supplementation interventions expected to influence EIMD identified dozens of compounds, some of which may have a more significant effect, including omega-3s, cherry and pomegranate polyphenols, curcumin, and beetroot (Harty et al., 2019). EIMD nutrition-based interventions have been considered, and the majority have a positive evidence base; however, most are not of high quality to justify their application across all athletic situations (Barnes, 2023). However, there are rare anti-inflammatory foods that have been integrated in a complementary manner with the already formulated recovery (sleep) supplementation (Suzuki, 2021).

Table 2. Selected anti-inflammatory nutrients and bioactive compounds with sports evidence

Nutrient/ compound	Principal food sources	Proposed mechanisms in inflammation and recovery	Sport-relevant outcomes reported	Key evidence
EPA + DHA (long-chain omega-3)	Oily fish, fish oil, algal oil	Reduced arachidonic acid–derived eicosanoids, increased pro-resolving mediators, and modulation of membrane fluidity and cell signaling.	Reduced IL-6, TNF-α, CRP; lower CK; improved perceived recovery; some improvements in VO_2max and cardiorespiratory function; mixed effects on strength and power	Mohammadi et al. (2025); Silva et al. (2024); Harty et al. (2019); Simopoulos (2020).
Tart cherry polyphenols	Tart cherry juice, concentrates, whole fruit	Antioxidant effects; downregulation of NF-κB; reduced oxidative stress and secondary muscle damage	Reduced post-exercise CK, attenuated strength loss, reduced oxidative and inflammatory markers; inconsistent effects on DOMS.	Rojano-Ortega et al. (2020).
Pomegranate polyphenols	Pomegranate juice, concentrate, arils	Antioxidant and anti-inflammatory properties; improved endothelial function	Reduced strength loss and soreness; improved oxidative stress markers; evidence heterogeneous	Trombold et al. (2011); Lynn et al. (2019).
Curcumin	Turmeric, curcumin extracts	Inhibition of NF-κB and COX pathways; modulation of cytokines; antioxidant actions	Reduced DOMS and inflammatory markers after eccentric exercise; variable effects on performance.	McFarlin et al. (2016). Nicol et al. (2015
Mixed polyphenols (berries, cocoa, green tea)	Berries, grapes, cocoa/dark chocolate, green tea	Antioxidant defense, vasodilation, endothelial support	Potential improvements in blood flow, oxidative balance, and recovery; limited direct athletic performance data	Crum et al. (2023); Suzuki (2021).
Antioxidant vitamins C and E (food-based)	Citrus, berries, peppers, nuts, seeds, vegetable oils	Support endogenous antioxidant systems, collagen synthesis, and membrane protection.	Moderate attenuation of oxidative stress; high-dose supplements may blunt training adaptations	Paulsen et al. (2014); Pingitore et al. (2015).

continued on following page

Table 2. Continued

Nutrient/ compound	Principal food sources	Proposed mechanisms in inflammation and recovery	Sport-relevant outcomes reported	Key evidence
Vitamin D	Sun exposure, fortified dairy/plant milks, fatty fish	Immune regulation, muscle function, and bone health	Low status is associated with increased risk of illness and injury; supplementation normalizes deficits.	Close et al. (2016); Jeukendrup (2017).
Selenium, zinc, magnesium	Seafood, nuts, seeds, whole grains	Cofactors for antioxidant enzymes; immune modulation	Deficiency impairs antioxidant capacity and immunity; correction supports recovery	Close et al. (2016); Maughan et al. (2018).

Table 2 provides a detailed characterization of microplastic contamination across diverse food categories, including seafood, salt, and drinking water. It specifies microplastic concentrations, polymer types, and the primary environmental or processing sources responsible for the contamination.

Table 3. Selected reviews and trials on anti-inflammatory nutrition and exercise-induced inflammation

Study/article type	Population/context	Intervention or focus	Primary outcomes related to inflammation and recovery	Citations
Systematic review of RCTs (Mohammadi et al., 2025)	Physically healthy adults	Omega-3 supplementation vs. control	Reduced IL-6, TNF-α, CRP, and oxidative stress markers; some improvements in performance and recovery indices	Mohammadi et al. (2025).
Meta-analysis (Silva et al., 2024)	Healthy subjects	Omega-3 intake vs. control	Significant reductions in systemic inflammatory markers: relevance for EIMD recovery	Silva et al. (2024).
Brief review (Harty et al., 2019)	Athletes and active individuals	Multiple nutritional strategies for EIMD	Summarizes evidence for omega-3, tart cherry, pomegranate, curcumin, beetroot, etc., in reducing muscle damage and soreness	Harty et al. (2019).

continued on following page

Table 3. Continued

Study/article type	Population/context	Intervention or focus	Primary outcomes related to inflammation and recovery	Citations
Editorial/special issue (Barnes, 2023)	EIMD in various settings	Nutrition-based strategies to reduce EIMD and soreness	Highlights tart cherry and omega-3 as promising, but notes overall limited and heterogeneous evidence	Barnes (2023).
Systematic review and meta-analysis	Athletes consuming tart cherry	Tart cherry supplementation vs. placebo	Significant reductions in post-exercise CK; inconsistent effects on DOMS	Devrim-Lanpir et al.,2024).
Systematic review (Rojano-Ortega et al., 2020)	Athletes using tart cherry or pomegranate	Polyphenol-rich juice supplementation	Suggests that both fruits accelerate recovery of strength and perceptual variables; pomegranate may better support recovery from oxidative stress.	Rojano-Ortega et al. (2020).
RCT (Lynn et al., 2019)	Non-resistance-trained men	Tart cherry vs. pomegranate vs. placebo	No significant differences in strength recovery or soreness; demonstrates heterogeneity of responses.	Lynn et al. (2019).
Editorial (Akbari-Fakhrabadi et al., 2024)	Diet and exercise-induced inflammation	Dietary modulation of post-exercise inflammation	Highlights the importance of diet in shaping acute and chronic inflammatory responses to exercise	Akbari-Fakhrabadi et al. (2024).
Narrative review (Suzuki, 2021)	Exercise immunology and sports nutrition	Multiple supplements and dietary patterns	Summarizes anti-inflammatory and antioxidant strategies to mitigate training-related stress and fatigue	Suzuki (2021).
Review (Crum et al., 2023)	Polyphenols and performance	Curcumin, resveratrol, quercetin, others	Describes antioxidant and anti-inflammatory effects; notes limited sport-specific outcome data.	Crum et al. (2023).

Table 3 summarizes bioactive compounds, including curcumin and vitamin C, that can mitigate microplastic-induced toxicity. It highlights the protective mech-

anisms and the current level of scientific evidence supporting the effectiveness of these nutritional interventions.

6. CONCLUSIONS

A growing body of evidence supports anti-inflammatory diets and foods as a biologically viable option for supporting athletic performance, recovery, and long-term health, and for modifying exercise-induced inflammation and redox signaling. Their combination with the base of the necessary energy, the necessary proportion of macronutrients, and the necessary adequacy of micronutrients, the directed consumption of omega-3-enriched food and polyphenol-enriched food and beverages, and other bioactives delivered by food will allow the athletes to cope with EIMD and low-grade systemic inflammation without being deprived of the adaptive benefits of training.

Nutrition is a crucial foundation of athletic performance, and a balanced, anti-inflammatory diet serves as a "natural recovery" mechanism for athletes. Herein lies the rationale: The Role of Nutrition in Performance: Adequate nutrition provides the energy and nutrients essential for athletes to perform at their best, recover effectively, and maintain overall health. Insufficient nutrition can severely impair performance and recuperation. The advantages of an anti-inflammatory diet: Rigorous physical activity may induce inflammation and elevate indicators like C-reactive protein by as much as 50%. Chronic inflammation can impede recovery and elevate the likelihood of injury or illness. Ingesting nutrient-rich, anti-inflammatory foods—such as fruits, vegetables, whole grains, fatty fish, nuts, and seeds—can mitigate inflammation, alleviate muscle discomfort, and facilitate tissue repair. A diet rich in antioxidants and anti-inflammatory agents not only facilitates immediate recovery but also promotes athletes' long-term cardiovascular, metabolic, and immunological health. Scientific Evidence: Numerous studies indicate that diets rich in processed foods and deficient in micronutrients are associated with heightened inflammation and prolonged healing times. Diets that prioritize complete, plant-based meals and healthy fats are linked to improved recovery and less inflammation. Conclusion: An equilibrated, anti-inflammatory diet is an essential recovery tool for athletes, helping manage physiological stress from training, accelerate recovery, and promote long-term health. This method is supported by empirical evidence and is frequently endorsed by sports nutrition specialists.

7. LIMITATIONS AND RECOMMENDATIONS

Further studies are recommended to include surveys, such as interviews and questionnaires, to gather respondents' perceptions for in-depth insight, and could explain the general situation.

REFERENCES

Akbari-Fakhrabadi, M., Kaviani, M., & Fernández-Lázaro, D. (2024). Diet and exercise-induced inflammation. *Frontiers in Nutrition*, *11*, 1438832. DOI: 10.3389/fnut.2024.1438832 PMID: 38953046

Amawi, A., Khataybeh, B., Al Aqaili, R., Ababneh, N., Alnimer, L., Qoqazeh, A., Oukal, F., Jahrami, H., Mousa Ay, K., Al Saoud, H., & Ghazzawi, H. (2024). Junior athletes' nutritional demands: A narrative review of consumption and prevalence of eating disorders. *Frontiers in Nutrition*, *11*, 1390204. DOI: 10.3389/fnut.2024.1390204 PMID: 39381351

Andriani, A. D., & Siripipatthanakul, S. (2026, a). Technology-Driven Organization Policies: E-Waste Governance Framework. In *Technology Policy and Its Impact on Green Governance and Sustainability* (pp. 31–62). IGI Global Scientific Publishing. DOI: DOI: 10.4018/979-8-3373-6821-4.ch002

Andriani, A. D., & Siripipatthanakul, S. (2026, b). Communicating Green Governance: Strategic Communication for Sustainable Digital Organizations. In *Green Governance of Digital Organizations* (pp. 187–216). IGI Global Scientific Publishing. DOI: DOI: 10.4018/979-8-3373-6736-1.ch007

Andriani, A. D., & Siripipatthanakul, S. (2026, c). Communicating Human Resource Management (HRM) for Recognized Sustainable Green Governance Universities. In *Green Governance of Digital Organizations* (pp. 157–186). IGI Global Scientific Publishing. DOI: DOI: 10.4018/979-8-3373-6736-1.ch006

Barnes, M. J. (2023). Nutrition-based strategies to reduce exercise-induced muscle damage and soreness. *Nutrients*, *15*(11), 2523. https://www.mdpi.com/2072-6643/15/11/2523. DOI: 10.3390/nu15112523 PMID: 37299486

Benson, D. (2025). UNLEASHING THE POWER OF Krill Oil. *Alternative Medicine*, (79), 42–47.

Bezuglov, E., Morgans, R., Lazarev, A., Kalinin, E., Butovsky, M., Savin, E., Tzgoev, E., Pirmakhanov, B., Emanov, A., Zholinsky, A., & Talibov, O. (2022). The effect of a single dose of citrulline on the physical performance of soccer-specific exercise in adult elite soccer players (a pilot randomized double-blind trial). *Nutrients*, *14*(23), 5036. https://www.mdpi.com/2072-6643/14/23/5036. DOI: 10.3390/nu14235036 PMID: 36501066

Caballero-García, A., Noriega-González, D., Roche, E., Córdova, A., & Córdova, A. (2023). Effects of L-Carnitine Intake on Exercise-Induced Muscle Damage and Oxidative Stress: A Narrative Scoping Review. *Nutrients, 15*(11), 2587. https://www.mdpi.com/2072-6643/15/11/2587. DOI: 10.3390/nu15112587 PMID: 37299549

Calder, P. C. (2015). Marine omega-3 fatty acids and inflammatory processes: Effects, mechanisms and clinical relevance. *Biochimica et Biophysica Acta, 1851*(4), 469–484. DOI: 10.1016/j.bbalip.2014.08.010 PMID: 25149823

Calder, P. C. (2017). Omega-3 fatty acids and inflammatory processes: From molecules to man. *Biochemical Society Transactions, 45*(5), 1105–1115. https://eprints.soton.ac.uk/415428/. DOI: 10.1042/BST20160474 PMID: 28900017

Clean Eatz Kitchen. (2026). *Athlete's guide to anti-inflammatory eating*. Clean Eatz Kitchen Blog.

Close, G. L., Hamilton, D. L., Philp, A., Burke, L. M., & Morton, J. P. (2016). New strategies in sports nutrition to increase exercise performance. *Free Radical Biology & Medicine, 98*, 144–158. DOI: 10.1016/j.freeradbiomed.2016.01.016 PMID: 26855422

Close, G. L., Kasper, A. M., Walsh, N. P., & Maughan, R. J. (2022). "Food first but not always food only": Recommendations for using dietary supplements in sport. *International Journal of Sport Nutrition and Exercise Metabolism, 32*(5), 371–386. DOI: 10.1123/ijsnem.2021-0335 PMID: 35279015

Close, G. L., & Peake, J. M. (2018). Exercise-induced muscle damage: What is it, what causes it and what are the nutritional solutions? *European Journal of Sport Science, 18*(8), 1127–1144.

Córdova, A., Caballero-García, A., Noriega-González, D., Bello, H. J., Pons, A., & Roche, E. (2022). Nitric-oxide-inducing factors on vitamin D changes in older people susceptible to suffer from sarcopenia. *International Journal of Environmental Research and Public Health, 19*(10), 5938. https://www.mdpi.com/1660-4601/19/10/5938. DOI: 10.3390/ijerph19105938 PMID: 35627475

Craddock, J. C., Probst, Y. C., & Peoples, G. E. (2016). Vegetarian and omnivorous nutrition—Comparing physical performance. *International Journal of Sport Nutrition and Exercise Metabolism, 26*(3), 212–220. DOI: 10.1123/ijsnem.2015-0231 PMID: 26568522

Craig, W. J., Mangels, A. R., & Fresán, U. (2021). The safe and effective use of plant-based diets in sports and exercise. *Nutrients, 13*(9), 3004. PMID: 34578880

Crum, A. J., Barnes, M. J., & Funnell, M. P. (2023). Deciphering the role of polyphenols in sports performance. *Nutrients*, *15*(6), 1354. PMID: 36986083

DeJong Lempke, A. F., Reece, L. M., & Whitney, K. E. (2025). Nutrition educational interventions for athletes related to low energy availability: A systematic review. *PLoS One*, *20*(2), e0314506. DOI: 10.1371/journal.pone.0314506 PMID: 39951403

Deru, L., Deru, L., Chamberlain, C., Lance, G., Gipson, E., Bikman, B., Davidson, L., Tucker, L., Coleman, J., & Bailey, B. (2023). The Effects of Exercise on Appetite-Regulating Hormone Concentrations over a 36-h Fast in Healthy Young Adults: A Randomized Crossover Study. *Nutrients*, *15*(8), 1911. DOI: 10.3390/nu15081911 PMID: 37111130

Devrim-Lanpir, A., Ihász, F., Demcsik, M., Horváth, A. C., Góczán, P., Czepek, P., Takács, J., Kimble, R., Zare, R., Gunes, F. E., Knechtle, B., Weiss, K., Rosemann, T., & Heinrich, K. M. (2024). Effects of acute citrulline malate supplementation on CrossFit® exercise performance: A randomized, double-blind, placebo-controlled, cross-over study. *Nutrients*, *16*(19), 3235. DOI: 10.3390/nu16193235 PMID: 39408204

Estruch, R., Ros, E., Salas-Salvadó, J., Covas, M. I., Corella, D., Arós, F., Gómez-Gracia, E., Ruiz-Gutiérrez, V., Fiol, M., Lapetra, J., Lamuela-Raventos, R. M., Serra-Majem, L., Pintó, X., Basora, J., Muñoz, M. A., Sorlí, J. V., Martínez, J. A., Fitó, M., Gea, A., & Martínez-González, M. A. (2018). Primary prevention of cardiovascular disease with a Mediterranean diet supplemented with extra-virgin olive oil or nuts. *The New England Journal of Medicine*, *378*(25), e34. https://www.nejm.org/doi/full/10.1056/NEJMoa1800389. DOI: 10.1056/NEJMoa1800389 PMID: 29897866

Fernández-Lázaro, D., Arribalzaga, S., Gutiérrez-Abejón, E., Azarbayjani, M. A., Mielgo-Ayuso, J., & Roche, E. (2024). Omega-3 fatty acid supplementation on post-exercise inflammation, muscle damage, oxidative response, and sports performance in physically healthy adults—A systematic review of randomized controlled trials. *Nutrients*, *16*(13), 2044. https://www.mdpi.com/2072-6643/11/7/1593. DOI: 10.3390/nu16132044 PMID: 38999792

Ferrer, M., & Lamprecht, M. (2015). Inflammation and immune function. In Lamprecht, M. (Ed.), *Antioxidants in sport nutrition* (pp. 1–40). CRC Press., DOI: 10.3389/fpsyg.2021.685082

Furley, P., & Goldschmied, N. (2021). Systematic vs. narrative reviews in sport and exercise psychology: Is either approach superior to the other? *Frontiers in Psychology*, *12*, 685082. DOI: 10.3389/fpsyg.2021.685082 PMID: 34305741

Gamba, M., Pano, O., Raguindin, P. F., Roa-Diaz, Z. M., Muka, T., Glisic, M., Franco, O. H., & Marques-Vidal, P. (2023). Association between total dietary phytochemical intake and cardiometabolic health outcomes—Results from a 10-year follow-up on a middle-aged cohort population. *Nutrients*, *15*(22), 4793. https://www.mdpi.com/2072-6643/15/22/4793. DOI: 10.3390/nu15224793 PMID: 38004187

Harty, P. S., Cottet, M. L., Malloy, J. K., & Kerksick, C. M. (2019). Nutritional and supplementation strategies to prevent and attenuate exercise-induced muscle damage: A brief review. *Sports Medicine - Open*, *5*(1), 1–17. https://link.springer.com/article/10.1186/s40798-018-0176-6. DOI: 10.1186/s40798-018-0176-6 PMID: 30617517

Jeukendrup, A. E. (2017). Periodized nutrition for athletes. *Sports Medicine*, *47*(S1, Suppl 1), 51–63. https://link.springer.com/article/10.1007/s40279-017-0694-2. DOI: 10.1007/s40279-017-0694-2 PMID: 28332115

Maughan, R. J., Burke, L. M., Dvorak, J., Larson-Meyer, D. E., Peeling, P., Phillips, S. M., Rawson, E. S., Walsh, N. P., Garthe, I., Geyer, H., Meeusen, R., van Loon, L., Shirreffs, S. M., Spriet, L. L., Stuart, M., Vernec, A., Currell, K., Ali, V. M., Budgett, R. G. M., & Engebretsen, L. (2018). IOC consensus statement: Dietary supplements and the high-performance athlete. *International Journal of Sport Nutrition and Exercise Metabolism*, *28*(2), 104–125. DOI: 10.1123/ijsnem.2018-0020 PMID: 29589768

McFarlin, B. K., Venable, A. S., Henning, A. L., Sampson, J. N. B., Pennel, K., Vingren, J. L., & Hill, D. W. (2016). Reduced inflammatory and muscle damage biomarkers following oral supplementation with bioavailable curcumin. *BBA Clinical*, *5*, 72–78. DOI: 10.1016/j.bbacli.2016.02.003 PMID: 27051592

Minihane, A. M., Vinoy, S., Russell, W. R., Baka, A., Roche, H. M., Tuohy, K. M., Teeling, J. L., Blaak, E. E., Fenech, M., Vauzour, D., McArdle, H. J., Kremer, B. H. A., Sterkman, L., Vafeiadou, K., Benedetti, M. M., Williams, C. M., & Calder, P. C. (2015). Low-grade inflammation, diet composition, and health: Current research evidence and its translation. *The British Journal of Nutrition*, *114*(7), 999–1012. DOI: 10.1017/S0007114515002093 PMID: 26228057

Mohammadi, I., Farahani, S., Karimi, A., Jahanian, S., Firouzabadi, S. R., Alinejadfard, M., Fatemi, A., Hajikarimloo, B., & Akhlaghpasand, M. (2025). Mortality prediction of heart transplantation using machine learning models: A systematic review and meta-analysis. *Frontiers in Artificial Intelligence*, *8*, 1551959. DOI: 10.3389/frai.2025.1551959 PMID: 40256322

Mountjoy, M., Sundgot-Borgen, J. K., Burke, L. M., Ackerman, K. E., Blauwet, C., Constantini, N., & Budgett, R. (2018). IOC consensus statement on relative energy deficiency in sport (RED-S): 2018 update. *British Journal of Sports Medicine*, *52*(11), 687–697. DOI: 10.1136/bjsports-2018-099193 PMID: 29773536

NESR (Nutrition Evidence Systematic Review). (2019). Nutrition evidence systematic review methodology infographic.

Nicol, L. M., Rowlands, D. S., Fazakerly, R., & Kellett, J. (2015). Curcumin supplementation likely attenuates delayed onset muscle soreness (DOMS). *European Journal of Applied Physiology*, *115*(8), 1769–1777. https://link.springer.com/article/10.1007/s00421-015-3152-6. DOI: 10.1007/s00421-015-3152-6 PMID: 25795285

Nieman, D. C., & Wentz, L. M. (2019). The compelling link between physical activity and the body's defense system. *Journal of Sport and Health Science*, *8*(3), 201–217. DOI: 10.1016/j.jshs.2018.09.009 PMID: 31193280

Nutrition Evidence Systematic Review (NESR). (2019). *Nutrition evidence systematic review methodology infographic.*

Page, M. J.. (2021). The PRISMA 2020 statement: An updated guideline for reporting systematic reviews. *BMJ (Clinical Research Ed.)*, *372*(71). PMID: 33782057

Paulsen, G., Cumming, K. T., Holden, G., Hallén, J., Rønnestad, B. R., Sveen, O., Skaug, A., Paur, I., Bastani, N. E., Østgaard, H. N., Buer, C., Midttun, M., Freuchen, F., Wiig, H., Ulseth, E. T., Garthe, I., Blomhoff, R., Benestad, H. B., & Raastad, T. (2014). Vitamin C and E supplementation hampers cellular adaptation to endurance training in humans: A double-blind, randomised, controlled trial. *The Journal of Physiology*, *592*(8), 1887–1901. https://physoc.onlinelibrary.wiley.com/doi/abs/10.1113/jphysiol.2013.267419. DOI: 10.1113/jphysiol.2013.267419 PMID: 24492839

Peake, J. M., Neubauer, O., Della Gatta, P. A., & Nosaka, K. (2017). Muscle damage and inflammation during recovery from exercise. *Journal of Applied Physiology (Bethesda, Md.)*, *122*(3), 559–570. https://journals.physiology.org/doi/full/10.1152/japplphysiol.00971.2016. DOI: 10.1152/japplphysiol.00971.2016 PMID: 28035017

Pingitore, A., Lima, G. P. P., Mastorci, F., Quinones, A., Iervasi, G., & Vassalle, C. (2015). Exercise and oxidative stress: Potential effects of antioxidant dietary strategies in sports. *Nutrition (Burbank, Los Angeles County, Calif.)*, *31*(7–8), 916–922. DOI: 10.1016/j.nut.2015.02.005 PMID: 26059364

Powers, S. K., Nelson, W. B., & Hudson, M. B. (2011). Exercise-induced oxidative stress in humans: Cause and consequences. *Free Radical Biology & Medicine*, *51*(5), 942–950. DOI: 10.1016/j.freeradbiomed.2010.12.009 PMID: 21167935

Ristow, M., & Schmeisser, K. (2014). Mitohormesis: promoting health and lifespan by increased levels of reactive oxygen species (ROS). *Dose-response, 12*(2), dose-response. https://doi.org/DOI: 10.2203/dose-response.13-035.Ristow

Rojano-Ortega, D., & Ortega, D. R.. (2020). Tart cherry and pomegranate supplementations enhance recovery from exercise-induced muscle damage: A systematic review. *Sports Medicine*, *50*(11), 1–20.

San Juan, A. F., López-Samanes, Á., Jodra, P., Valenzuela, P. L., Rueda, J., Veiga-Herreros, P., Pérez-López, A., & Domínguez, R. (2019). Caffeine supplementation improves anaerobic performance, neuromuscular efficiency, and fatigue in Olympic-level boxers. *Nutrients*, *11*(9), 2120. https://www.mdpi.com/2072-6643/11/9/2120. DOI: 10.3390/nu11092120 PMID: 31492050

Schek, A. (2025). 'Food First', Not ' Food Only ' in Competitive Sports: A Mini-Review. *The Open Sports Sciences Journal*, *18*(1), e1875399X378498. Advance online publication. DOI: 10.2174/011875399X378498250508065801

Schwingshackl, L., & Hoffmann, G. (2015). Adherence to Mediterranean diet and risk of cancer: An updated systematic review and meta-analysis of observational studies. *Cancer Medicine*, *4*(12), 1933–1947. https://onlinelibrary.wiley.com/doi/full/10.1002/cam4.539. DOI: 10.1002/cam4.539 PMID: 26471010

Silva, R. A., Santos, R., & Pereira, L. (2024). Effect of omega-3 fatty acids supplementation on inflammatory markers in healthy subjects: A meta-analysis. *Clinical Nutrition : Official Journal of the European Society of Parenteral and Enteral Nutrition*, *43*(5), 1034–1046.

Simopoulos, A. P. (2015). Anti-inflammatory dietary interventions and supplements to improve health. *Molecular Nutrition & Food Research*, *59*(1), 19–35.

Smith, J. D.. (2023). Popular dietary trends' impact on athletic performance: A review of ketogenic, plant-based, intermittent fasting, and Mediterranean diets. *Sports Medicine - Open*, *9*(1), 67. PMID: 37526793

Suzuki, K. (2021). Recent progress in applicability of exercise immunology and inflammation research to sports nutrition. *Nutrients*, *13*(12), 4299. https://www.mdpi.com/2072-6643/13/12/4299. DOI: 10.3390/nu13124299 PMID: 34959851

Tanabe, Y., Maeda, S., Akazawa, N., Zempo-Miyaki, A., Choi, Y., Ra, S. G., Imaizumi, A., Otsuka, Y., & Nosaka, K. (2015). Attenuation of indirect markers of eccentric exercise-induced muscle damage by curcumin. *European Journal of Applied Physiology*, *115*(9), 1949–1957. https://link.springer.com/article/10.1007/s00421-015-3170-4. DOI: 10.1007/s00421-015-3170-4 PMID: 25921600

Thielecke, F., & Blannin, A. (2020). Omega-3 fatty acids for sport performance—Are they equally beneficial for athletes and amateurs? A narrative review. *Nutrients, 12*(12), 3712. https://www.mdpi.com/2072-6643/12/12/3712. DOI: 10.3390/nu12123712 PMID: 33266318

Tipton, K. D. (2011). Nutrition for acute exercise-induced injuries. *Annals of Nutrition & Metabolism, 57*(Suppl. 2), 43–53. DOI: 10.1159/000322703 PMID: 21346336

Trombold, J. R., Reinfeld, A. S., Casler, J. R., & Coyle, E. F. (2011). The effect of acute pomegranate juice supplementation on exercise performance and markers of oxidative stress. *Applied Physiology, Nutrition, and Metabolism, 36*(6), 1018–1025.

Vitale, K. C., Hueglin, S., & Broad, E. (2017). Tart cherry juice in athletes: A literature review and commentary. *Current Sports Medicine Reports, 16*(4), 230–239. DOI: 10.1249/JSR.0000000000000385 PMID: 28696985

Willett, W., Rockström, J., Loken, B., Springmann, M., Lang, T., Vermeulen, S., & Murray, C. J. (2019). Food in the Anthropocene: The EAT–Lancet Commission on healthy diets from sustainable food systems. *Lancet, 393*(10170), 447–492. https://www.thelancet.com/journals/lancet/article/PIIS0140-6736(18)31788-4/fulltext. DOI: 10.1016/S0140-6736(18)31788-4 PMID: 30660336

Wingrove, K., Lawrence, M. A., & McNaughton, S. A. (2022). A systematic review of the methods used to assess and report dietary patterns. *Frontiers in Nutrition, 9*, 892351. DOI: 10.3389/fnut.2022.892351 PMID: 35694166

Xiong, Y.. (2024). Overview of anti-inflammatory diets and their promising effects on chronic disease prevention. *The British Journal of Nutrition, 132*(4), 601–625.

Yu, X., Pu, H., & Voss, M. (2024). Overview of anti-inflammatory diets and their promising effects on non-communicable diseases. *The British Journal of Nutrition, 132*(7), 898–918. DOI: 10.1017/S0007114524001405 PMID: 39411832

Zouhal, H., Bagheri, R., Triki, R., Saeidi, A., Wong, A., Hackney, A. C., Laher, I., Suzuki, K., & Ben Abderrahman, A. (2020). Effects of Ramadan intermittent fasting on gut hormones and body composition in males with obesity. *International Journal of Environmental Research and Public Health, 17*(15), 5600. https://www.mdpi.com/1660-4601/17/15/5600. DOI: 10.3390/ijerph17155600 PMID: 32756479

KEY TERMS AND DEFINITIONS

Anti-Inflammatory Foods: Antioxidants, polyphenols, and good fats included in anti-inflammatory diets help fight chronic inflammation. Fatty fish (salmon, mackerel), berries (blueberries, cherries), leafy greens (kale, spinach), olive oil, almonds, and spices (turmeric, ginger) are popular options that are largely in line with the Mediterranean diet.

Athletes' Performance: The ability to successfully carry out physical tasks while integrating strength, speed, endurance, talent, and mental toughness to win competitions is known as athletic performance. It is a complex, multifaceted idea shaped by genetic, environmental, and psychological factors. To achieve the best outcomes, one must practice ideal physical fitness, a healthy diet, and mental techniques.

Athletes' Recovery: To heal tissues, improve performance, and avoid injury, athletes must recover with a combination of 7-9 hours of good sleep, adequate protein and carbohydrate intake, and sufficient water. To increase circulation and lessen discomfort, effective methods include massage, foam rolling, active rehabilitation (mild, low-intensity activity), and immersion in cold water.

PRISMA Method: The PRISMA (Preferred Reporting Items for Systematic Reviews and Meta-Analyses) 2020 checklist and flow diagram were created to ensure accurate, thorough, and transparent reporting of systematic reviews and meta-analyses. To assess bias, it provides writers with guidance on describing the identification, screening, and synthesis of studies.

Compilation of References

Abdel-Rahman, A., Anyangwe, N., Carlacci, L., Casper, S., Danam, R. P., Enongene, E., Erives, G., Fabricant, D., Gudi, R., Hilmas, C. J., Hines, F., Howard, P., Levy, D., Lin, Y., Moore, R. J., Pfeiler, E., Thurmond, T. S., Turujman, S., & Walker, N. J. (2011). The safety and regulation of natural products used as foods and food ingredients. *Toxicological Sciences : An Official Journal of the Society of Toxicology*, *123*(2), 333–348. DOI: 10.1093/toxsci/kfr198 PMID: 21821733

Abeltino, A., Riente, A., Bianchetti, G., Serantoni, C., Spirito, M. D., Capezzone, S., Esposito, R., & Maulucci, G. (2025). Digital applications for diet monitoring, planning, and precision nutrition for citizens and professionals: A state of the art. *Nutrition Reviews*, *83*(2), e574–e601. DOI: 10.1093/nutrit/nuae035 PMID: 38722240

Ackland, T. R., Lohman, T. G., Sundgot-Borgen, J., Maughan, R. J., Meyer, N. L., Stewart, A. D., & Müller, W. (2012). Current status of body composition assessment in sport: Review and position statement on behalf of the ad hoc research working group on body composition health and performance, under the auspices of the I.O.C. Medical Commission. *Sports Medicine*, *42*(3), 227–249. DOI: 10.2165/11597140-000000000-00000 PMID: 22303996

Addolorato, S. (2025). Can Wearable and Digital Technologies Augment Business-to-Consumer Data Driven Outcomes in Health and Fitness Industry? *Sport i Turystyka, 8*(1), 161–175. https://www.ceeol.com/search/article-detail?id=1327735

Adebisi, E., Balogun, T. N., Oguntuase, S. B., & Olajide, F. O. (2025). Leveraging Artificial Intelligence (AI) for Stress Management in Peak Athletic Performance: An Integrative Review. *Scientific Journal of Engineering and Technology, 2*(2), 94–106. https://journals.stecab.com/sjet/article/view/999

Adu, M. D., Malabu, U. H., Malau-Aduli, A. E., Drovandi, A., & Malau-Aduli, B. S. (2020). User retention and engagement with a mobile app intervention to support self-management in Australians with type 1 or type 2 diabetes (My Care Hub): Mixed methods study. *JMIR mHealth and uHealth*, *8*(6), e17802. DOI: 10.2196/17802 PMID: 32525491

Aekplakorn, W., Chariyalertsak, S., Kessomboon, P., Sangthong, R., Inthawong, R., Putwatana, P., & Taneepanichskul, S. (2011). Prevalence and management of diabetes and metabolic risk factors in Thai adults: The Thai national health examination survey IV, 2009. *Diabetes Care*, *34*(9), 1980–1985. DOI: 10.2337/dc11-0099 PMID: 21816976

Afaghi, A., O'Connor, H., & Chow, C. M. (2007). High-glycemic-index carbohydrate meals shorten sleep onset. *The American Journal of Clinical Nutrition*, *85*(2), 426–430. DOI: 10.1093/ajcn/85.2.426 PMID: 17284739

Afshar Naseri, M. B. (2025). Beyond performance: A narrative review of prioritizing recovery and mental conditioning of athletes in times of crisis. *Journal of Sports and Rehabilitation Sciences*, *3*(1), 26–38. https://www.jsportrs.com/article_229674.html. DOI: 10.32598/JSRS.2505.1083

Aggarwal, A. K., & Travers, S. (2001). E-commerce in healthcare: Changing the traditional landscape. *Journal of Healthcare Information Management*, *15*(1), 25–36. https://pubmed.ncbi.nlm.nih.gov/11338906/ PMID: 11338906

Agrawal, K., Goktas, P., Kumar, N., & Leung, M. F. (2025). Artificial intelligence in personalized nutrition and food manufacturing: A comprehensive review of methods, applications, and future directions. *Frontiers in Nutrition*, *12*, 1636980. DOI: 10.3389/fnut.2025.1636980 PMID: 40771216

Ahmad, M., Naqvi, R., & Ashfaq, Q. (2025). Developing a performance-based nutrition mobile application design and implementation. *Insights-Journal of Health and Rehabilitation*, *3*(2), 772–779. DOI: 10.71000/z873q831

Ajibesin, A. A. G., N., & Thangavel, S. K. (Eds.). (2025). *Synergizing data envelopment analysis and machine learning for performance optimization in healthcare.* IGI Global Scientific Publishing. DOI: 10.4018/979-8-3373-0081-8

Ajiye, O. T., Olajide, F. O., Ologunja, Y. S., Bamidele, S. O., Badmus, Y. K., & Appah, O. H. (2025). The impact of digital technologies, recreation, and nutrition on stress management and mental well-being in athletes. *Journal of Education, Learning, and Management*, *2*(2), 364–382. DOI: 10.69739/jelm.v2i2.1209

Akbari-Fakhrabadi, M., Kaviani, M., & Fernández-Lázaro, D. (2024). Diet and exercise-induced inflammation. *Frontiers in Nutrition, 11*, 1438832. DOI: 10.3389/fnut.2024.1438832 PMID: 38953046

Al Naabi, Y., Ibrahim, N., & Dhillon, J. S. (2024). Designing sustainable mobile weight management applications: Information technology (IT) experts perspectives. *mHealth, 10*, 25. DOI: 10.21037/mhealth-24-4 PMID: 39114463

Alghannam, A. F., Jedrzejewski, D., Bilzon, J., Thompson, D., Tsintzas, K., & Betts, J. A. (2016). Influence of post-exercise carbohydrate-protein ingestion on muscle glycogen metabolism in recovery and subsequent running exercise. *International Journal of Sport Nutrition and Exercise Metabolism, 26*(6), 572–580. DOI: 10.1123/ijsnem.2016-0021 PMID: 27097042

Alojail, M., & Khan, S. B. (2023). Impact of digital transformation toward sustainable development. *Sustainability (Basel), 15*(20), 14697. DOI: 10.3390/su152014697

Al-Shareeda, M. A., Obaid, A. A., & Almajid, A. A. H. (2025). The role of artificial intelligence in bodybuilding: A systematic review of applications, challenges, and future prospects. *Jordanian Journal of Informatics and Computing, 2025*(1), 16–26. DOI: 10.63180/jjic.thestap.2025.1.3

Alves Bersot, C. D., Ferreira Gomes Pereira, L., Goncho, V. G. V., Pereira, J. E. G., & Falcão, L. F. D. R. (2024). Enhancing recovery and reducing inflammation: The impact of enhanced recovery after surgery recommendations on inflammatory markers in laparoscopic surgery—A scoping review. *Frontiers in Surgery, 11*, 1450434. DOI: 10.3389/fsurg.2024.1450434 PMID: 39717352

Amanollahnejad, A., Fosso-Wamba, S., Shabbir, M. S., & Pakseresht, A. (2026). Aligning socio-technical systems: Rethinking AI adoption and digital transformation in SMEs. *Information Systems Management, 43*(2), 1–15. DOI: 10.1080/10580530.2025.2612175

Amawi, A., AlKasasbeh, W., Jaradat, M., Almasri, A., Alobaidi, S., Hammad, A. A., Bishtawi, T., Fataftah, B., Turk, N., Saoud, H. A., Jarrar, A., & Ghazzawi, H. (2024). Athletes' nutritional demands: A narrative review of nutritional requirements. *Frontiers in Nutrition, 10*, 1331854. DOI: 10.3389/fnut.2023.1331854 PMID: 38328685

Amawi, A., Khataybeh, B., Al Aqaili, R., Ababneh, N., Alnimer, L., Qoqazeh, A., Oukal, F., Jahrami, H., Mousa Ay, K., Al Saoud, H., & Ghazzawi, H. (2024). Junior athletes' nutritional demands: A narrative review of consumption and prevalence of eating disorders. *Frontiers in Nutrition, 11*, 1390204. DOI: 10.3389/fnut.2024.1390204 PMID: 39381351

Amornkitvikai, Y., Tham, S. Y., Harvie, C., & Buachoom, W. W. (2022). Barriers and factors affecting the e-commerce sustainability of Thai micro-, small-and medium-sized enterprises (MSMEs). *Sustainability (Basel), 14*(14), 8476. DOI: 10.3390/su14148476

Andriani, A. D., & Siripipatthanakul, S. (2026). Communicating Human Resource Management (HRM) for Recognized Sustainable Green Governance Universities. In *Green Governance of Digital Organizations* (pp. 157–186, b). IGI Global Scientific Publishing. https://www.igi-global.com/chapter/communicating-human-resource-management-hrm-for-recognized-sustainable-green-governance-universities/401459

Andriani, A. D., & Siripipatthanakul, S. (2026). Technology-Driven Organization Policies: E-Waste Governance Framework. In *Technology Policy and Its Impact on Green Governance and Sustainability* (pp. 31–62). IGI Global Scientific Publishing. DOI: DOI: 10.4018/979-8-3373-6821-4.ch002

Andriani, A. D., & Siripipatthanakul, S. (2026, a). Communicating Green Governance: Strategic Communication for Sustainable Digital Organizations. In *Green Governance of Digital Organizations* (pp. 187–216). IGI Global Scientific Publishing. https://www.igi-global.com/chapter/communicating-green-governance/401460

Andriani, A. D., & Siripipatthanakul, S. (2026, a). Technology-Driven Organization Policies: E-Waste Governance Framework. In *Technology Policy and Its Impact on Green Governance and Sustainability* (pp. 31–62). IGI Global Scientific Publishing. https://www.igi-global.com/chapter/technology-driven-organization-policies/401080

Andriani, A. D., & Siripipatthanakul, S. (2026, b). Communicating Green Governance: Strategic Communication for Sustainable Digital Organizations. In *Green Governance of Digital Organizations* (pp. 187–216). IGI Global Scientific Publishing. DOI: DOI: 10.4018/979-8-3373-6736-1.ch007

Andriani, A. D., & Siripipatthanakul, S. (2026, b). Communicating Green Governance: Strategic Communication for Sustainable Digital Organizations. In *Green Governance of Digital Organizations* (pp. 187–216). IGI Global Scientific Publishing. https://www.igi-global.com/chapter/communicating-green-governance/401460

Andriani, A. D., & Siripipatthanakul, S. (2026, c). Communicating Human Resource Management (HRM) for Recognized Sustainable Green Governance Universities. In *Green Governance of Digital Organizations* (pp. 157–186). IGI Global Scientific Publishing. DOI: DOI: 10.4018/979-8-3373-6736-1.ch006

Aparicio-Pascual, D., Clemente-Suárez, V. J., Tornero-Aguilera, J. F., & Rubio-Zarapuz, A. (2025). The effect of probiotic supplementation on cytokine modulation in athletes after a bout of exercise: A systematic review and meta-analysis. *Sports Medicine - Open, 11*(1), 58. https://link.springer.com/article/10.1186/s40798-025-00860-7. DOI: 10.1186/s40798-025-00860-7 PMID: 40402402

Aragon, A. A., & Schoenfeld, B. J. (2013). Nutrient timing revisited: Is there a post-exercise anabolic window? *Journal of the International Society of Sports Nutrition, 10*(1), 5. https://www.tandfonline.com/doi/full/10.1186/1550-2783-10-5. DOI: 10.1186/1550-2783-10-5 PMID: 23360586

Arenas-Jal, M., Suñé-Negre, J. M., Pérez-Lozano, P., & García-Montoya, E. (2020). Trends in the food and sports nutrition industry: A review. *Critical Reviews in Food Science and Nutrition, 60*(14), 2405–2421. DOI: 10.1080/10408398.2019.1643287 PMID: 31352832

Areta, J. L., Burke, L. M., Ross, M. L., Camera, D. M., West, D. W., Broad, E. M., Jeacocke, N. A., Moore, D. R., Stellingwerff, T., Phillips, S. M., Hawley, J. A., & Coffey, V. G. (2013). Timing and distribution of protein ingestion during prolonged recovery from resistance exercise alters myofibrillar protein synthesis. *The Journal of Physiology, 591*(9), 2319–2331. DOI: 10.1113/jphysiol.2012.244897 PMID: 23459753

Armand, T. P. T., Nfor, K. A., Kim, J. I., & Kim, H. C. (2024). Applications of artificial intelligence, machine learning, and deep learning in nutrition: A systematic review. *Nutrients, 16*(7), 1073. DOI: 10.3390/nu16071073 PMID: 38613106

Armstrong, L. E., Maresh, C. M., Castellani, J. W., Bergeron, M. F., Kenefick, R. W., LaGasse, K. E., & Riebe, D. (1994). Urinary indices of hydration status. *International Journal of Sport Nutrition and Exercise Metabolism, 4*(3), 265–279. DOI: 10.1123/ijsn.4.3.265 PMID: 7987361

Arnarson, A., Gudny Geirsdottir, O., Ramel, A., Briem, K., Jonsson, P. V., & Thorsdottir, I. (2013). Effects of whey proteins and carbohydrates on the efficacy of resistance training in elderly people: Double blind, randomised controlled trial. *European Journal of Clinical Nutrition, 67*(8), 821–826. https://www.nature.com/articles/ejcn201340. DOI: 10.1038/ejcn.2013.40 PMID: 23486511

Arshad, M. T., Ali, M. K. M., Maqsood, S., Ikram, A., Ahmed, F., Aljameel, A. I., Al-Farga, A., & Hossain, M. S. (2025). Personalized nutrition in the era of digital health: A new frontier for managing diabetes and obesity. *Food Science & Nutrition, 13*(10), e71006. DOI: 10.1002/fsn3.71006 PMID: 41019177

Arslan, S. (2025). The Future of Nutrition in Esports: Integrating AI, Personalized Diets, and Holistic Approaches. In *Esports Nutrition: Enhancing Cognitive and Physical Performance in Competitive Gaming* (pp. 171–180). Cham: Springer Nature Switzerland. https://doi.org/DOI: 10.1007/978-3-031-99625-2_10

Arslan, S. (2025). The Future of Nutrition in Esports: Integrating AI, Personalized Diets, and Holistic Approaches. In *Esports Nutrition: Enhancing Cognitive and Physical Performance in Competitive Gaming* (pp. 171-180). Cham: Springer Nature Switzerland. https://link.springer.com/chapter/10.1007/978-3-031-99625-2_10

Arslan, S. (2025). Artificial intelligence in food safety and nutrition practices: Opportunities and risks. *Academia Nutrition and Dietetics*, *2*(3), 1–11. DOI: 10.20935/AcadNutr7904

Arunruangsirilert, T., & Intanant, S. (2021). Measuring social return on investment: A case study of a social project of a company in Thailand. *Journal of Federation of Accounting Professions*, *3*(7), 34–47. https://so02.tci-thaijo.org/index.php/JFAC/article/view/248043

Asanprakit, S., & Limna, P. (2023). Understanding the role of social influence in consumers' intention to use social commerce. *Rom Yoong Thong Journal, 1*(2), 103-121. https://so08.tci-thaijo.org/index.php/romyoongthong/article/view/2188

Aurora, W. I. D. (2026). Micronutrient Deficiencies and Their Public Health Impact: An Epidemiological Narrative Review. *Journal of Tropical Community And One Health, 1*(1), 23–35. https://jtco.org/index.php/journal/article/view/3

Aydın, S. K., Ali, R. H., Faiz, S., & Khan, T. A. (2025). An integrated AI framework for personalized nutrition using machine learning and natural language processing for dietary recommendations. *Applied Sciences (Basel, Switzerland), 15*(17), 9283. DOI: 10.3390/app15179283

Babault, N., Deley, G., Le Ruyet, P., Morgan, F., & Allaert, F. A. (2014). Effects of soluble milk protein or casein supplementation on muscle fatigue following resistance training program: A randomized, double blind, and placebo-controlled study. *Journal of the International Society of Sports Nutrition, 11*(1), 36. DOI: 10.1186/1550-2783-11-36 PMID: 25057266

Balaji, D. P., Kalayci, P. D., & Ramkumar, S. S. (Eds.). (2025). *Advances in sports science and technology* (1st ed.). CRC Press., DOI: 10.1201/9781003616283

Bangsbo, J., Hostrup, M., Hellsten, Y., Hansen, M. H., Melin, A., Kjær, M., Burr, J. F., Engebretsen, L., Egan, B., Hackney, A. C., Chambers, T. L., Jones, A. M., Pitsiladis, Y., Magnusson, S. P., Petersen, J., Deshmukh, A. S., Calbet, J. A. L., Elliott-Sale, K. J., Joyner, M. J., & Moesgaard, L. (2025). Consensus statements—Optimizing performance of the elite athlete. *Scandinavian Journal of Medicine & Science in Sports*, *35*(8), e70112. DOI: 10.1111/sms.70112 PMID: 40781883

Barnes, M. J. (2023). Nutrition-based strategies to reduce exercise-induced muscle damage and soreness. *Nutrients*, *15*(11), 2523. https://www.mdpi.com/2072-6643/15/11/2523. DOI: 10.3390/nu15112523 PMID: 37299486

Bartlett, J. D., Hawley, J. A., & Morton, J. P. (2015). Carbohydrate availability and exercise training adaptation: Too much of a good thing? *European Journal of Sport Science*, *15*(1), 3–12. DOI: 10.1080/17461391.2014.920926 PMID: 24942068

Bassaganya-Riera, J., Berry, E. M., Blaak, E. E., Burlingame, B., Le Coutre, J., Van Eden, W., El-Sohemy, A., German, J. B., Knorr, D., Lacroix, C., Muscaritoli, M., Nieman, D. C., Rychlik, M., Scholey, A., & Serafini, M. (2021). Goals in nutrition science 2020-2025. *Frontiers in Nutrition*, *7*, 606378. DOI: 10.3389/fnut.2020.606378 PMID: 33665201

Beck, K. L., Thomson, J. S., Swift, R. J., & von Hurst, P. R. (2015). Role of nutrition in performance enhancement and postexercise recovery. *Open Access Journal Of Sports Medicine, 6*, 259-267. DOI: 10.2147/OAJSM.S33605

Bell, P. G., Walshe, I. H., Davison, G. W., Stevenson, E., & Howatson, G. (2014). Montmorency cherries reduce the oxidative stress and inflammatory responses to repeated days high-intensity stochastic cycling. *Nutrients*, *6*(2), 829–843. DOI: 10.3390/nu6020829 PMID: 24566440

Benson, D. (2025). UNLEASHING THE POWER OF Krill Oil. *Alternative Medicine*, (79), 42–47.

Berciano, S., Figueiredo, J., Brisbois, T. D., Alford, S., Koecher, K., Eckhouse, S., Ciati, R., Kussmann, M., Ordovas, J. M., Stebbins, K., & Blumberg, J. B. (2022). Precision nutrition: Maintaining scientific integrity while realizing market potential. *Frontiers in Nutrition*, *9*, 979665. DOI: 10.3389/fnut.2022.979665 PMID: 36118748

Bergström, J., Hermansen, L., Hultman, E., & Saltin, B. (1967). Diet, muscle glycogen and physical performance. *Acta Physiologica Scandinavica*, *71*(2-3), 140–150. DOI: 10.1111/j.1748-1716.1967.tb03720.x PMID: 5584523

Bergström, J., & Hultman, E. (1966). Muscle glycogen synthesis after exercise: An enhancing factor localized to the muscle cells in man. *Nature*, *210*(5033), 309–310. DOI: 10.1038/210309a0 PMID: 5954569

Berry, E. M., Cardoso, B. R., Cash, S. B., Cifuentes, A., Collado, M. C., le Coutre, J., German, J. B., Ibáñez, E., Lawrence, M., Nieman, D. C., Pravst, I., Raubenheimer, D., Rychlik, M., Scholey, A., Terranegra, A., & Zivkovic, A. M. (2026). Goals in Nutrition Science 2025–2030. *Frontiers in Nutrition*, *13*, 1784021. https://pmc.ncbi.nlm.nih.gov/articles/PMC13006240/. DOI: 10.3389/fnut.2026.1784021 PMID: 41878571

Betts, J. A., & Williams, C. (2010). Short-term recovery from prolonged exercise: Exploring the potential for protein ingestion to accentuate the benefits of carbohydrate supplements. Sports Medicine, 40(11), 941 959. https://doi.org/DOI: 10.2165/11536900-000000000-00000

Bezuglov, E., Morgans, R., Lazarev, A., Kalinin, E., Butovsky, M., Savin, E., Tzgoev, E., Pirmakhanov, B., Emanov, A., Zholinsky, A., & Talibov, O. (2022). The effect of a single dose of citrulline on the physical performance of soccer-specific exercise in adult elite soccer players (a pilot randomized double-blind trial). *Nutrients*, *14*(23), 5036. https://www.mdpi.com/2072-6643/14/23/5036. DOI: 10.3390/nu14235036 PMID: 36501066

Bickel, C. S., Cross, J. M., & Bamman, M. M. (2005). Exercise dosing to retain resistance training adaptations in young and older adults. *Medicine and Science in Sports and Exercise*, *43*(7), 1177–1187. DOI: 10.1249/MSS.0b013e318207c15d PMID: 21131862

Big Data Institute. (2021). *Digital transformation of healthcare services*. Ministry of Digital Economy and Society.

Boland, M., Alam, F., & Bronlund, J. (2019). Modern technologies for personalized nutrition. In Galanakis, C. M. (Ed.), *Trends in Personalized Nutrition* (pp. 195–222). Academic Press., DOI: 10.1016/B978-0-12-816403-7.00006-4

Boland, M., & Bronlund, J. (2019). eNutrition-The next dimension for eHealth? *Trends in Food Science & Technology*, *91*, 634–639. DOI: 10.1016/j.tifs.2019.08.001

Bompa, T. O., & Haff, G. G. (2009). *Periodization: Theory and methodology of training* (5th ed.). Human Kinetics.

Bongiovanni, T., Genovesi, F., Nemmer, M., Carling, C., Alberti, G., & Howatson, G. (2020). Nutritional interventions for reducing the signs and symptoms of exercise-induced muscle damage and accelerate recovery in athletes: Current knowledge, practical application and future perspectives. *European Journal of Applied Physiology, 120*(9), 1965–1996. DOI: 10.1007/s00421-020-04432-3 PMID: 32661771

Bonilla, D. A., Stout, J. R., Gleeson, M., Campbell, B. I., Escalante, G., Rojas-Valverde, D., Petro, J. L., Kreider, R. B., & Odriozola-Martínez, A. (2025). The 4Rs framework of sports nutrition: An update with recommendations to evaluate allostatic load in athletes. *Life (Basel, Switzerland), 15*(6), 867. DOI: 10.3390/life15060867 PMID: 40566521

Borecki, M. (2025). Legal and ethical analysis of dietary supplement use in the light of anti-doping regulations. *Quality in Sport, 39*, 58988-58988. https://orcid.org/0009-0009-4678-5986

Bose, A., & Sharma, S. (2025). Global regulatory trends and comparative insights: Nutraceuticals in the USA, India, and Europe. *PharmaNutrition, 31*, 100430. DOI: 10.1016/j.phanu.2025.100430

Bo, Z. (2026). *Effect of Ketogenic Diet on Athletic Performance of Men's Basketball Players in Petaling Jaya.*, DOI: 10.6007/IJARPED/v15-i1/27578

Breen, L., Philp, A., Witard, O. C., Jackman, S. R., Selby, A., Smith, K., Baar, K., & Tipton, K. D. (2011). The influence of carbohydrate-protein co-ingestion following endurance exercise on myofibrillar and mitochondrial protein synthesis. *The Journal of Physiology, 589*(16), 4011–4025. DOI: 10.1113/jphysiol.2011.211888 PMID: 21746787

Brewer, S., Pearson, S., Maull, R., Godsiff, P., Frey, J. G., Zisman, A., Parr, G., McMillan, A., Cameron, S., Blackmore, H., Manning, L., & Bidaut, L. (2021). A trust framework for digital food systems. *Nature Food, 2*(8), 543–545. DOI: 10.1038/s43016-021-00346-1 PMID: 37118166

Bryndin, E. G., & Bryndina, I. E. (2017). Formation of public health care on basis of healthy lifestyle. *International Journal of Psychological and Brain Sciences, 2*(3), 63–68. DOI: 10.11648/j.ijpbs.20170203.11

Buceta, A. J. (2025). Nutritional Strategies in the Injury and Recovery Process in Athletes. In *Evaluating the Effectiveness of Functional Ingredients in Sports Nutrition* (pp. 75–90). IGI Global Scientific Publishing., DOI: 10.4018/979-8-3693-8699-6.ch003

Budhiraja, A. (2025). The winning edge: Leveraging data-driven decision making in modern sports management. *International Journal For Multidisciplinary Research*, *7*(4), 1–9. DOI: 10.36948/ijfmr.2025.v07i04.43883

Burke, L. M., Collier, G. R., & Hargreaves, M. (1993). Muscle glycogen storage after prolonged exercise: Effect of the glycemic index of carbohydrate feedings. *Journal of Applied Physiology (Bethesda, Md.)*, *75*(2), 1019–1023. DOI: 10.1152/jappl.1993.75.2.1019 PMID: 8226443

Burke, L. M., Hawley, J. A., Wong, S. H. S., & Jeukendrup, A. E. (2011). Carbohydrates for training and competition. *Journal of Sports Sciences*, *29*(sup1, Suppl 1), S17–S27. DOI: 10.1080/02640414.2011.585473 PMID: 21660838

Burke, L. M., van Loon, L. J., & Hawley, J. A. (2017). Postexercise muscle glycogen resynthesis in humans. *Journal of Applied Physiology (Bethesda, Md.)*, *122*(5), 1055–1067. Advance online publication. DOI: 10.1152/japplphysiol.00860.2016 PMID: 27789774

Caballero-García, A., Noriega-González, D., Roche, E., Córdova, A., & Córdova, A. (2023). Effects of L-Carnitine Intake on Exercise-Induced Muscle Damage and Oxidative Stress: A Narrative Scoping Review. *Nutrients*, *15*(11), 2587. https://www.mdpi.com/2072-6643/15/11/2587. DOI: 10.3390/nu15112587 PMID: 37299549

Cai, Z. J. (2024). The Regulation of Slow-Wave Sleep on Growth Hormone Secretion and Homeostatic Aging: A Pure Model in Man. *OAlib*, *11*(9), e12041. DOI: 10.4236/oalib.1112041

Calder, P. C. (2013). Omega-3 polyunsaturated fatty acids and inflammatory processes: Nutrition or pharmacology? *British Journal of Clinical Pharmacology*, *75*(3), 645–662. DOI: 10.1111/j.1365-2125.2012.04374.x PMID: 22765297

Calder, P. C. (2015). Marine omega-3 fatty acids and inflammatory processes: Effects, mechanisms and clinical relevance. *Biochimica et Biophysica Acta*, *1851*(4), 469–484. DOI: 10.1016/j.bbalip.2014.08.010 PMID: 25149823

Calder, P. C. (2017). Omega-3 fatty acids and inflammatory processes: From molecules to man. *Biochemical Society Transactions*, *45*(5), 1105–1115. https://eprints.soton.ac.uk/415428/. DOI: 10.1042/BST20160474 PMID: 28900017

Campbell, S., Greenwood, M., Prior, S., Shearer, T., Walkem, K., Young, S., Bywaters, D., & Walker, K. (2020). Purposive sampling: Complex or simple? Research case examples. *Journal of Research in Nursing : JRN*, *25*(8), 652–661. DOI: 10.1177/1744987120927206 PMID: 34394687

Can, S., & Can, H. (Eds.). (2025). *Evaluating the effectiveness of functional ingredients in sports nutrition*. IGI Global Scientific Publishing., DOI: 10.4018/979-8-3693-8699-6

Casey, M. M., Payne, W. R., & Eime, R. M. (2012). Organisational readiness and capacity building strategies of sporting organisations to promote health. *Sport Management Review, 15*(1), 109–124. DOI: 10.1016/j.smr.2011.01.001

Chambers, R., & Conway, G. (1991). Sustainable rural livelihoods: Practical concepts for the 21st century. Retrieved from https://opendocs.ids.ac.uk/opendocs/bitstream/handle/123456789/775/Dp296.pdf? sequence=1&isAllowed=y

Charfare, R., Desai, A., Keni, N., Nambiar, A., & Cherian, M. (2025). Smart healthcare framework: Real-time vital monitoring and personalized diet and fitness recommendations using IoT and machine learning. *International Journal of Robotics and Control Systems, 5*(2), 1254–1277. DOI: 10.31763/ijrcs.v5i2.1839

Chatterjee, A., & Sarkar, T. (Eds.). (2025). *Examining physiology, nutrition, and body composition in sports science*. IGI Global Scientific Publishing., DOI: 10.4018/979-8-3693-6317-1

Chaudhry, B. M., Siek, K. A., & Connelly, K. (2024). The usability and feasibility of a dietary intake self-monitoring application in a population with varying literacy levels. *Journal of Personalized Medicine, 14*(9), 1001. DOI: 10.3390/jpm14091001 PMID: 39338255

Chauhan, V., & Sagar, M. (2023). Healthcare decision making and choice: An empirical model of patient confusion. *Management Decision, 61*(11), 3454–3474. DOI: 10.1108/MD-11-2022-1488

Chen, Z. (2025). Empowering sports in the digital economy: Change, opportunity and the future. *Highlights in Business. Economics and Management, 59*, 34–39. DOI: 10.54097/ddqnsm75

Cherian, R. (2019). Health benefits of basil seeds. *International Journal of Scientific Research in Science, Engineering and Technology, 511–515*, 511–515. Advance online publication. DOI: 10.32628/IJSRSET1962145

Chhabra, G., Kumar, S., Gupta, S., & Nagpal, P. (2023). Technology for nutrition, fitness, and sports. In *Artificial Intelligence to Analyze Psychophysical and Human Lifestyle* (pp. 105–112). Springer Nature Singapore., DOI: 10.1007/978-981-99-3039-5_9

Chhabra, N., Shiriskar, J., & Srinivasan, G. (2025). Current and future market of the dietary supplements and nutraceuticals in the global Economy. In *Dietary Supplements and Nutraceuticals* (pp. 1–48). Springer Nature Singapore., https://link.springer.com/rwe/10.1007/978-981-97-9936-7_29-1

Cho, H., Chi, C., & Chiu, W. (2020). Understanding sustained usage of health and fitness apps: Incorporating the technology acceptance model with the investment model. *Technology in Society*, *63*, 101429. DOI: 10.1016/j.techsoc.2020.101429

Choi, D. H., Cho, J. Y., Koo, J. H., & Kim, T. K. (2021). Effects of electrolyte supplements on body water homeostasis and exercise performance during exhaustive exercise. *Applied Sciences (Basel, Switzerland)*, *11*(19), 9093. https://www.mdpi.com/2076-3417/11/19/9093?uid=680b54f39b. DOI: 10.3390/app11199093

Chopvitayakun, S., Rattanasiriwongwut, M., & Ketcham, M. (2025). Factors influencing mobile platform adoption for nutritional tracking among Thai elderly: A unified UTAUT and STAM approach. *Journal of Open Innovation*, *11*(3), 100606. DOI: 10.1016/j.joitmc.2025.100606

Choudhury, T., Arya, P., Kotecha, K., Sharma, A., & Um, J. (Eds.). (2025). *AI and machine learning applications in sports analytics*. IGI Global Scientific Publishing., DOI: 10.4018/979-8-3693-5385-1

Christ, A. S., Carl, K. V., Kurtz, C., Lobschat, L., Mueller, B., & Zimmer, M. P. (2025). Taking digital responsibility for data: Toward a governance model for user-generated data. *Schmalenbachs Zeitschrift für Betriebswirtschaftliche Forschung = Schmalenbach Journal of Business Research*, *77*(3), 527–556. DOI: 10.1007/s41471-025-00225-6

Christodimitropoulou, M., Choustoulakis, E., & Antonopoulou, P. (2025). Digital transformation in sports management: Technologies, trends, and strategic implications. *European Journal of Management and Marketing Studies*, *10*(2), 135–152. DOI: 10.46827/ejmms.v10i2.2031

Clark, K. L., Sebastianelli, W., Flechsenhar, K. R., Aukermann, D. F., Meza, F., Millard, R. L., Deitch, J. R., Sherbondy, P. S., & Albert, A. (2008). 24-week study on the use of collagen hydrolysate as a dietary supplement in athletes with activity-related joint pain. *Current Medical Research and Opinion*, *24*(5), 1485–1496. DOI: 10.1185/030079908X291967 PMID: 18416885

Clarkson, P. M., & Hubal, M. J. (2002). Exercise-induced muscle damage in humans. *American Journal of Physical Medicine & Rehabilitation, 81*(11, Supplement), S52–S69. https://journals.lww.com/ajpmr/abstract/2002/11001/exercise_induced_muscle_damage_in_humans.7.aspx. DOI: 10.1097/00002060-200211001-00007 PMID: 12409811

Clayton, D. J., Burbeary, R., Hennis, P. J., James, R. M., Saward, C., Colledge, A., Scott, R., Gilpin, S., McMahon, R., & Varley, I. (2023). Turmeric supplementation improves markers of recovery in elite male footballers: A pilot study. *Frontiers in Nutrition, 10*, 1175622. DOI: 10.3389/fnut.2023.1175622 PMID: 37293669

Clean Eatz Kitchen. (2026). *Athlete's guide to anti-inflammatory eating*. Clean Eatz Kitchen Blog.

Close, G. L., Hamilton, D. L., Philp, A., Burke, L. M., & Morton, J. P. (2016). New strategies in sports nutrition to increase exercise performance. *Free Radical Biology & Medicine, 98*, 144–158. DOI: 10.1016/j.freeradbiomed.2016.01.016 PMID: 26855422

Close, G. L., Kasper, A. M., Walsh, N. P., & Maughan, R. J. (2022). "Food first but not always food only": Recommendations for using dietary supplements in sport. *International Journal of Sport Nutrition and Exercise Metabolism, 32*(5), 371–386. DOI: 10.1123/ijsnem.2021-0335 PMID: 35279015

Close, G. L., Leckey, J., Patterson, M., Bradley, W., Owens, D. J., Fraser, W. D., & Morton, J. P. (2013). The effects of vitamin D3 supplementation on serum total 25[OH]D concentration and physical performance: A randomised dose-response study. *British Journal of Sports Medicine, 47*(11), 692–696. DOI: 10.1136/bjsports-2012-091735 PMID: 23410885

Close, G. L., & Peake, J. M. (2018). Exercise-induced muscle damage: What is it, what causes it and what are the nutritional solutions? *European Journal of Sport Science, 18*(8), 1127–1144.

Close, G. L., Sale, C., Baar, K., & Bermon, S. (2019). Nutrition for the prevention and treatment of injuries in track and field athletes. *International Journal of Sport Nutrition and Exercise Metabolism, 29*(2), 189–197. DOI: 10.1123/ijsnem.2018-0290 PMID: 30676133

Coelho, R. R., Bonato, S. V., Pacheco, D. A. D. J., & Brito, P. D. S. (2025). Moving Health 4.0 forward: A systematic literature review, challenges and future research agenda. *The TQM Journal*. Advance online publication. DOI: 10.1108/TQM-07-2024-0269

Córdova, A., Caballero-García, A., Noriega-González, D., Bello, H. J., Pons, A., & Roche, E. (2022). Nitric-oxide-inducing factors on vitamin D changes in older people susceptible to suffer from sarcopenia. *International Journal of Environmental Research and Public Health, 19*(10), 5938. https://www.mdpi.com/1660-4601/19/10/5938. DOI: 10.3390/ijerph19105938 PMID: 35627475

Cossich, V. R., Carlgren, D., Holash, R. J., & Katz, L. (2023). Technological breakthroughs in sport: Current practice and future potential of artificial intelligence, virtual reality, augmented reality, and modern data visualization in performance analysis. *Applied Sciences (Basel, Switzerland), 13*(23), 12965. DOI: 10.3390/app132312965

Craddock, J. C., Probst, Y. C., & Peoples, G. E. (2016). Vegetarian and omnivorous nutrition—Comparing physical performance. *International Journal of Sport Nutrition and Exercise Metabolism, 26*(3), 212–220. DOI: 10.1123/ijsnem.2015-0231 PMID: 26568522

Craig, W. J., Mangels, A. R., & Fresán, U. (2021). The safe and effective use of plant-based diets in sports and exercise. *Nutrients, 13*(9), 3004. PMID: 34578880

Crum, A. J., Barnes, M. J., & Funnell, M. P. (2023). Deciphering the role of polyphenols in sports performance. *Nutrients, 15*(6), 1354. PMID: 36986083

Daniel Vasile, P. R., Patricia, M. L., Marta, M. S., & Laura, E. (2024). Evaluation of curcumin intake in reducing exercise-induced muscle damage in athletes: A systematic review. *Journal of the International Society of Sports Nutrition, 21*(1), 2434217. DOI: 10.1080/15502783.2024.2434217 PMID: 39623590

Das, S. K., Miki, A. J., Blanchard, C. M., Sazonov, E., Gilhooly, C. H., Dey, S., Wolk, C. B., Khoo, C. S. H., Hill, J. O., & Shook, R. P. (2022). Perspective: opportunities and challenges of technology tools in dietary and activity assessment: bridging stakeholder viewpoints. *Advances in Nutrition, 13*(1), 1–15. DOI: 10.1093/advances/nmab103 PMID: 34545392

de Oliveira, T. V. P. (2025). Genetics and Sports Nutrition. In Genetics and Sports Performance (pp. 47-60). Cham: Springer Nature Switzerland. https://link.springer.com/chapter/10.1007/978-3-032-11647-5_4

de Oliveira, D. M., Silva, A. K. A. C., Macedo, A. G., Fernandes, M. B., & Fernandes, E. V. (2025). Global Research Trends in Sports Nutrition and Football over the Last 20 Years (2004–2024). *Sports (Basel, Switzerland), 13*(10), 365. DOI: 10.3390/sports13100365 PMID: 41150500 de Souza, L. C., Moris, J. M., Gordon, P. M., Heileson, J. L., & Funderburk, L. K. (2025). From fish oil to resolution: A narrative review on the potential of SPM-enriched marine oil for exercise-induced muscle damage recovery. *Nutrients, 17*(12), 2014. DOI: 10.3390/nu17122014 PMID: 40573125

De Souza, M. J., Nattiv, A., Joy, E., Misra, M., Williams, N. I., Mallinson, R. J., Gibbs, J. C., Olmsted, M., Goolsby, M., & Matheson, G. (2014). 2014 Female Athlete Triad Coalition consensus statement on treatment and return to play of the female athlete triad. *British Journal of Sports Medicine, 48*(4), 289. DOI: 10.1136/bjsports-2013-093218 PMID: 24463911

DeJong Lempke, A. F., Reece, L. M., & Whitney, K. E. (2025). Nutrition educational interventions for athletes related to low energy availability: A systematic review. *PLoS One, 20*(2), e0314506. DOI: 10.1371/journal.pone.0314506 PMID: 39951403

Delany, L. V., Costello, N., Jones, B., & Backhouse, S. H. (2025). Dietary Recommendations for Body Mass and Composition Manipulation in Male and Female Athletes: a Scoping Review of Consensus Statements, Position Stands and Practice Guidelines from International Expert Groups: LV Delany et al. *Sports Medicine, 55*(10), 2445–2487. https://link.springer.com/article/10.1007/s40279-025-02285-4

Deru, L., Deru, L., Chamberlain, C., Lance, G., Gipson, E., Bikman, B., Davidson, L., Tucker, L., Coleman, J., & Bailey, B. (2023). The Effects of Exercise on Appetite-Regulating Hormone Concentrations over a 36-h Fast in Healthy Young Adults: A Randomized Crossover Study. *Nutrients, 15*(8), 1911. DOI: 10.3390/nu15081911 PMID: 37111130

Desbrow, B., McCormack, J., Burke, L. M., Cox, G. R., Fallon, K., Hislop, M., Logan, R., Marino, N., Sawyer, S. M., Shaw, G., Star, A., Vidgen, H., & Leveritt, M. (2014). Sports Dietitians Australia position statement: Sports nutrition for the adolescent athlete. *International Journal of Sport Nutrition and Exercise Metabolism, 24*(5), 570–584. DOI: 10.1123/ijsnem.2014-0031 PMID: 24668620

Devrim-Lanpir, A., Ihász, F., Demcsik, M., Horváth, A. C., Góczán, P., Czepek, P., Takács, J., Kimble, R., Zare, R., Gunes, F. E., Knechtle, B., Weiss, K., Rosemann, T., & Heinrich, K. M. (2024). Effects of acute citrulline malate supplementation on CrossFit® exercise performance: A randomized, double-blind, placebo-controlled, cross-over study. *Nutrients, 16*(19), 3235. DOI: 10.3390/nu16193235 PMID: 39408204

Dima-Cozma, C., Gavrilută, C., Mitrea, G., & Cojocaru, D. C. (2014). The importance of healthy lifestyle in modern society: A medical, social and spiritual perspective. *European Journal of Science and Theology*, *10*(3), 111–120. https://www.ejst.tuiasi.ro/Files/45/12_Dima-Cozma%20et%20al.pdf

Dogra, N., Bakshi, S., & Gupta, A. (2023). Exploring the switching intention of patients to e-health consultations platforms: Blending inertia with push–pull–mooring framework. *Journal of Asia Business Studies*, *17*(1), 15–37. DOI: 10.1108/JABS-02-2021-0066

Domínguez Díaz, L., Fernández-Ruiz, V., & Cámara, M. (2020). The frontier between nutrition and pharma: The international regulatory framework of functional foods, food supplements and nutraceuticals. *Critical Reviews in Food Science and Nutrition*, *60*(10), 1738–1746. DOI: 10.1080/10408398.2019.1592107 PMID: 30924346

Dressler, P., Gehring, D., Zdzieblik, D., Oesser, S., Gollhofer, A., & König, D. (2018). Improvement of functional ankle properties following supplementation with specific collagen peptides in athletes with chronic ankle instability. *Journal of Sports Science & Medicine*, *17*(2), 298–304. https://pmc.ncbi.nlm.nih.gov/articles/PMC5950747/ PMID: 29769831

Drummond, M. J., & Rasmussen, B. B. (2008). Leucine-enriched nutrients and the regulation of mammalian target of rapamycin signaling and human skeletal muscle protein synthesis. *Current Opinion in Clinical Nutrition and Metabolic Care*, *11*(3), 222–226. DOI: 10.1097/MCO.0b013e3282fa17fb PMID: 18403916

Duda, G. N., Geissler, S., Checa, S., Tsitsilonis, S., Petersen, A., & Schmidt-Bleek, K. (2023). The decisive early phase of bone regeneration. *Nature Reviews. Rheumatology*, *19*(2), 78–95. https://www.nature.com/articles/s41584-022-00887-0. DOI: 10.1038/s41584-022-00887-0 PMID: 36624263

Dunne, D. M., Lefevre-Lewis, C., Cunniffe, B., Impey, S. G., Tod, D., Close, G. L., Morton, J. P., & Murphy, R. (2022). Athlete experiences of communication strategies in applied sports nutrition and future considerations for mobile app supportive solutions. *Frontiers in Sports and Active Living*, *4*, 911412. DOI: 10.3389/fspor.2022.911412 PMID: 36172339

Du, T., & Bi, N. (2025). Application of artificial intelligence advances in athletics industry: A review. *Concurrency and Computation*, *37*(3), e8372. DOI: 10.1002/cpe.8372

Efstathiou, E., Akam, L., & Mastana, S. (2026). Opinions and attitudes on genetic testing for personalised nutrition among professional footballers and sports nutritionists. *Performance Enhancement & Health, 14*(1), 100385. DOI: 10.1016/j.peh.2025.100385

Esco, M. R., Fields, A. D., Mohammadnabi, M. A., & Kliszczewicz, B. M. (2025). Monitoring training adaptation and recovery status in athletes using heart rate variability via mobile devices: A narrative review. *Sensors (Basel), 26*(1), 3. DOI: 10.3390/s26010003 PMID: 41516438

Estruch, R., Ros, E., Salas-Salvadó, J., Covas, M. I., Corella, D., Arós, F., Gómez-Gracia, E., Ruiz-Gutiérrez, V., Fiol, M., Lapetra, J., Lamuela-Raventos, R. M., Serra-Majem, L., Pintó, X., Basora, J., Muñoz, M. A., Sorlí, J. V., Martínez, J. A., Fitó, M., Gea, A., & Martínez-González, M. A. (2018). Primary prevention of cardiovascular disease with a Mediterranean diet supplemented with extra-virgin olive oil or nuts. *The New England Journal of Medicine, 378*(25), e34. https://www.nejm.org/doi/full/10.1056/NEJMoa1800389. DOI: 10.1056/NEJMoa1800389 PMID: 29897866

Evans, G. H., James, L. J., Shirreffs, S. M., & Maughan, R. J. (2017). Optimizing the restoration and maintenance of fluid balance after exercise-induced dehydration. *Journal of Applied Physiology*. https://journals.physiology.org/doi/full/10.1152/japplphysiol.00745.2016?utm_

Fajrin, F. I., Nikmah, K., & Ningsih, E. S. (2022). The Effect of Spinach Consumption on the Incidence of Anemia in Pregnant Women. *Azerbaijan Medical Journal, 62*(09), 5115–5121.

Fanani, L., Az-Zahra, H. M., Akbar, M. A., & Sianturi, R. S. (2023). User experience design for nutrition information applications using design thinking. *MATICS: Jurnal Ilmu Komputer dan Teknologi Informasi, 15*(1), 43-50. DOI: 10.18860/mat.v15i1.23025

Fang, W., Fan, S., Zheng, H., Fang, Z., You, Y., Yin, B., Li, B., & Ye, X. (2025). How to improve mental health in the older adults through AI-enhanced physical activity: An emerging research topic. *Humanities & Social Sciences Communications, 12*(1), 1–15. https://www.nature.com/articles/s41599-025-05155-6. DOI: 10.1057/s41599-025-05155-6

Feng, L. B. (2025). The correlation between different lifestyles and body composition focuses on eating habits, nutritional status, and physical exercise components. *Hormones : International Journal of Endocrinology and Metabolism, 24*(3), 621–641. https://link.springer.com/article/10.1007/s42000-025-00661-3. DOI: 10.1007/s42000-025-00661-3 PMID: 40266535

Fernández-Lázaro, D., Arribalzaga, S., Gutiérrez-Abejón, E., Azarbayjani, M. A., Mielgo-Ayuso, J., & Roche, E. (2024). Omega-3 fatty acid supplementation on post-exercise inflammation, muscle damage, oxidative response, and sports performance in physically healthy adults—A systematic review of randomized controlled trials. *Nutrients*, *16*(13), 2044. DOI: 10.3390/nu16132044 PMID: 38999792

Fernández-Lázaro, D., Sánchez-Serrano, N., Rabail, R., Aadil, R. M., Mielgo-Ayuso, J., Radesca Fabiano, K., & Garrosa, E. (2023). Is probiotics supplementation an appropriate strategy to modulate inflammation in physically active healthy adults or athletes? A systematic review. *Applied Sciences (Basel, Switzerland)*, *13*(6), 3448. DOI: 10.3390/app13063448

Fernandez, R. M. (2019). SDG3 good health and well-being: integration and connection with other SDGs. In *Good health and well-being* (pp. 629–636). Springer International Publishing., https://link.springer.com/rwe/10.1007/978-3-319-95681-7_64

Ferrer, M., & Lamprecht, M. (2015). Inflammation and immune function. In Lamprecht, M. (Ed.), *Antioxidants in sport nutrition* (pp. 1–40). CRC Press., DOI: 10.3389/fpsyg.2021.685082

Figueiredo, T., Alcântara, L., Carrilho, J., Paúl, C., & Costa, E. (2025). Understanding adherence to digital health technologies: Systematic review of predictive factors. *Journal of Medical Internet Research*, *27*, e77362. DOI: 10.2196/77362 PMID: 41248309

Filho, E. M. A. A. (2024). O papel do nutricionista no acompanhamento de atletas: como a nutrição pode auxiliar na melhora do desempenho atlético e na recuperação pós-exercício. 12–13. https://doi.org/DOI: 10.69849/revistaft/fa10202408241812

Fraschetti, E. C., Abdul-Sater, A. A., Perry, C. G., & Josse, A. R. (2025). Resistance exercise training and Greek yogurt consumption modulate markers of systemic inflammation in healthy young males—A Secondary Analysis of a Randomized Controlled Trial. *Nutrients*, *17*(17), 2816. DOI: 10.3390/nu17172816 PMID: 40944203

Fu, T., Liu, H., Shi, C., Zhao, H., Liu, F., & Xia, Y. (2024). Global hotspots and trends of nutritional supplements in sport and exercise from 2000 to 2024: A bibliometric analysis. *Journal of Health, Population and Nutrition*, *43*(1), 146. DOI: 10.1186/s41043-024-00638-9 PMID: 39267150

Gabrišová, I., Koman, G., Soviar, J., & Holubčík, M. (2025). The adoption of modern sports technologies from professional settings to everyday life. *Administrative Sciences*, *15*(7), 249. DOI: 10.3390/admsci15070249

Gamba, M., Pano, O., Raguindin, P. F., Roa-Diaz, Z. M., Muka, T., Glisic, M., Franco, O. H., & Marques-Vidal, P. (2023). Association between total dietary phytochemical intake and cardiometabolic health outcomes—Results from a 10-year follow-up on a middle-aged cohort population. *Nutrients, 15*(22), 4793. https://www.mdpi.com/2072-6643/15/22/4793. DOI: 10.3390/nu15224793 PMID: 38004187

Ganio, M. S., Klau, J. F., Casa, D. J., Armstrong, L. E., & Maresh, C. M. (2009). Effect of caffeine on sport-specific endurance performance: A systematic review. *Journal of Strength and Conditioning Research, 23*(1), 315–324. DOI: 10.1519/JSC.0b013e31818b979a PMID: 19077738

García-Montero, C., de Castro-Martínez, P., Liviu Boaru, D., Ortega, M. A., & Fraile-Martínez, Ó. (2026). An Overview of the Impact of the Menstrual Cycle on Nutrient Metabolism: An Integrative Perspective. *Nutrients, 18*(7), 1063. https://www.mdpi.com/2072-6643/18/7/1063. DOI: 10.3390/nu18071063 PMID: 41978114

Gattani, M., & Kumari, V. (2023). Comprehensive evaluation of nutrient and phytochemical profile of bok choy (Brassica rapa subsp. chinensis) at different growth stages. *Sustainability, Agri. Food and Environmental Research, 11*. Advance online publication. DOI: 10.7770/safer-V11N1-art622

Gavurova, B., & Megyesiova, S. (2022). Sustainable health and wellbeing in the European Union. *Frontiers in Public Health, 10*, 851061. DOI: 10.3389/fpubh.2022.851061 PMID: 35372223

Ghanem, M. R. (2025). The Impact of an AI-Supported Smart HIIT Program on Cardiovascular Fitness and Physical Performance. *Modern Sport, 24*(3), 370–384. DOI: 10.54702/2708-3454.2083

Ghazzawi, H. A., Hussain, M. A., Raziq, K. M., Alsendi, K. K., Alaamer, R. O., Jaradat, M., Alobaidi, S., Al Aqili, R., Trabelsi, K., & Jahrami, H. (2023). Exploring the relationship between micronutrients and athletic performance: A comprehensive scientific systematic review of the literature in sports medicine. *Sports (Basel, Switzerland), 11*(6), 109. DOI: 10.3390/sports11060109 PMID: 37368559

Ghazzawi, H., Al Aqaili, R., Khataybeh, B., Al-Aittan, F., Hamaideh, S., Alhalaiqah, T., Amawi, A., Trabelsi, K., Jahrami, H., & Hasan, M. A. (2025). Tailored nutrition strategies for Paralympic athletes: Addressing unique energy, nutrients, and hydration needs to enhance performance and health. *Frontiers in Nutrition, 12*, 1572961. https://www.frontiersin.org/journals/nutrition/articles/10.3389/fnut.2025.1572961/full. DOI: 10.3389/fnut.2025.1572961 PMID: 40693203

Giraldo-Vallejo, J. E., Cardona-Guzmán, M. Á., Rodríguez-Alcivar, E. J., Kočí, J., Petro, J. L., Kreider, R. B., Cannataro, R., & Bonilla, D. A. (2023). Nutritional strategies in the rehabilitation of musculoskeletal injuries in athletes: A systematic integrative review. *Nutrients*, *15*(4), 819. DOI: 10.3390/nu15040819 PMID: 36839176

Gleeson, M. (2006). Can nutrition limit exercise-induced immunodepression? *Nutrition Reviews*, *64*(3), 119–131. DOI: 10.1111/j.1753-4887.2006.tb00195.x PMID: 16572599

Govindasamy, K., Parpa, K., Katanic, B., Clark, C. C., Elayaraja, M., Kambitta Valappil, I. N., Dulceanu, C., Geantă, V. A., Tolan, G. A., & Zouhal, H. (2025). Effect of Plant-Based Proteins on Recovery from Resistance Exercise-Induced Muscle Damage in Healthy Young Adults—A Systematic Review. *Nutrients*, *17*(15), 2571. DOI: 10.3390/nu17152571 PMID: 40806155

Grabia, M., Perkowski, J., Socha, K., & Markiewicz-Żukowska, R. (2024). Female athlete triad and relative energy deficiency in sport (REDs): Nutritional management. *Nutrients*, *16*(3), 359. https://www.mdpi.com/2072-6643/16/3/359. DOI: 10.3390/nu16030359 PMID: 38337644

Grivas, G. V., & Safari, K. (2025). Artificial intelligence in endurance sports: Metabolic, recovery, and nutritional perspectives. *Nutrients*, *17*(20), 3209. https://www.mdpi.com/2072-6643/17/20/3209. DOI: 10.3390/nu17203209 PMID: 41156462

Grosso, F. D., & Turco, D. (2026). Nutrition in sport: An opportunity to balance performance, sustainability and Preventive Medicine. *Research in Sports Medicine*, *34*(1), 61–70. https://www.tandfonline.com/doi/abs/10.1080/15438627.2025.2525854. DOI: 10.1080/15438627.2025.2525854 PMID: 40590526

Guest, N. S., Horne, J., Vanderhout, S. M., & El-Sohemy, A. (2019). Sport nutrigenomics: Personalized nutrition for athletic performance. *Frontiers in Nutrition*, *6*, 8. DOI: 10.3389/fnut.2019.00008 PMID: 30838211

Guo, S., Guo, X., & Wang, P. (2024). Optimizing nutrition strategies for women's soccer players' seasonal recovery and performance in the context of big data. *Journal of Biotech Research*, •••, 19.

Hales, R., & Birdthistle, N. (2023). The Sustainable Development Goal–SDG# 3 Good Health and Well-Being. In *Attaining the 2030 Sustainable Development Goal of Good Health and Well-Being* (pp. 1–12). Emerald Publishing Limited. https://doi.org/DOI: 10.1108/978-1-80455-209-420231001

Hansen, A. K., Fischer, C. P., Plomgaard, P., Andersen, J. L., Saltin, B., & Pedersen, B. K. (2005). Skeletal muscle adaptation: Training twice every second day vs. training once daily. *Journal of Applied Physiology (Bethesda, Md.)*, *98*(1), 93–99. DOI: 10.1152/japplphysiol.00163.2004 PMID: 15361516

Hargreaves, M. (2015). Exercise, muscle, and carbohydrate metabolism. *Progress in Molecular Biology and Translational Science*, *135*, 129–152. DOI: 10.1016/bs.pmbts.2015.07.016

Harty, P. S., Cottet, M. L., Malloy, J. K., & Kerksick, C. M. (2019). Nutritional and supplementation strategies to prevent and attenuate exercise-induced muscle damage: A brief review. *Sports Medicine - Open*, *5*(1), 1. DOI: 10.1186/s40798-018-0176-6 PMID: 30617517

Hausswirth, C., & Le Meur, Y. (2011). Physiological and nutritional aspects of post-exercise recovery: Specific recommendations for female athletes. *Sports Medicine*, *41*(10), 861–882. https://link.springer.com/article/10.2165/11593180-000000000-00000. DOI: 10.2165/11593180-000000000-00000 PMID: 21923203

Hawley, J. A., & Burke, L. M. (2010). Carbohydrate availability and training adaptation: Effects on cell metabolism. *Exercise and Sport Sciences Reviews*, *38*(4), 152–160. DOI: 10.1097/JES.0b013e3181f44dd9 PMID: 20871231

Hawley, J. A., Schabort, E. J., Noakes, T. D., & Dennis, S. C. (1997). Carbohydrate-loading and exercise performance. *Sports Medicine*, *24*(2), 73–81. DOI: 10.2165/00007256-199724020-00001 PMID: 9291549

Heaton, L. E., Davis, J. K., Rawson, E. S., Nuccio, R. P., Witard, O. C., Stein, K. W., Baar, K., Carter, J. M., & Baker, L. B. (2017). Selected in-season nutritional strategies to enhance recovery for team sport athletes: A practical overview. *Sports Medicine*, *47*(11), 2201–2218. DOI: 10.1007/s40279-017-0759-2 PMID: 28702900

Heikura, I. A. (2020). *Dietary periodisation for health and performance in world-class endurance athletes* (Doctoral dissertation, Australian Catholic University). DOI: DOI: 10.26199/e8tq-dh06

Helder, T. A., Condon, S., Grant, I., Lewis, N. A., Hill, J., Pedlar, C. R., & Hughes, L. (2025). The dose–response effects of hydrolyzed curcumin on recovery, inflammation, and oxidative stress following exercise-induced muscle damage in males. *Physiological Reports*, *13*(15), e70504. DOI: 10.14814/phy2.70504 PMID: 40781899

Hermes, S., Riasanow, T., Clemons, E. K., Böhm, M., & Krcmar, H. (2020). The digital transformation of the healthcare industry: Exploring the rise of emerging platform ecosystems and their influence on the role of patients. *Business Research, 13*(3), 1033–1069. DOI: 10.1007/s40685-020-00125-x

Hexis. (2023, December 7). *Technology unlocks the future of sports nutrition.* https://www.hexis.live/blog/technology-unlocks-the-future-of-sports-nutrition

Hillen, B., Oestreicher, G., Schwab, L., Enders, K., Simon, P., Elme, A., Ben-Aharon, I., Goshenlago, T., Neuzillet, C., Sclafani, F., Beltran, E. E. M., Schuster, M., Doncheva, H., Ruckes, C., Karlecik, M., Petrowski, K., Rosenbaum, D., Diou, C., Ballas, A., & Moehler, M. (2025). Digital and AI-assisted multimodal supportive care, combining physical activity, nutrition, and pain management during chemotherapy for advanced pancreatic cancer patients: Study protocol of the European multicenter randomized controlled trial of the RELEVIUM project. *BMC Cancer, 25*(1), 1610. DOI: 10.1186/s12885-025-14867-6 PMID: 41109944

Hobson, R. M., Saunders, B., Ball, G., Harris, R. C., & Sale, C. (2012). Effects of β-alanine supplementation on exercise performance: A meta-analysis. *Amino Acids, 43*(1), 25–37. DOI: 10.1007/s00726-011-1200-z PMID: 22270875

Hongsuchon, T., Chen, S. C., & Khan, A. (2025). Applying the S-O-R model to explore impulsive buying behavior driven by influencers on social commerce websites. *PeerJ. Computer Science, 11*, e3113. DOI: 10.7717/peerj-cs.3113 PMID: 40989320

Houlden, V., Jani, A., & Hong, A. (2021). Is biodiversity of greenspace important for human health and wellbeing? A bibliometric analysis and systematic literature review. *Urban Forestry & Urban Greening, 66*, 127385. DOI: 10.1016/j.ufug.2021.127385

Howatson, G., McHugh, M. P., Hill, J. A., Brouner, J., Jewell, A. P., van Someren, K. A., Shave, R. E., & Howatson, S. A. (2010). Influence of tart cherry juice on indices of recovery following marathon running. *Scandinavian Journal of Medicine & Science in Sports, 20*(6), 843–852. DOI: 10.1111/j.1600-0838.2009.01005.x PMID: 19883392

Howden-Chapman, P., Siri, J., Chisholm, E., Chapman, R., Doll, C. N., & Capon, A. (2017). *SDG 3: Ensure healthy lives and promote wellbeing for all at all ages. A guide to SDG interactions: from science to implementation.* International Council for Science.

Hoxha, S. (2025). Technological innovations in sports: Advancing performance, accuracy, and global impact. *The Journal of Bio based Marketing©*, 135.

Huang, M., & Yongquan, T. (2025). Tech-driven excellence: A quantitative analysis of cutting-edge technology impact on professional sports training. *Journal of Computer Assisted Learning, 41*(1), e13082. https://onlinelibrary.wiley.com/doi/abs/10.1111/jcal.13082. DOI: 10.1111/jcal.13082

Hunter, D. J. (2009). Leading for health and wellbeing: The need for a new paradigm. *Journal of Public Health (Oxford, England), 31*(2), 202–204. DOI: 10.1093/pubmed/fdp036 PMID: 19372148

Hwang, D. J., & Yang, H. J. (2024). Nutritional strategies for enhancing performance and training adaptation in weightlifters. *International Journal of Molecular Sciences, 26*(1), 240. DOI: 10.3390/ijms26010240 PMID: 39796095

Ihsan, F., Nasrulloh, A., Kozina, Z., Hidayat, R. A., Perdana, S., & Sukendro, S. (2024). Nutritional strategies for rapid recovery in sport: A literature review. *Retos: nuevas tendencias en educación física, deporte y recreación*, (57), 153–164. https://doi.org/DOI: 10.47197/retos.v57.105622

Impey, S. G., Hearris, M. A., Hammond, K. M., Bartlett, J. D., Louis, J., Close, G. L., & Morton, J. P. (2018). Fuel for the work required: A theoretical framework for carbohydrate periodization and the glycogen threshold hypothesis. *Sports Medicine, 48*(5), 1031–1048. DOI: 10.1007/s40279-018-0867-7 PMID: 29453741

Ionescu, G. H., Firoiu, D., Tănasie, A., Sorin, T., Pîrvu, R., & Manta, A. (2020). Assessing the Achievement of the SDG Targets for Health and Well-Being at EU Level by 2030. *Sustainability (Basel), 12*(14), 5829. DOI: 10.3390/su12145829

Ismail, H., McVicar, J., Lewandowski, A. J., Sherwood, A., Lwin, M. O., & Makin, S. (2020). Continuous glucose monitoring in sport: A systematic review. *Frontiers in Sports and Active Living, 2*, 570324. DOI: 10.3389/fspor.2020.570324

Ivy, J. L., Katz, A. L., Cutler, C. L., Sherman, W. M., & Coyle, E. F. (1988). Muscle glycogen synthesis after exercise: Effect of time of carbohydrate ingestion. *Journal of Applied Physiology (Bethesda, Md.), 64*(4), 1480–1485. DOI: 10.1152/jappl.1988.64.4.1480 PMID: 3132449

Jacobsson, J., Kowalski, J., Timpka, T., Hansson, P. O., Spreco, A., & Dahlstrom, O. (2023). Universal prevention through a digital health platform reduces injury incidence in youth athletics (track and field): A cluster randomised controlled trial. *British Journal of Sports Medicine, 57*(6), 364–371. DOI: 10.1136/bjsports-2021-105332 PMID: 36564148

Jäger, R., Kerksick, C. M., Campbell, B. I., Cribb, P. J., Wells, S. D., Skwiat, T. M., Purpura, M., Ziegenfuss, T. N., Ferrando, A. A., Arent, S. M., Smith-Ryan, A. E., Stout, J. R., Arciero, P. J., Ormsbee, M. J., Taylor, L. W., Wilborn, C. D., Kalman, D. S., Kreider, R. B., Willoughby, D. S., & Antonio, J. (2017). International Society of Sports Nutrition position stand: Protein and exercise. *Journal of the International Society of Sports Nutrition, 14*(1), 20. https://www.tandfonline.com/doi/abs/10.1186/s12970-017-0177-8. DOI: 10.1186/s12970-017-0177-8 PMID: 28642676

Jalonen, H., Tuominen, S., Ryömä, A., Haltia, J., Nenonen, J., & Kuikka, A. (2018). How does value creation manifest itself in the nexus of sport and business? A systematic literature review. *Open Journal of Business and Management, 6*(1), 103–138. DOI: 10.4236/ojbm.2018.61008

Jangjarat, K., Shaengchart, Y., Limna, P., Suradinkura, S., & Bhumpenpein, N. (2026). The role of the 4Es in driving business performance and competitive advantage for cosmetic industry SMEs in emerging economies. *Business Performance Review, 4*(1), 33–44. DOI: 10.22495/bprv4i1p3

Jaswal, R. S., Stergiou, P., & Katz, L. (2022). How Canadian high-performance coaches adopt and implement technology: Exploring the antecedents of intra- and interorganizational trust, technological proficiency, and subjective norms and social influence on technology adoption. *International Sport Coaching Journal, 9*(2), 234–243. DOI: 10.1123/iscj.2020-0088

Jessup-Varnum, M. (2018). Food security and the sustainable livelihood approach to development in Uganda.

Jeukendrup, A. E. (2017). Periodized nutrition for athletes. *Sports Medicine, 47*(S1, Suppl 1), 51–63. DOI: 10.1007/s40279-017-0694-2 PMID: 28332115

Jiang, X., Timmons, M., Boroda, E., & Onakomaiya, M. (2025). Impact of platform design and usability on adherence and retention: Randomized web- and mobile-based longitudinal study. *Journal of Participatory Medicine, 17*, e50225. DOI: 10.2196/50225 PMID: 40152343

Jones, R. L., Stellingwerff, T., Artioli, G. G., Saunders, B., Cooper, S., & Sale, C. (2016). Dose-response of sodium bicarbonate ingestion highlights individuality in experience of side-effects. *International Journal of Sport Nutrition and Exercise Metabolism, 26*(5), 445–453. DOI: 10.1123/ijsnem.2015-0286 PMID: 27098290

Jouris, K. B., McDaniel, J. L., & Weiss, E. P. (2011). The effect of omega-3 fatty acid supplementation on The inflammatory response to eccentric strength exercise. *Journal of Sports Science & Medicine, 10*(3), 432–438. https://pmc.ncbi.nlm.nih.gov/articles/PMC3737804/ PMID: 24150614

Jovanovski, E., Bosco, L., Khan, K., Au-Yeung, F., Ho, H., Zurbau, A., Jenkins, A. L., & Vuksan, V. (2015). Effect of spinach, a high dietary nitrate source, on arterial stiffness and related hemodynamic measures: A randomized, controlled trial in healthy adults. *Clinical Nutrition Research*, *4*(3), 160–167. DOI: 10.7762/cnr.2015.4.3.160 PMID: 26251834

Jud, M., & Thalmann, S. (2025). AI in digital sports coaching–a systematic review. *Managing Sport and Leisure*, *30*(6), 1577–1593. DOI: 10.1080/23750472.2024.2449016

Kanabur, V., & Reddy, R. L. (2014). Bioactive components of spinach and their effect on some pathophysiological conditions: A review. *International Journal of Current Research and Review*, *6*(9), 156–166.

Kanwal, S., Ahsan, M. T, Khan, R. N., & Khan, A. (2025). Load management and injury prevention in elite athletes: A narrative review. *Premier Journal of Science*, 1-7. DOI: 10.70389/PJS.100088

Karnika, S., Sharma, S., Singh, A., Batth, S. S., & Sharma, A. (2025). From data to diet: The impact of artificial intelligence on nutritional science. *Journal of Scientific Research and Reports*, *31*(8), 449–458. DOI: 10.9734/jsrr/2025/v31i83388

Kassem, H., Beevi, A. A., Basheer, S., Lutfi, G., Cheikh Ismail, L., & Papandreou, D. (2025). Investigation and assessment of ai's role in nutrition—An updated narrative review of the evidence. *Nutrients*, *17*(1), 190. DOI: 10.3390/nu17010190 PMID: 39796624

Kaufman, M., Nguyen, C., Shetty, M., Oppezzo, M., Barrack, M., & Fredericson, M. (2023). Popular dietary trends' impact on athletic performance: A critical analysis review. *Nutrients*, *15*(16), 3511. https://www.mdpi.com/2072-6643/15/16/3511. DOI: 10.3390/nu15163511 PMID: 37630702

Kenefick, R. W., & Sawka, M. N. (2007). Hydration at the work site. *Journal of the American College of Nutrition*, *26*(sup5, Suppl 5), 597S–603S. DOI: 10.1080/07315724.2007.10719665 PMID: 17921472

Kerksick, C. M., Arent, S., Schoenfeld, B. J., Stout, J. R., Campbell, B., Wilborn, C. D., Taylor, L., Kalman, D., Smith-Ryan, A. E., Kreider, R. B., Willoughby, D., Arciero, P. J., VanDusseldorp, T. A., Ormsbee, M. J., Wildman, R., Greenwood, M., Ziegenfuss, T. N., Aragon, A. A., & Antonio, J. (2017). International Society of Sports Nutrition position stand: Nutrient timing. *Journal of the International Society of Sports Nutrition*, *14*(1), 33. https://www.tandfonline.com/doi/full/10.1186/s12970-017-0189-4. DOI: 10.1186/s12970-017-0189-4 PMID: 28919842

Knutsson, P. (2006). The sustainable livelihoods approach: A framework for knowledge integration assessment. *Human Ecology Review*, *13*(1), 90–99. https://www.jstor.org/stable/24707559

Koo, A., Chew, D. X., Ghate, V., & Zhou, W. (2023). Residual polyphenol oxidase and peroxidase activities in high pressure processed bok choy (Brassica rapa subsp. chinensis) juice did not accelerate nutrient degradation during storage. *Innovative Food Science & Emerging Technologies*, *84*, 103284. DOI: 10.1016/j.ifset.2023.103284

Kotler, P. (2017). Philip Kotler: Some of my adventures in marketing. *Journal of Historical Research in Marketing*, *9*(2), 203–208. DOI: 10.1108/JHRM-11-2016-0027

Kraiwanit, T., Limna, P., & Siripipatthanakul, S. (2023). NVivo for social sciences and management studies: A systematic review. *Advance Knowledge for Executives, 2*(3), 1-11. https://papers.ssrn.com/sol3/papers.cfm?abstract_id=4523829

Kreher, J. B., & Schwartz, J. B. (2012). Overtraining syndrome: A practical guide. *Sports Health*, *4*(2), 128–138. DOI: 10.1177/1941738111434406 PMID: 23016079

Kretschmer, T., Leiponen, A., Schilling, M., & Vasudeva, G. (2022). Platform ecosystems as meta-organizations: Implications for platform strategies. *Strategic Management Journal*, *43*(3), 405–424. DOI: 10.1002/smj.3250

Kumar, S. S., Muthukumaran, V., Devi, A., Geetha, V., & Yadav, P. N. (2023). A quantitative approach of purposive sampling techniques for security and privacy issues in IoT healthcare applications. In Zhao, J., Kumar, V., Natarajan, R., & Mahesh, T. (Eds.), *Handbook of Research on Advancements in AI and IoT Convergence Technologies* (pp. 281–299). IGI Global Scientific Publishing., DOI: 10.4018/978-1-6684-6971-2.ch016

Lane, S. C., Camera, D. M., Lassiter, D. G., Areta, J. L., Bird, S. R., Yeo, W. K., Jeacocke, N. A., Krook, A., Zierath, J. R., Burke, L. M., & Hawley, J. A. (2015). Effects of sleeping with reduced carbohydrate availability on acute training responses. *Journal of Applied Physiology (Bethesda, Md.)*, *119*(6), 643–655. DOI: 10.1152/japplphysiol.00857.2014 PMID: 26112242

Lanhers, C., Pereira, B., Naughton, G., Trousselard, M., Lesage, F. X., & Dutheil, F. (2017). Creatine supplementation and upper limb strength performance: A systematic review and meta-analysis. *Sports Medicine*, *47*(1), 163–173. DOI: 10.1007/s40279-016-0571-4 PMID: 27328852

Larson-Meyer, D. E., & Willis, K. S. (2010). Vitamin D and athletes. *Current Sports Medicine Reports*, *9*(4), 220–226. DOI: 10.1249/JSR.0b013e3181e7dd45 PMID: 20622540

Lasya, C. S. (2022). Spinach and its health benefits: A review. *The Pharma Innovation Journal*, 1232-1239.

Lee, E. C., Fragala, M. S., Kavouras, S. A., Queen, R. M., Pryor, J. L., & Casa, D. J. (2017). Biomarkers in sports and exercise: Tracking health, performance, and recovery in athletes. *Journal of Strength and Conditioning Research*, *31*(10), 2920–2937. DOI: 10.1519/JSC.0000000000002122 PMID: 28737585

Lee, P. C. (2026). A Cardiologist's [Dietary Guidelines and Contemporary Nutrition Research.]. *VIEW*, •••, 2025–2030.

Lee, Y. K., Yoon, E. J., Kim, T. H., Kim, J. I., & Kim, J. H. (2025). Musculoskeletal digital therapeutics and digital health rehabilitation: A global paradigm shift in orthopedic care. *Journal of Clinical Medicine*, *14*(23), 8467. DOI: 10.3390/jcm14238467 PMID: 41375770

Lemire, J. (2023, April 12). *How Hexis is aiming to help athletes optimize performance with their AI-powered nutrition app.* Sports Business Journal. https://www.sportsbusinessjournal.com/Journal/Issues/2023/04/10/Technology/hexis/

Lillis, J. B., Willmott, A. G., Chichger, H., & Roberts, J. D. (2025). The application of olive-derived polyphenols on exercise-induced inflammation: A scoping review. *Nutrients*, *17*(2), 223. DOI: 10.3390/nu17020223 PMID: 39861354

Limna, P. (2023). The digital transformation of healthcare in the digital economy: A systematic review. *International Journal of Advanced Health Science and Technology*, *3*(2), 127–132. DOI: 10.35882/ijahst.v3i2.244

Limna, P., Shaengchart, Y., Kraiwanit, T., Asanprakit, S., & Nivornusit, R. (2025). Muketing: The fusion of *Mutelu* and marketing in e-commerce—Trends in Thailand's faith economy. *Frontiers in Communication*, *10*, 1662524. DOI: 10.3389/fcomm.2025.1662524

Limna, P., & Siripipattanakul, S. (2026). Sustainable clinic management based on practices and human resource management (HRM). In Siripipatthanakul, S. (Ed.), *Sustainable Development for Hospitals and Clinics* (pp. 65–96). IGI Global Scientific Publishing., DOI: 10.4018/979-8-3693-9800-5.ch003

Limna, P., Siripipattanakul, S., Sitthipon, T., Jaipong, P., & Auttawechasakoon, P. (2022). Telemedicine consultations among healthcare providers and patients during the COVID-19 pandemic: A review article. *Review of Advanced Multidisciplinary Sciences, Engineering & Innovation, 1*(1), 1-8. https://ssrn.com/abstract=4080873

Link, L. (2024). *Nutrient timing: fueling strategies to unlock peak performance.* Human Kinetics.

Liu, H., & Liu, G. (2019). Bok Choy, an Asian Leafy Green Vegetable Emerging in Florida: HS1337, 11/2019. *EDIS*, *2019*(6), 5–5. DOI: 10.32473/edis-hs1337-2019

Liu, J., Mao, S., Lu, L., Jing, Y., Yang, X., Xu, H., & Ren, Y. (2025). The impact of digital economy on the supply chain resilience of cross-border healthcare e-commerce. *Frontiers in Public Health*, *13*, 1570338. DOI: 10.3389/fpubh.2025.1570338 PMID: 40487520

Liu, J., Yu, H., Cheung, W. C., Bleakney, A., & Jan, Y. K. (2025). Societal attitudes and structural barriers in coaching para-athletes: A mixed-methods systematic review. *PLoS One*, *20*(6), e0326585. DOI: 10.1371/journal.pone.0326585 PMID: 40560855

Liu, X., Xu, M., Wang, H., & Zhu, L. (2025). Integrating precision medicine and digital health in personalized weight management: The central role of nutrition. *Nutrients*, *17*(16), 2695. https://www.mdpi.com/2072-6643/17/16/2695. DOI: 10.3390/nu17162695 PMID: 40871725

Liu, Y., Lu, X., Zhao, G., Li, C., & Shi, J. (2022). Adoption of mobile health services using the unified theory of acceptance and use of technology model: Self-efficacy and privacy concerns. *Frontiers in Psychology*, *13*, 944976. DOI: 10.3389/fpsyg.2022.944976 PMID: 36033004

Li, X., Qiao, Y., Yu, C., Guo, Y., Bian, Z., Yang, L., Chen, Y., Yan, S., Xie, X., Huang, D., Chen, J., Chen, Z., Lv, J., & Li, L.China Kadoorie Biobank Collaborative Group. (2019). Tea consumption and bone health in Chinese adults: A population-based study. *Osteoporosis International : A Journal Established as Result of Cooperation between the European Foundation for Osteoporosis and the National Osteoporosis Foundation of the USA*, *30*(2), 333–341. DOI: 10.1007/s00198-018-4767-3 PMID: 30443748

Li, Z., & Jia, L. (2025). Bridging the virtual and the real: The impact of metaverse sports event characteristics on event marketing communication effectiveness. *Communication & Sport*, *13*(6), 1090–1123. DOI: 10.1177/21674795251321754

Lomiwes, D., Barnes, M., Shaw, O., Ngametua, N., Sawyer, G., Burr, N., Hedderley, D., Kanon, A., Bear, T., Carroll, A., Bentley-Hewitt, K., Tian, H. S., & Miller, M. R. (2023). The Efficacy of New Zealand Greenshell™ Mussel Powder Supplementation in Supporting Muscle Recovery Following Eccentric Exercise-Induced Muscle Damage in Healthy, Untrained Adult Males. *Nutrients*, *15*(10), 2316. DOI: 10.3390/nu15102316 PMID: 37242198

Loucks, A. B. (2004). Energy balance and body composition in sports and exercise. *Journal of Sports Sciences*, *22*(1), 1–14. DOI: 10.1080/0264041031000140518 PMID: 14974441

Loucks, A. B., Kiens, B., & Wright, H. H. (2011). Energy availability in athletes. *Journal of Sports Sciences*, *29*(sup1, Suppl 1), S7–S15. DOI: 10.1080/02640414.2011.588958 PMID: 21793767

Luczak, T., Burch, R., Lewis, E., Chander, H., & Ball, J. (2020). State-of-the-art review of athletic wearable technology: What 113 strength and conditioning coaches and athletic trainers from the USA said about technology in sports. *International Journal of Sports Science & Coaching*, *15*(1), 26–40. DOI: 10.1177/1747954119885244

Luo, P., & Song, J. (2025). Beyond raw data: AI-driven biosensor fusion for enhancing athletic performance. *Array (New York, N.Y.)*, *26*, 100418. DOI: 10.1016/j.array.2025.100418

Lu, Y., Stathopoulou, T., Vasiloglou, M. F., Pinault, L. F., Kiley, C., Spanakis, E. K., & Mougiakakou, S. (2020). goFOODTM: An artificial intelligence system for dietary assessment. *Sensors (Basel)*, *20*(15), 4283. https://www.mdpi.com/1424-8220/20/15/4283. DOI: 10.3390/s20154283 PMID: 32752007

Macassa, G. (2022). Can Sustainable Health Behaviour Contribute to Ensure Healthy Lives and Well-being for All at All Ages (Sdg 3)? A Viewpoint. *Journal of Public Health Research*, *10*(3), jphr.2021.2051. Advance online publication. DOI: 10.4081/jphr.2021.2051 PMID: 33870681

Macedo, A. G., Almeida, T. A. F., Massini, D. A., de Oliveira, D. M., Espada, M. C., Robalo, R. A. M., Hernández-Beltrán, V., Gamonales, J. M., Vilela Terra, A. M. S., & Pessôa Filho, D. M. (2024). Load monitoring methods for controlling training effectiveness on physical conditioning and planning involvement: A narrative review. *Applied Sciences (Basel, Switzerland)*, *14*(22), 10465. DOI: 10.3390/app142210465

MacGregor, E. A. (2024). The Regulatory Effects of Vitamin C, Vitamin E, and Natural Antioxidants on Oxidative Stress and Muscle Inflammation Induced by High-Intensity Exercise. *Studies in Sports Science and Physical Education*, *2*(4), 1–5. DOI: 10.56397/SSSPE.2024.12.01

Mach, N., & Fuster-Botella, D. (2017). Endurance exercise and gut microbiota: A review. *Journal of Sport and Health Science*, *6*(2), 179–197. DOI: 10.1016/j.jshs.2016.05.001 PMID: 30356594

Macnaughton, L. S., Wardle, S. L., Witard, O. C., McGlory, C., Hamilton, D. L., Jeromson, S., Lawrence, C. E., Wallis, G. A., & Tipton, K. D. (2016). The response of muscle protein synthesis following whole-body resistance exercise is greater following 40 g than 20 g of ingested whey protein. *Physiological Reports*, *4*(15), e12893. https://physoc.onlinelibrary.wiley.com/doi/10.14814/phy2.12893. DOI: 10.14814/phy2.12893 PMID: 27511985

Madhumanchi, C. (2025). AI-powered personalized nutrition: Transforming grocery retail into a public health partner. *International Journal of Computing and Engineering*, *7*(12), 11–23. DOI: 10.47941/ijce.2974

Madrigal-Cerezo, R., Domínguez-Sanz, N., & Martín-Rodríguez, A. (2026). Wearable Biosensing and Machine Learning for Data-Driven Training and Coaching Support. *Biosensors (Basel)*, *16*(2), 97. https://www.mdpi.com/2079-6374/16/2/97. DOI: 10.3390/bios16020097 PMID: 41744715

Mamta. (2025). The Role of Artificial Intelligence in Modern Healthcare: Transforming Diagnosis, Treatment and Rehabilitation. *AI-driven Innovations in Physiotherapy and Oncology 2*, 335–358. https://doi.org/DOI: 10.1002/9781394423552.ch17

Mănescu, D. C. (2025). Big data analytics framework for decision-making in sports performance optimization. *Data*, *10*(7), 116. DOI: 10.3390/data10070116

Marinescu, M. R., Ionescu, O. N., Pachiu, C. I., Dinescu, M. A., Muller, R., & uchea, M. P. (2025). Next-gen healthcare devices: Evolution of MEMS and BioMEMS in the era of the Internet of bodies for personalized medicine. *Micromachines*, *16*(10), 1182. DOI: 10.3390/mi16101182 PMID: 41156428

Marinescu, . A., Oncioiu, I., & Ghibanu, A.-I. (2025). The digital transformation of healthcare through intelligent technologies: A path dependence-augmented–Unified theory of acceptance and use of technology model for clinical decision support systems. *Health Care*, *13*(11), 1222. DOI: 10.3390/healthcare13111222 PMID: 40508836

Martín-Rodríguez, A., Belinchón-deMiguel, P., Rubio-Zarapuz, A., Tornero-Aguilera, J. F., Martínez-Guardado, I., Villanueva-Tobaldo, C. V., & Clemente-Suárez, V. J. (2024). Advances in understanding the interplay between dietary practices, body composition, and sports performance in athletes. *Nutrients*, *16*(4), 571. DOI: 10.3390/nu16040571 PMID: 38398895

Maughan, R. J., Burke, L. M., Dvorak, J., Larson-Meyer, D. E., Peeling, P., Phillips, S. M., Rawson, E. S., Walsh, N. P., Garthe, I., Geyer, H., Meeusen, R., van Loon, L. J. C., Shirreffs, S. M., Spriet, L. L., Stuart, M., Vernec, A., Currell, K., Ali, V. M., Budgett, R. G. M., & Engebretsen, L. (2018). IOC consensus statement: Dietary supplements and the high-performance athlete. *British Journal of Sports Medicine*, *52*(7), 439–455. DOI: 10.1136/bjsports-2018-099027 PMID: 29540367

Maughan, R. J., Burke, L. M., Dvorak, J., Larson-Meyer, D. E., Peeling, P., Phillips, S. M., Rawson, E. S., Walsh, N. P., Garthe, I., Geyer, H., Meeusen, R., van Loon, L., Shirreffs, S. M., Spriet, L. L., Stuart, M., Vernec, A., Currell, K., Ali, V. M., Budgett, R. G. M., & Engebretsen, L. (2018). IOC consensus statement: Dietary supplements and the high-performance athlete. *International Journal of Sport Nutrition and Exercise Metabolism*, *28*(2), 104–125. DOI: 10.1123/ijsnem.2018-0020 PMID: 29589768

Maughan, R. J., & Shirreffs, S. M. (2019). Muscle cramping during exercise: Causes, solutions, and questions remaining. *Sports Medicine*, *49*(2), 115–124. DOI: 10.1007/s40279-019-01162-1 PMID: 31696455

Maughan, R. J., Shirreffs, S. M., & Leiper, J. B. (2007). Errors in the estimation of hydration status from changes in body mass. *Journal of Sports Sciences*, *25*(7), 797–804. DOI: 10.1080/02640410600875143 PMID: 17454547

McFarlin, B. K., Venable, A. S., Henning, A. L., Sampson, J. N. B., Pennel, K., Vingren, J. L., & Hill, D. W. (2016). Reduced inflammatory and muscle damage biomarkers following oral supplementation with bioavailable curcumin. *BBA Clinical*, *5*, 72–78. DOI: 10.1016/j.bbacli.2016.02.003 PMID: 27051592

Melin, A., Tornberg, Å. B., Skouby, S., Faber, J., Ritz, C., Sjödin, A., & Sundgot-Borgen, J. (2014). The LEAF questionnaire: A screening tool for the identification of female athletes at risk for the female athlete triad. *British Journal of Sports Medicine*, *48*(7), 540–545. DOI: 10.1136/bjsports-2013-093240 PMID: 24563388

Minihane, A. M., Vinoy, S., Russell, W. R., Baka, A., Roche, H. M., Tuohy, K. M., Teeling, J. L., Blaak, E. E., Fenech, M., Vauzour, D., McArdle, H. J., Kremer, B. H. A., Sterkman, L., Vafeiadou, K., Benedetti, M. M., Williams, C. M., & Calder, P. C. (2015). Low-grade inflammation, diet composition, and health: Current research evidence and its translation. *The British Journal of Nutrition*, *114*(7), 999–1012. DOI: 10.1017/S0007114515002093 PMID: 26228057

Mohammadi, I., Farahani, S., Karimi, A., Jahanian, S., Firouzabadi, S. R., Alinejadfard, M., Fatemi, A., Hajikarimloo, B., & Akhlaghpasand, M. (2025). Mortality prediction of heart transplantation using machine learning models: A systematic review and meta-analysis. *Frontiers in Artificial Intelligence*, *8*, 1551959. DOI: 10.3389/frai.2025.1551959 PMID: 40256322

Moore, D. R. (2019). Maximizing post-exercise anabolism: The case for relative protein intakes. *Frontiers in Nutrition*, *6*, 485822. DOI: 10.3389/fnut.2019.00147 PMID: 31552263

Moore, D. R., Camera, D. M., Areta, J. L., & Hawley, J. A. (2014). Beyond muscle hypertrophy: Why dietary protein is important for endurance athletes. *Applied Physiology, Nutrition, and Metabolism*, *39*(9), 987–997. DOI: 10.1139/apnm-2013-0591 PMID: 24806440

Moore, D. R., Churchward-Venne, T. A., Witard, O., Breen, L., Burd, N. A., Tipton, K. D., & Phillips, S. M. (2015). Protein ingestion to stimulate myofibrillar protein synthesis requires greater relative protein intakes in healthy older versus younger men. *The Journals of Gerontology. Series A, Biological Sciences and Medical Sciences*, *70*(1), 57–62. DOI: 10.1093/gerona/glu103 PMID: 25056502

Moore, D. R., Robinson, M. J., Fry, J. L., Tang, J. E., Glover, E. I., Wilkinson, S. B., Prior, T., Tarnopolsky, M. A., & Phillips, S. M. (2009). Ingested protein dose response of muscle and albumin protein synthesis after resistance exercise in young men. *The American Journal of Clinical Nutrition*, *89*(1), 161–168. DOI: 10.3945/ajcn.2008.26401 PMID: 19056590

Moreira, Y. S., de Carvalho Simões, M. A., & Borba, É. L. (2024). O uso de estratégias nutricionais na prevenção e recuperação de lesões em atletas: Uma revisão de literatura. *Research. Social Development*, *13*(5), e6813545807–e6813545807. DOI: 10.33448/rsd-v13i5.45807

Morton, J. P., Hearris, M., Fell, M. J., Owens, D. J., Halson, S., & Trommelen, J. (2025). UCI sports nutrition project: Nutritional periodization: Strategies to enhance training adaptation and recovery. *International Journal of Sport Nutrition and Exercise Metabolism*, •••, 1–26. DOI: 10.1123/ijsnem.2025-0073 PMID: 41130458

Morton, R. W., Murphy, K. T., McKellar, S. R., Schoenfeld, B. J., Henselmans, M., Helms, E., Aragon, A. A., Devries, M. C., Banfield, L., Krieger, J. W., & Phillips, S. M. (2018). A systematic review, meta-analysis and meta-regression of the effect of protein supplementation on resistance training-induced gains in muscle mass and strength in healthy adults. *British Journal of Sports Medicine*, *52*(6), 376–384. DOI: 10.1136/bjsports-2017-097608 PMID: 28698222

Mountjoy, M., Sundgot-Borgen, J. K., Burke, L. M., Ackerman, K. E., Blauwet, C., Constantini, N., Lebrun, C., Lundy, B., Melin, A. K., Meyer, N. L., Sherman, R. T., Tenforde, A. S., Torstveit, M. K., & Budgett, R. (2018). IOC consensus statement on relative energy deficiency in sport (RED-S): 2018 update. *British Journal of Sports Medicine*, *52*(11), 687–697. DOI: 10.1136/bjsports-2018-099193 PMID: 29773536

Mountjoy, M., Sundgot-Borgen, J., Burke, L., Carter, S., Constantini, N., Lebrun, C., Meyer, N., Sherman, R., Steffen, K., Budgett, R., & Ljungqvist, A. (2014). The IOC consensus statement: Beyond the Female Athlete Triad, Relative Energy Deficiency in Sport (RED-S). *British Journal of Sports Medicine*, *48*(7), 491–497. DOI: 10.1136/bjsports-2014-093502 PMID: 24620037

Moussa, M. A., El-Safty, S. M., & Mahmoud, Y. A. H. (2026). Enhancing Psychological Well-being Through AI-Assisted Nutrition: A Study on Female University Students. *Port Said Journal of Educational Research, 5*(1), 30–58. https://journals.ekb.eg/article_477829.html

Mujika, I., & Padilla, S. (2000). Detraining: Loss of training-induced physiological and performance adaptations. Part I. *Sports Medicine, 30*(2), 79–87. https://link.springer.com/article/10.2165/00007256-200030020-00002. DOI: 10.2165/00007256-200030020-00002 PMID: 10966148

Munarso, S. J., Elmatsani, H. M., Djafar, M. J., Kailaku, S. I., Lukas, A., Susetyo, E. B., Setianto, W. B., & Warsono, S. Y. (2026). Global Trends and Innovations in Anti-Inflammatory Functional Beverages: A Bibliometric and Consumer Insights Analysis (2006–2025). *Beverages*, *12*(1), 7. DOI: 10.3390/beverages12010007

Mundt, C., Yusufoğlu, B., Kudenko, D., Mertoğlu, K., & Esatbeyoglu, T. (2025). AI-driven personalized nutrition: Integrating omics, ethics, and digital health. *Molecular Nutrition & Food Research*, *69*(24), e70293. DOI: 10.1002/mnfr.70293 PMID: 41163310

Naderi, A., Rothschild, J. A., Santos, H. O., Hamidvand, A., Koozehchian, M. S., Ghazzagh, A., Berjisian, E., & Podlogar, T. (2025). Nutritional strategies to improve post-exercise recovery and subsequent exercise performance: A narrative review. *Sports Medicine*, *55*(7), 1559–1577. DOI: 10.1007/s40279-025-02213-6 PMID: 40221559

Nasb, M., Zhang, Y., & Chen, N. (2025). The role of artificial intelligence in precision exercise nutrition: A shift from data to diets. *Food Science and Human Wellness*. https://www.sciopen.com/local/article_pdf/10.26599/FSHW.2025.9250623.pdf

Natalucci, V., Spinello, G., Moro, T., Pavei, G., Boccia, G., La Torre, A., & Bonato, M. (2026). Menstrual Cycle and Hormonal Contraceptives in Female Athletes: Should Symptoms and Nutrition Matter More Than Cycle Phase? A Narrative Review. *Nutrients*, *18*(7), 1144. https://www.mdpi.com/2072-6643/18/7/1144. DOI: 10.3390/nu18071144 PMID: 41978194

Nattiv, A., Loucks, A. B., Manore, M. M., Sanborn, C. F., Sundgot-Borgen, J., & Warren, M. P. (2007). American College of Sports Medicine position stand: The female athlete triad. *Medicine and Science in Sports and Exercise*, *39*(10), 1867–1882. DOI: 10.1249/mss.0b013e318149f111 PMID: 17909417

NESR (Nutrition Evidence Systematic Review). (2019). Nutrition evidence systematic review methodology infographic.

Nicholls, J., Lawlor, E., Neitzert, E., & Goodspeed, T. (2009). *A guide to social return on investment*. Cabinet Office.

Nicol, L. M., Rowlands, D. S., Fazakerly, R., & Kellett, J. (2015). Curcumin supplementation likely attenuates delayed onset muscle soreness (DOMS). *European Journal of Applied Physiology*, *115*(8), 1769–1777. https://link.springer.com/article/10.1007/s00421-015-3152-6. DOI: 10.1007/s00421-015-3152-6 PMID: 25795285

Nieman, D. C., & Pedersen, B. K. (1999). Exercise and immune function. *Sports Medicine*, *27*(2), 73–80. DOI: 10.2165/00007256-199927020-00001 PMID: 10091272

Nieman, D. C., & Wentz, L. M. (2019). The compelling link between physical activity and the body's defense system. *Journal of Sport and Health Science*, *8*(3), 201–217. DOI: 10.1016/j.jshs.2018.09.009 PMID: 31193280

Nikitjuk, D. B., Korosteleva, M. M., & Tarmaeva, I. Y. (2025). Sports nutrition as an example of effective implementation of innovative trends in nutrition: Personalization and digitalization (Literature review). *Healthcare of the Russian Federation*, *69*(1), 65–69. DOI: 10.47470/0044-197X-2025-69-1-65-69

Nomura, K., Nakayama, M., & Okizaki, A. (2023). Benefits of basil tea for patients with differentiated thyroid cancer during radioiodine therapy: A randomized controlled trial. *Heliyon*, *9*(10), e20691. https://www.cell.com/heliyon/fulltext/S2405-8440(23)07899-4. DOI: 10.1016/j.heliyon.2023.e20691 PMID: 37829808

Nongbet, A., Chettry, U., Upadhaya, S., & Mohapatra, S. (2026). The future of personalized nutrition: AI, genomics, and precision medicine. In *Nanomedicine and Nutrigenomics* (pp. 269–285). Academic Press., DOI: 10.1016/B978-0-443-26761-1.00005-3

Norton, L. E., & Layman, D. K. (2006). Leucine regulates translation initiation of protein synthesis in skeletal muscle after exercise. *The Journal of Nutrition*, *136*(2), 533S–537S. DOI: 10.1093/jn/136.2.533S PMID: 16424142

Nuszkiewicz, J., Wróblewska, J., Wróblewski, M., & Woźniak, A. (2025). Anthocyanin-Rich Purple Plant Foods: Bioavailability, Antioxidant Mechanisms, and Functional Roles in Redox Regulation and Exercise Recovery. *Nutrients*, *17*(15), 2453. DOI: 10.3390/nu17152453 PMID: 40806038

Nutrition Evidence Systematic Review (NESR). (2019). *Nutrition evidence systematic review methodology infographic*.

Office of the Personal Data Protection Commission. (2021). *Guideline on personal data protection*. PDPA.

Okolo, C. A., Babawarun, O., Arowoogun, J. O., Adeniyi, A. O., & Chidi, R. (2024). The role of mobile health applications in improving patient engagement and health outcomes: A critical review. *International Journal of Science and Research Archive*, *11*(1), 2566–2574. DOI: 10.30574/ijsra.2024.11.1.0334

Okon, J. J. (2025). Leveraging Artificial Intelligence in Sports and Business Management for Enhanced Health and Performance Outcomes. *Applied Sciences, Computing, and Energy, 3*(2), 252-266. https://cemrj.com/index.php/volumes/article/view/58

Olagoke, O. (2018). Phytochemical analysis and antibacterial activities of spinach leaf. *Am. J. Phytomed. Clin. Ther*, *6*, 8. DOI: 10.21767/2321-2748.100344

Oliver, J. M., Jones, M. T., Kirk, K. M., Gable, D. A., Repshas, J. T., Johnson, T. A., Andreasen, U., Doyle, N., Benotmane, Z., & Oliver, N. (2016). Effect of docosahexaenoic acid on a biomarker of head trauma in American football. *Medicine and Science in Sports and Exercise*, *48*(6), 974–982. DOI: 10.1249/MSS.0000000000000875 PMID: 26765633

Owens, D. J., Allison, R., & Close, G. L. (2018). Vitamin D and the athlete: Current perspectives and new challenges. *Sports Medicine*, *48*(S1, Suppl 1), 3–16. DOI: 10.1007/s40279-017-0841-9 PMID: 29368183

Page, M. J.. (2021). The PRISMA 2020 statement: An updated guideline for reporting systematic reviews. *BMJ (Clinical Research Ed.)*, *372*(71). PMID: 33782057

Page, M. J., McKenzie, J. E., Bossuyt, P. M., Boutron, I., Hoffmann, T. C., Mulrow, C. D., Shamseer, L., Tetzlaff, J. M., & Moher, D. (2021). Updating guidance for reporting systematic reviews: Development of the PRISMA 2020 statement. *Journal of Clinical Epidemiology*, *134*, 103–112. DOI: 10.1016/j.jclinepi.2021.02.003 PMID: 33577987

Panayotova, G. G. (2025, October). Artificial Intelligence in Nutrition and Dietetics: A Comprehensive Review of Current Research. In *Healthcare* (Vol. 13, No. 20, p. 2579). MDPI. https://www.mdpi.com/2227-9032/13/20/2579

Panayotova, G. G. (2025). Artificial intelligence in nutrition and dietetics: A comprehensive review of current research. *Health Care, 13*(20), 2579. DOI: 10.3390/healthcare13202579 PMID: 41154258

Pan, C. W., Ma, Q., Sun, H. P., Xu, Y., Luo, N., & Wang, P. (2017). Tea consumption and health-related quality of life in older adults. *The Journal of Nutrition, Health & Aging, 21*(5), 480–486. DOI: 10.1007/s12603-016-0784-0 PMID: 28448076

Pandya, N. N., Limbani, D. P., Ajmera, T., Prajapati, A., Kodwani, M., & Dadhania, A. J. (2026). AI-Driven Personalization of Sports Nutrition Supplements for Performance Optimization. *Advances in Consumer Research. Association for Consumer Research (U. S.), 3*(2).

Papadopoulou, S. K. (2020). Rehabilitation nutrition for injury recovery of athletes: The role of macronutrient intake. *Nutrients, 12*(8), 2449. DOI: 10.3390/nu12082449 PMID: 32824034

Paria, D., Banik, T. D., Manna, S., & Pal, S. (2026). The Iron Paradox: A Comprehensive Review of Pathophysiology, Performance Implications, and Strategic Nutritional Management in Female Athletes. *Journal of Research in Allied Life Sciences, 2*(2), 1–14. https://jralsjournal.com/index.php/jrals/article/view/20

Park, J. I., Lee, H. Y., Kim, H., Lee, J., Shinn, J., & Kim, H. S. (2021). Lack of acceptance of digital healthcare in the medical market: Addressing old problems raised by various clinical professionals and developing possible solutions. *Journal of Korean Medical Science, 36*(37), e253. DOI: 10.3346/jkms.2021.36.e253 PMID: 34581521

Patel, R. V., Mistry, B. M., Shinde, S. K., Syed, R., Singh, V., & Shin, H. S. (2018). Therapeutic potential of quercetin as a cardiovascular agent. *European Journal of Medicinal Chemistry, 155*, 889–904. DOI: 10.1016/j.ejmech.2018.06.053 PMID: 29966915

Patra, E., Kokkinopoulou, A., Wilson-Barnes, S., Hart, K., Gymnopoulos, L. P., Tsatsou, D., Solachidis, V., Dimitropoulos, K., Rouskas, K., Argiriou, A., Lalama, E., Csanalosi, M., Pfeiffer, A. F. H., Cornelissen, V., Decorte, E., Dias, S. B., Oikonomidis, Y., María Botana, J., Leoni, R., & Pagkalos, I. (2024). Personal goals, user engagement, and meal adherence within a personalised AI-based mobile application for nutrition and physical activity. *Life (Basel, Switzerland), 14*(10), 1238. DOI: 10.3390/life14101238 PMID: 39459538

Paul, J., Ueno, A., Dennis, C., Alamanos, E., Curtis, L., Foroudi, P., Kacprzak, A., Kunz, W. H., Liu, J., Marvi, R., Nair, S. L. S., Ozdemir, O., Pantano, E., Papadopoulos, T., Petit, O., Tyagi, S., & Wirtz, J. (2024). Digital transformation: A multidisciplinary perspective and future research agenda. *International Journal of Consumer Studies*, *48*(2), e13015. DOI: 10.1111/ijcs.13015

Paulsen, G., Cumming, K. T., Holden, G., Hallén, J., Rønnestad, B. R., Sveen, O., Skaug, A., Paur, I., Bastani, N. E., Østgaard, H. N., Buer, C., Midttun, M., Freuchen, F., Wiig, H., Ulseth, E. T., Garthe, I., Blomhoff, R., Benestad, H. B., & Raastad, T. (2014). Vitamin C and E supplementation hampers cellular adaptation to endurance training in humans: A double-blind, randomised, controlled trial. *The Journal of Physiology*, *592*(8), 1887–1901. https://physoc.onlinelibrary.wiley.com/doi/abs/10.1113/jphysiol.2013.267419. DOI: 10.1113/jphysiol.2013.267419 PMID: 24492839

Peake, J. M., Neubauer, O., Della Gatta, P. A., & Nosaka, K. (2017). Muscle damage and inflammation during recovery from exercise. *Journal of Applied Physiology (Bethesda, Md.)*, *122*(3), 559–570. DOI: 10.1152/japplphysiol.00971.2016 PMID: 28035017

Peeling, P., Castell, L. M., Derave, W., de Hon, O., & Burke, L. M. (2019). Sports foods and dietary supplements for optimal function and performance enhancement in track-and-field athletes. *International Journal of Sport Nutrition and Exercise Metabolism*, *29*(2), 198–209. DOI: 10.1123/ijsnem.2018-0271 PMID: 30299192

Peeling, P., Dawson, B., Goodman, C., Landers, G., & Trinder, D. (2008). Athletic induced iron deficiency: New insights into the role of inflammation, cytokines and hormones. *European Journal of Applied Physiology*, *103*(4), 381–391. DOI: 10.1007/s00421-008-0726-6 PMID: 18365240

Pereira, D. M., Dos Santos, V. T., Vilela, M. M., De Oliveira, T. M., Oliveira, D. C., & Junior, J. K. K. (2024). *Contribuição da nutrição para a prevenção e recuperação da Síndrome do Overtraining em atletas*. Brazilian Journal of Health Review., DOI: 10.34119/bjhrv7n1-560

Perez-Uribe, R., Ocampo-Guzman, D., & Lozano-Correa, L. J. (Eds.). (2025). *Models, strategies, and tools for competitive SMEs*. IGI Global Scientific Publishing., DOI: 10.4018/979-8-3693-4046-2

Persistence Market Research. (2025, October 29). *Sports nutrition market size, share, growth, and regional forecast, 2025–2032* (Report No. PMRREP2889). https://www.persistencemarketresearch.com/market-research/sports-nutrition-market.asp

Petpiamsiri, C., Siritientong, T., Kangsadalampai, K., & Tongyonk, L. (2018). The nitrate content in some green leafy vegetables with different cultivation methods in Thailand. *Thai Journal of Public Health, 48*(3), 385–397. https://he02.tci-thaijo.org/index.php/jph/article/view/133167

Phalle, A., & Gokhale, D. (2025). Navigating next-gen nutrition care using artificial intelligence-assisted dietary assessment tools—A scoping review of potential applications. *Frontiers in Nutrition, 12*, 1518466. DOI: 10.3389/fnut.2025.1518466 PMID: 39917741

Phillips, S. M. (2014). A brief review of critical processes in exercise-induced muscular hypertrophy. *Sports Medicine, 44*(S1, Suppl 1), 71–77. https://link.springer.com/article/10.1007/s40279-014-0152-3. DOI: 10.1007/s40279-014-0152-3 PMID: 24791918

Phillips, S. M., & Van Loon, L. J. C. (2011). Dietary protein for athletes: From requirements to optimum adaptation. *Journal of Sports Sciences, 29*(sup1, Suppl 1), S29–S38. DOI: 10.1080/02640414.2011.619204 PMID: 22150425

Phuangsuwan, P., Siripipatthanakul, S., Chaiprakarn, S., & Rakpathum, W. Muthmainnha, Pariwongkhuntorn, N., & Wattanakul, P. (2024, June). Sustainable Development Adopting Artificial Intelligence (AI) in Marketing and Consumer Behaviour Analysis. In *International Conference on Data Analytics & Management* (pp. 569–587). Singapore: Springer Nature Singapore. https://link.springer.com/chapter/10.1007/978-981-96-3372-2_39

Phuangsuwan, P., Siripipatthanakul, S., Limna, P., & Pariwongkhuntorn, N. (2024). *The impact of google maps application on the digital economy. Corporate and Business Strategy Review, 5 (1), 192–203.* https://virtusinterpress.org/IMG/pdf/cbsrv5i1art18.pdf

Phuangsuwan, P., Siripipatthanakul, S., Limna, P., & Pariwongkhuntorn, N. (2024). The impact of Google Maps application on the digital economy. *Phuangsuwan, P., Siripipatthanakul, S., Limna, P., & Pariwongkhuntorn*, (2024), 192-203. https://virtusinterpress.org/IMG/pdf/cbsrv5i1art18.pdf

Phuangsuwan, P., Siripipatthanakul, S., Siripipattanakul, S., & Jaipong, P. (2025). The impact of community participation in sustainable learning resource development: A case of Bangkok, Thailand. *Sustainability (Basel), 17*(10), 4620. https://www.mdpi.com/2071-1050/17/10/4620. DOI: 10.3390/su17104620

Pingitore, A., Lima, G. P. P., Mastorci, F., Quinones, A., Iervasi, G., & Vassalle, C. (2015). Exercise and oxidative stress: Potential effects of antioxidant dietary strategies in sports. *Nutrition (Burbank, Los Angeles County, Calif.)*, *31*(7–8), 916–922. DOI: 10.1016/j.nut.2015.02.005 PMID: 26059364

Piskorz-Ryń, O., Ballester-Ripoll, R., Gottschlich, D., Rostami, M., & Bulut, S. (2025). Understanding user perceptions of personalized feedback in digital health tools. *Health Nexus*, *3*(4), 1–10. DOI: 10.61838/kman.hn.3.4.2

Powers, S. K., Deruisseau, K. C., Quindry, J., & Hamilton, K. L. (2004). Dietary antioxidants and exercise. *Journal of Sports Sciences*, *22*(1), 81–94. DOI: 10.1080/0264041031000140563 PMID: 14971435

Powers, S. K., Nelson, W. B., & Hudson, M. B. (2011). Exercise-induced oxidative stress in humans: Cause and consequences. *Free Radical Biology & Medicine*, *51*(5), 942–950. DOI: 10.1016/j.freeradbiomed.2010.12.009 PMID: 21167935

Prasad, S., Gupta, E., Yadav, S., Babulal, K. S., & Mishra, S. (2025). Plant-based food industry: overview and trends. *The future of plant protein: innovations, challenges, and opportunities*, 73-97. https://link.springer.com/chapter/10.1007/978-981-96-4190-1_4

Prasad, G., Padhiary, M., Hoque, A., & Kumar, K. (2025). AI-driven personalized nutrition apps and platforms for enhanced diet and wellness. In Alhussaini Hamad, A., & Soni, R. (Eds.), *Food in the Metaverse and Web 3.0 Era: Intersecting Food, Technology, and Culture* (pp. 125–158). IGI Global Scientific Publishing., DOI: 10.4018/979-8-3693-9025-2.ch006

Precedence Research. (2025, December 18). *Sports nutrition market size, share and trends 2026 to 2035* (Report No. 1737). https://www.precedenceresearch.com/sports-nutrition-market

Pritchett, K., & Pritchett, R. (2012). Chocolate milk: A post-exercise recovery beverage for endurance sports. *Medicine and Sport Science*, *59*, 127–134. DOI: 10.1159/000341954 PMID: 23075563

Puce, L., Ceylan, H., Trompetto, C., Cotellessa, F., Schenone, C., Marinelli, L., Zmijewski, P., Bragazzi, N., & Mori, L. (2024). Optimizing athletic performance through advanced nutrition strategies: Can AI and digital platforms have a role in ultraendurance sports? *Biology of Sport*, *41*(4), 305–313. DOI: 10.5114/biolsport.2024.141063 PMID: 39416500

Purcell, L. K. (2013). Sport nutrition for young athletes. *Paediatrics & Child Health*, *18*(4), 200–205. DOI: 10.1093/pch/18.4.200 PMID: 24421690

Puspitasari, R. D., & Arfajah, A. A. (2026). The Role of Nutrition in Optimizing Athletic Performance and Recovery: A Literature Review. *Journal of Nutrition and Health Care*, 1–5. https://junic.professorline.com/index.php/journal/article/view/39

Putra, I. P. O. D. J., Purnami, C. T., & Kartini, A. (2024). Overview of user experience in using nutrition information system: Scoping review. *Jurnal Multidisiplin Madani*, *4*(1), 45–56. DOI: 10.55927/mudima.v4i1.7670

PwC. (2025). *Sports industry outlook: Insights and opportunities for the Middle East.* https://www.pwc.com/m1/en/publications/2025/docs/sports-industry-outlook-2025-eng.pdf

Qi, Y., Sajadi, S. M., Baghaei, S., Rezaei, R., & Li, W. (2024). Digital technologies in sports: Opportunities, challenges, and strategies for safeguarding athlete wellbeing and competitive integrity in the digital era. *Technology in Society*, *77*, 102496. DOI: 10.1016/j.techsoc.2024.102496

Quan, W., Zhou, J., Wang, J., Huang, J., & Du, L. (2026). Machine learning-driven precision nutrition: A paradigm evolution in dietary assessment and intervention. *Nutrients*, *18*(1), 45. DOI: 10.3390/nu18010045 PMID: 41515163

Rakshit, D. (2025). Mobile applications in e-commerce and healthcare prescription management: Integrating AI-driven personalization, accessibility, and multi-domain services. *Journal of Computer Science and Technology Studies*, *7*(12), 46–54. https://al-kindipublishers.org/index.php/jcsts/article/view/11485

Raleigh, C. (2025). *An exploration of low carbohydrate dietary intake in endurance athletes: prevalence, knowledge and the potential effect on bone health and remodelling* (Doctoral dissertation). https://hdl.handle.net/10344/14017

Ranchordas, M. K., Dawson, J. T., & Russell, M. (2017). Practical nutritional recovery strategies for elite soccer players when limited time separates repeated matches. *Journal of the International Society of Sports Nutrition*, *14*(1), 35. DOI: 10.1186/s12970-017-0193-8 PMID: 28919844

Rao, S., & Rao, F. (2026). Transforming Health Education: AI-Driven Games and Simulations for Mental Health, Nutrition, and Physical Well-Being. In *AI-Powered Educational Games and Simulations* (pp. 273–306). IGI Global Scientific Publishing. DOI: DOI: 10.4018/979-8-3373-0035-1.ch008

Rao, S., & Neethirajan, S. (2025). Computational architectures for precision dairy nutrition digital twins: A technical review and implementation framework. *Sensors (Basel)*, *25*(16), 4899. DOI: 10.3390/s25164899 PMID: 40871763

Rasińska, A., Jachimczak, J., Rzyczniok, P., Bala, P., Matusik, J., Rostkowska, A., Grydź, F., Filipow, J., Kupisiak, S., Pasierb, N., & Kopczyński, M. (2025). The impact of omega-3 fatty acids supplementation on reducing exercise-induced muscle damage: A review. *Archiv EuroMedica, 15*(3). Advance online publication. DOI: 10.35630/2025/15/3.321

Ratten, V., & Thompson, A. J. (2020). Digital sport entrepreneurial ecosystems. *Thunderbird International Business Review, 62*(5), 565–578. DOI: 10.1002/tie.22160

Rauscher, O., Grünhaus, C., & Millner, R. (2012). *Social impact measurement and social return on investment (SROI)-analysis.* Vienna University of Economics and Business. https://www.researchgate.net/publication/357335567

Rawson, E. S., & Volek, J. S. (2003). Effects of creatine supplementation and resistance training on muscle strength and weightlifting performance. *Journal of Strength and Conditioning Research, 17*(4), 822–831. DOI: 10.1519/1533-4287(2003)017<0822:EOCSAM>2.0.CO;2 PMID: 14636102

Research and Markets. (2026, January). *B2B sports nutrition market - Global forecast 2026-2032.* https://www.researchandmarkets.com/report/b2b-sports-nutrition

Res, P. T., Groen, B., Pennings, B., Beelen, M., Wallis, G. A., Gijsen, A. P., Senden, J. M., & van Loon, L. J. C. (2012). Protein ingestion before sleep improves postexercise overnight recovery. *Medicine and Science in Sports and Exercise, 44*(8), 1560–1569. DOI: 10.1249/MSS.0b013e31824cc363 PMID: 22330017

Richter, E. A., & Hargreaves, M. (2013). Exercise, GLUT4, and skeletal muscle glucose uptake. *Physiological Reviews, 93*(3), 993–1017. DOI: 10.1152/physrev.00038.2012 PMID: 23899560

Righetti, S., Medoro, A., Graziano, F., Mondazzi, L., Martegani, S., Chiappero, F., Casiraghi, E., Petroni, P. A., Corbi, G., Pina, R., Scapagnini, G., Davinelli, S., & Ricordi, C. (2024). Effects of Maltodextrin–Fructose Supplementation on Inflammatory Biomarkers and Lipidomic Profile Following Endurance Running: A Randomized Placebo-Controlled Cross-Over Trial. *Nutrients, 16*(18), 3078. DOI: 10.3390/nu16183078 PMID: 39339678

Ristow, M., & Schmeisser, K. (2014). Mitohormesis: promoting health and lifespan by increased levels of reactive oxygen species (ROS). *Dose-response, 12*(2), dose-response. https://doi.org/DOI: 10.2203/dose-response.13-035.Ristow

Rivera-Brown, A. M., Ramírez-Marrero, F. A., Wilk, B., & Bar-Or, O. (2006). Voluntary drinking and hydration in trained, heat-acclimatized girls exercising in a hot and humid climate. *European Journal of Applied Physiology*, *96*(2), 109–117. DOI: 10.1007/s00421-005-0060-0 PMID: 18247043

Rohilla, R., & Therattil, P. (2024). Optimising Bone Health in Female Athletes: A Narrative Review. *Sports Science & Health Advances, 2*(2), 316–321. https://sshajournal.com/index.php/1/article/view/143

Rojano-Ortega, D., & Ortega, D. R.. (2020). Tart cherry and pomegranate supplementations enhance recovery from exercise-induced muscle damage: A systematic review. *Sports Medicine*, *50*(11), 1–20.

Rojas, A. S., & Cisterna, M. Z. (2026). Dialogue and sports supplementation: reflections from the social sciences: a systematic review. *Frontiers in Sports and Active Living*, *7*, 1719247. https://pmc.ncbi.nlm.nih.gov/articles/PMC12867773/. DOI: 10.3389/fspor.2025.1719247 PMID: 41647279

Romano, R., De Luca, L., Aiello, A., Pagano, R., Di Pierro, P., Pizzolongo, F., & Masi, P. (2022). Basil (Ocimum Basilicum L.) leaves as a source of bioactive compounds. *Foods*, *11*(20), 3212. DOI: 10.3390/foods11203212 PMID: 37430961

Roppelt, J. S., Kanbach, D. K., & Kraus, S. (2024). Artificial intelligence in healthcare institutions: A systematic literature review on influencing factors. *Technology in Society*, *76*, 102443. DOI: 10.1016/j.techsoc.2023.102443

Rosińska-Lewandoska, D., Lewandowska, D., Morawska, M., Jarosz, K., Wolff, A., Kożuchowska, K., Gruszka, S., Szewczyk, M., Pilarz, D., & Ufnal, J. (2024). The impact of curcumin supplementation on inflammatory processes and recovery in athletes. *Journal of Education, Health and Sport*, *76*, 56583. DOI: 10.12775/JEHS.2024.76.56583

Saadati, N., & Torres, M. (2024). Dimensions of trust in AI coaching assistants among elite athletes: Interviews with users and non-users. *Game Nexus, 1*(2), 1-11. https://game-nexus.org/index.php/gamenexus/article/view/7

Sah, D., Kumar, A., Bhatia, R., Singh, K., Thakur, U., & Kesharwani, R. (2024). Unveiling the power of personalization in health and fitness apps. *International Journal for Research in Applied Science and Engineering Technology*, *12*(11), 755–761. DOI: 10.22214/ijraset.2024.64980

San Juan, A. F., López-Samanes, Á., Jodra, P., Valenzuela, P. L., Rueda, J., Veiga-Herreros, P., Pérez-López, A., & Domínguez, R. (2019). Caffeine supplementation improves anaerobic performance, neuromuscular efficiency, and fatigue in Olympic-level boxers. *Nutrients, 11*(9), 2120. https://www.mdpi.com/2072-6643/11/9/2120. DOI: 10.3390/nu11092120 PMID: 31492050

Sandbakk, Ø., Herzog, S., McGawley, K., Pyne, D. B., Talsnes, R. K., Millet, G. P., & Sandbakk, S. B. (2025). Perspectives of World-Class Endurance Coaches on the Evolution of Athlete Training and Performance. *International Journal of Sports Physiology and Performance, 21*(1), 98–105. https://journals.humankinetics.com/view/journals/ijspp/21/1/article-p98.xml. DOI: 10.1123/ijspp.2025-0317 PMID: 41248624

Sandbakk, Ø., Spörri, J., Fridén, C., Melin, A., Zoppirolli, C., Sperlich, B., Skattebo, Ø., Fornasiero, A., Ørtenblad, N., & Holmberg, H. C. (2026). From Biological Foundations to Optimizing Performance and Health in Elite Female Winter Olympians. *Scandinavian Journal of Medicine & Science in Sports, 36*(3), e70263. https://onlinelibrary.wiley.com/doi/abs/10.1111/sms.70263. DOI: 10.1111/sms.70263 PMID: 41842718

Sansome, K., Conduit, J., & Wilkie, D. C. H. (2024). Consumer-based conceptualisation of brand transparency: Scope, characteristics and contextual determinants. *European Journal of Marketing, 58*(12), 2637–2669. DOI: 10.1108/EJM-12-2022-0885

Santomier, J. P. (2026). Digital transformation: The global sport industry. *International Encyclopedia of Business Management, 2*, 414-419. DOI: 10.1016/B978-0-443-13701-3.00209-7

Santos, R. V., Bassit, R. A., Caperuto, E. C., & Costa Rosa, L. F. (2004). The effect of creatine supplementation upon inflammatory and muscle soreness markers after a 30km race. *Life Sciences, 75*(16), 1917–1924. DOI: 10.1016/j.lfs.2003.11.036 PMID: 15306159

Sawka, M. N., Burke, L. M., Eichner, E. R., Maughan, R. J., Montain, S. J., & Stachenfeld, N. S. (2007). American College of Sports Medicine position stand: Exercise and fluid replacement. *Medicine and Science in Sports and Exercise, 39*(2), 377–390. DOI: 10.1249/mss.0b013e31802ca597 PMID: 17277604

Schek, A. (2025). 'Food First', Not ' Food Only ' in Competitive Sports: A Mini-Review. *The Open Sports Sciences Journal, 18*(1), e1875399X378498. Advance online publication. DOI: 10.2174/011875399X378498250508065801

Schneider, C., & Segre, T. (2009). Green tea: Potential health benefits. *American Family Physician*, *79*(7), 591–594. https://www.aafp.org/pubs/afp/issues/2009/0401/p591.html PMID: 19378876

Schoenfeld, B. J., & Aragon, A. A. (2018). Is there a post-workout anabolic window of opportunity for nutrient consumption? Clearing up controversies. *journal of orthopaedic & sports physical therapy*, 48(12), 911-914. https://www.jospt.org/doi/abs/10.2519/jospt.2018.0615

Schwellnus, M. P., Derman, W. E., & Noakes, T. D. (2011). Aetiology of skeletal muscle 'cramps' during exercise: A novel hypothesis. *Journal of Sports Sciences*, *15*(3), 277–285. DOI: 10.1080/026404197367281 PMID: 9232553

Schwingshackl, L., & Hoffmann, G. (2015). Adherence to Mediterranean diet and risk of cancer: An updated systematic review and meta-analysis of observational studies. *Cancer Medicine*, *4*(12), 1933–1947. https://onlinelibrary.wiley.com/doi/full/10.1002/cam4.539. DOI: 10.1002/cam4.539 PMID: 26471010

Selvi, M. K., Sowmya, B., Kannan, T., Latha, M., Jena, I., Kumar, V. A., & Vijayaraj, P. (2022). Advances in personalized food and nutrition. In Prakash, B. (Ed.), *Research and Technological Advances in Food Science* (pp. 31–60). Academic Press., DOI: 10.1016/B978-0-12-824369-5.00004-X

Serra, C. M., Aroca Tanarro, A., Cummings, C. M., Jimenez Fuertes, A., & Tomás Martínez, J. F. (2022). Impact on the reduction of CO2 emissions due to the use of telemedicine. *Scientific Reports*, *12*(1), 12507. DOI: 10.1038/s41598-022-16864-2 PMID: 35869274

Shaengchart, Y., Limna, P., Kraiwanit, T., Siripipatthanakul, S., & Jangjarat, K. (2026). Community Enterprise and Social Economy for Sustainability in a Developing Country. In *Technology Policy and Its Impact on Green Governance and Sustainability* (pp. 1–30). IGI Global Scientific Publishing., https://www.igi-global.com/chapter/community-enterprise-and-social-economy-for-sustainability-in-a-developing-country/401079

Shan, F., Liu, L., Li, L., Wang, W., Bi, Y., & Li, M. (2025). Management, safety, and efficacy evaluation of nutraceutical and functional food: A global perspective. *Comprehensive Reviews in Food Science and Food Safety*, *24*(4), e70222. https://ift.onlinelibrary.wiley.com/doi/full/10.1111/1541-4337.70222. DOI: 10.1111/1541-4337.70222 PMID: 40613254

Shanita, S. N., Rahman, A. H. A., Azimah, A., Izham, M. M., Othman, N. E., Chan, Y. T., Pushpa, B. S., Poh, B. K., & Ruzita, A. T. (2017). DietScore™: Sports nutrition-based mobile application for athletes and active individuals. In Ibrahim, F., Cheong, J., Usman, J., Ahmad, M., Razman, R., & Selvanayagam, V. (Eds.), *3rd International Conference on Movement, Health and Exercise (MoHE 2016)* (IFMBE Proceedings, Vol. 58). Springer. DOI: 10.1007/978-981-10-3737-5_1

Sharma, A. (2019). Development and nutritional assessment of selected snacks using basil leaves. *International Journal of Home Science*, *5*(2), 409–413.

Shaw, G., Lee-Barthel, A., Ross, M. L., Wang, B., & Baar, K. (2017). Vitamin C-enriched gelatin supplementation before intermittent activity augments collagen synthesis. *The American Journal of Clinical Nutrition*, *105*(1), 136–143. DOI: 10.3945/ajcn.116.138594 PMID: 27852613

Sherman, W. M., Costill, D. L., Fink, W. J., & Miller, J. M. (1981). Effect of exercise-diet manipulation on muscle glycogen and its subsequent utilization during performance. *International Journal of Sports Medicine*, *2*(2), 114–118. DOI: 10.1055/s-2008-1034594 PMID: 7333741

Shirreffs, S. M., & Sawka, M. N. (2011). Fluid and electrolyte needs for training, competition, and recovery. *Journal of Sports Sciences*, 29(sup1), S39-S46. https://doi.org/DOI: 10.1080/02640414.2011.614269

Shirreffs, S. M., Taylor, A. J., Leiper, J. B., & Maughan, R. J. (1996). Post-exercise rehydration in man: Effects of volume consumed and drink sodium content. *Medicine and Science in Sports and Exercise*, *28*(10), 1260–1271. DOI: 10.1097/00005768-199610000-00009 PMID: 8897383

Shlykov, S. N., Sycheva, O. V., Omarov, R. S., Trubina, I. A., & Skorbina, E. A. (2025). Sports Nutrition and Recovery: Key Nutrients and Supplements for Effective Regeneration. *Human Physiology*, *51*(2), 201–216. DOI: 10.1134/S036211972570032X

Siddika, M. A., Chakraborty, D., Noor, M. S., & Haque, M. N. (2024). Integrating business information systems in public health nutrition programs: Challenges and opportunities. *International Journal of Management Information Systems and Data Science*, *1*(04), 17–33. DOI: 10.62304/ijmisds.v1i04.178

Silpi, C. (2025). Nutraceuticals traditional practices, regulatory guidelines, opportunities and challenges. *Discover Food*, *5*(1), 191. https://link.springer.com/article/10.1007/s44187-025-00437-z. DOI: 10.1007/s44187-025-00437-z

Silva, R. A., Santos, R., & Pereira, L. (2024). Effect of omega-3 fatty acids supplementation on inflammatory markers in healthy subjects: A meta-analysis. *Clinical Nutrition : Official Journal of the European Society of Parenteral and Enteral Nutrition*, *43*(5), 1034–1046.

Simopoulos, A. P. (2015). Anti-inflammatory dietary interventions and supplements to improve health. *Molecular Nutrition & Food Research*, *59*(1), 19–35.

Singletary, K. W. (2018). Basil: A brief summary of potential health benefits. *Nutrition Today*, *53*(2), 92–97. DOI: 10.1097/NT.0000000000000267

Siri, P. (2025). *Evaluating the economic and social benefits of health application use in Thailand* (Doctoral dissertation). Rangsit University. DOI: 10.13140/RG.2.2.19760.67848

Siri, P., Kraiwanit, T., Keawngam, T., & Ponsri, R. (2025). The social impact of health applications: Transforming self-care and patient support. [Humanities and Social Sciences]. *Journal of Suvarnabhumi Institute of Technology*, *11*(2), 213–225. https://so04.tci-thaijo.org/index.php/svittj/article/view/277401

Siripipatthanakul, S., Phuangsuwan, P., & Jaipong, P. (2025, a). Mobile application security: A case study of Bank of Ayudhya PCL.(KMA), Thailand. In *International Conference on Data Processing and Networking* (pp. 479–493). Springer, Singapore. https://link.springer.com/chapter/10.1007/978-981-96-3102-5_36

Siripipatthanakul, S., Phuangsuwan, P., Jaipong, P., & Muthmainnha. (2025, September). Wi-Fi Networks and Security: A Systematic Review. In *International Conference on Artificial Intelligence and Networking* (pp. 81-92). Singapore: Springer Nature Singapore. https://link.springer.com/chapter/10.1007/978-981-96-2015-9_6

Siripipatthanakul, S., Phuangsuwan, P., Jaipong, P., & Muthmainnha. (2025,b, September). Wi-Fi Networks and Security: A Systematic Review. In *International Conference on Artificial Intelligence and Networking* (pp. 81–92). Singapore: Springer Nature Singapore. https://link.springer.com/chapter/10.1007/978-981-96-2015-9_6

Siripipatthanakul, S., Rakpathum, W., Siripipattanakul, S., Kaewnaknaew, C., Phuangsuwan, P., & Jaipong, P. (2025, a). The Future Artificial Intelligence (AI) for the Hotel and Hospitality Industry: The Case of Hotels' Human Resource Management (HRM). In *Best Practices for Human Resources Management in Tourism and Hospitality* (pp. 395–422). IGI Global Scientific Publishing.

Siripipatthanakul, S., Rungsiyanont, S., & Siripipattanakul, S. (2025, b). Sustainable dentistry using artificial intelligence (AI) for digital education and business among university dental hospitals. In *Sustainable development for hospitals and clinics* (pp. 33–64). IGI Global Scientific Publishing. DOI: DOI: 10.4018/979-8-3693-9800-5.ch002

Siripipatthanakul, S., Chaiprakarn, S., Rungsiyanont, S., & Phuangsuwan, P. (2025). A case study of sustainable development in hospitals in Thailand using ChatGPT. In *Sustainable development for hospitals and clinics* (pp. 1–32). IGI Global Scientific Publishing., DOI: 10.4018/979-8-3693-9800-5.ch001

Siripipatthanakul, S., Limna, P., Sriboonruang, P., & Kaewpuang, P. (2023). Applying the TPB and the UTAUT models predicting intentions to use telemedicine among Thai people during the COVID-19 pandemic. *International Journal of Computing Sciences Research*, *7*(1), 1362–1384. https://stepacademic.net/ijcsr/article/view/350. DOI: 10.25147/ijcsr.2017.001.1.107

Sitthipon, T., Siripipatthanakul, S., Phayaphrom, B., Siripipattanakul, S., & Limna, P. (2022). Determinants of customers' intention to use healthcare chatbots and apps in Bangkok, Thailand. *International Journal of Behavioral Analytics*, *2*(2), 1–15. https://ssrn.com/abstract=4045661

Smith, G. I., Atherton, P., Reeds, D. N., Mohammed, B. S., Rankin, D., Rennie, M. J., & Mittendorfer, B. (2011). Omega-3 polyunsaturated fatty acids augment the muscle protein anabolic response to hyperinsulinaemia-hyperaminoacidaemia in healthy young and middle-aged men and women. *Clinical Science (London, England)*, *121*(6), 267–278. DOI: 10.1042/CS20100597 PMID: 21501117

Smith, J. D.. (2023). Popular dietary trends' impact on athletic performance: A review of ketogenic, plant-based, intermittent fasting, and Mediterranean diets. *Sports Medicine - Open*, *9*(1), 67. PMID: 37526793

Snijders, T., Res, P. T., Smeets, J. S., van Vliet, S., van Kranenburg, J., Maase, K., Kies, A. K., Verdijk, L. B., & van Loon, L. J. C. (2015). Protein ingestion before sleep increases muscle mass and strength gains during prolonged resistance-type exercise training in healthy young men. *The Journal of Nutrition*, *145*(6), 1178–1184. DOI: 10.3945/jn.114.208371 PMID: 25926415

Sonnen, J. (2024). *Framework for mobile applications aiding the visualization of performance data: A case study in swimming* (Master's thesis, KTH Royal Institute of Technology). DiVA. https://www.diva-portal.org/smash/get/diva2:1878986/FULLTEXT01.pdf

Sousa, M., Teixeira, V. H., & Soares, J. (2014). Dietary strategies to recover from exercise-induced muscle damage. *International Journal of Food Sciences and Nutrition, 65*(2), 151–163. DOI: 10.3109/09637486.2013.849662 PMID: 24180469

Stellar Market Research. (2025, February 12). *Sport nutrition market overview* (Report No. SMR_330). https://www.stellarmr.com/report/Sports-Nutrition-Market/330

Suarez, C., & Adibi, S. (2025). Integrating traditional nutritional wisdom into digital nutrition platforms: Toward culturally adaptive and inclusive health technologies. *Nutrients, 17*(12), 1978. DOI: 10.3390/nu17121978 PMID: 40573089

Sun, S., Gu, B., & Tang, F. (2025). Cross-category innovation strategy and evolution of digital platform ecosystems: A technology-driven perspective. *Sustainability (Basel), 17*(11), 5113. DOI: 10.3390/su17115113

Sutehall, S., & Pitsiladis, Y. (2025). Personalized nutrition for the enhancement of elite athletic performance. *Scandinavian Journal of Medicine & Science in Sports, 35*(4), e70044. DOI: 10.1111/sms.70044 PMID: 40164953

Suzuki, K. (2021). Recent progress in applicability of exercise immunology and inflammation research to sports nutrition. *Nutrients, 13*(12), 4299. https://www.mdpi.com/2072-6643/13/12/4299. DOI: 10.3390/nu13124299 PMID: 34959851

Suzuki, T., Miyoshi, N., Hayakawa, S., Imai, S., Isemura, M., & Nakamura, Y. (2016). *Health benefits of tea consumption* (2nd ed.). Beverage Impacts on Health and Nutrition., https://link.springer.com/chapter/10.1007/978-3-319-23672-8_4 DOI: 10.1007/978-3-319-23672-8_4

Talebi, S., Zeraattalab-Motlagh, S., Arab, A., Ghoreishy, S. M., Amiri Khosroshahi, R., & Djafarian, K. (2023). Nutritional interventions for exercise-induced muscle damage: An umbrella review of systematic reviews and meta-analyses of randomized trials. *Nutrition Reviews*. Advance online publication. DOI: 10.1093/nutrit/nuad078 PMID: 37460208

Tanabe, Y., Maeda, S., Akazawa, N., Zempo-Miyaki, A., Choi, Y., Ra, S. G., Imaizumi, A., Ohmori, H., & Nosaka, K. (2015). Attenuation of indirect markers of eccentric exercise-induced muscle damage by curcumin. *European Journal of Applied Physiology, 115*(9), 1949–1957. DOI: 10.1007/s00421-015-3170-4 PMID: 25921600

Tangcharoensathien, V., Adulyanon, S., Supaka, N., Munkong, R., Viriyathorn, S., Sirithienthong, S., Kanhachon, S., & Marten, R. (2024). The Thai health promotion foundation: Two decades of joint contributions to addressing noncommunicable diseases and creating healthy populations. *Global Health, Science and Practice, 12*(2), e2300311. DOI: 10.9745/GHSP-D-23-00311 PMID: 38448166

Tarnopolsky, M. A. (2004). Protein requirements for endurance athletes. *Nutrition (Burbank, Los Angeles County, Calif.)*, *20*(7-8), 662–668. DOI: 10.1016/j.nut.2004.04.008 PMID: 15212749

Tasmurzayev, N., Amangeldy, B., Imanbek, B., Baigarayeva, Z., Imankulov, T., Dikhanbayeva, G., Amangeldi, I., & Sharipova, S. (2025). Digital cardiovascular twins, AI agents, and sensor data: A narrative review from system architecture to proactive heart health. *Sensors (Basel)*, *25*(17), 5272. DOI: 10.3390/s25175272 PMID: 40942702

Teamworks. (2024, July 2). *Teamworks acquires ZoneIn performance nutrition.* https://teamworks.com/blog/teamworks-acquires-zonein/

Teamworks. (2025, June 17). *Teamworks raises $235M to accelerate AI-powered innovation*. https://teamworks.com/blog/teamworks-series-f/

Tertipi, N., Sfyri, E., Grech, V. S., Kefala, V., & Rallis, E. (2025). Optimizing Skin Quality via AI-Enhanced Physical Activity. *Cosmetics*, *12*(3), 104. DOI: 10.3390/cosmetics12030104

Thielecke, F., & Blannin, A. (2020). Omega-3 fatty acids for sport performance—Are they equally beneficial for athletes and amateurs? A narrative review. *Nutrients*, *12*(12), 3712. https://www.mdpi.com/2072-6643/12/12/3712. DOI: 10.3390/nu12123712 PMID: 33266318

Thomas, D. T., Erdman, K. A., & Burke, L. M. (2016). American College of Sports Medicine joint position statement: Nutrition and athletic performance. *Medicine and Science in Sports and Exercise*, *48*(3), 543–568. DOI: 10.1249/MSS.0000000000000852 PMID: 26891166

Thomas, D. T., Erdman, K. A., & Burke, L. M. (2016). Position of the Academy of Nutrition and Dietetics, Dietitians of Canada, and the American College of Sports Medicine: Nutrition and athletic performance. *Journal of the Academy of Nutrition and Dietetics*, *116*(3), 501–528. DOI: 10.1016/j.jand.2015.12.006 PMID: 26920240

Tipton, K. D. (2011). Nutrition for acute exercise-induced injuries. *Annals of Nutrition & Metabolism*, *57*(Suppl. 2), 43–53. DOI: 10.1159/000322703 PMID: 21346336

Tipton, K. D., Borsheim, E., Wolf, S. E., Sanford, A. P., & Wolfe, R. R. (2004). Acute response of net muscle protein balance reflects 24-h balance after exercise and amino acid ingestion. *American Journal of Physiology. Endocrinology and Metabolism*, *284*(1), E76–E89. DOI: 10.1152/ajpendo.00234.2002 PMID: 12388164

Tipton, K. D., Elliott, T. A., Cree, M. G., Aarsland, A. A., Sanford, A. P., & Wolfe, R. R. (2007). Stimulation of net muscle protein synthesis by whey protein ingestion before and after exercise. *American Journal of Physiology. Endocrinology and Metabolism, 292*(1), E71–E76. DOI: 10.1152/ajpendo.00166.2006 PMID: 16896166

Tipton, K. D., & Witard, O. C. (2007). Protein requirements and recommendations for athletes: Relevance of ivory tower arguments for practical recommendations. *Clinics in Sports Medicine, 26*(1), 17–36. DOI: 10.1016/j.csm.2006.11.003 PMID: 17241913

Toledo, M. C. B., Brustoloni, J. G. F., Rocha, I., Faleiro, A. M. A., Costa, A. M., Dourado, A. R., Nunes, F., Takahagassi, R. H., Castro, A. V., & Rodrigues, M. S. (2025). A influência da nutrição lipídica em atletas de alto rendimento: Uma revisão sistemática. *Revista CPAQV, 17*(2), 9. DOI: 10.36692/V17N2-76R

Tossici, G., Zurloni, V., & Nitri, A. (2024). Stress and sport performance: A PNEI multidisciplinary approach. *Frontiers in Psychology, 15*, 1358771. DOI: 10.3389/fpsyg.2024.1358771 PMID: 38495423

Townsend, J. R., Kirby, T. O., Sapp, P. A., Gonzalez, A. M., Marshall, T. M., & Esposito, R. (2023). Nutrient synergy: Definition, evidence, and future directions. *Frontiers in Nutrition, 10*, 1279925. DOI: 10.3389/fnut.2023.1279925 PMID: 37899823

Tripkovic, L., Lambert, H., Hart, K., Smith, C. P., Bucca, G., Penson, S., Chope, G., Hyppönen, E., Berry, J., Vieth, R., & Lanham-New, S. (2012). Comparison of vitamin D2 and vitamin D3 supplementation in raising serum 25-hydroxyvitamin D status: A systematic review and meta-analysis. *The American Journal of Clinical Nutrition, 95*(6), 1357–1364. DOI: 10.3945/ajcn.111.031070 PMID: 22552031

Trombold, J. R., Reinfeld, A. S., Casler, J. R., & Coyle, E. F. (2011). The effect of acute pomegranate juice supplementation on exercise performance and markers of oxidative stress. *Applied Physiology, Nutrition, and Metabolism, 36*(6), 1018–1025.

Tsolakidis, D., Gymnopoulos, L. P., & Dimitropoulos, K. (2024). Artificial intelligence and machine learning technologies for personalized nutrition: A review. *Informatics (MDPI), 11*(3), 62. DOI: 10.3390/informatics11030062

Tungtrakul, C., Thawornsujaritkul, T., & Silpcharu, T. (2024). The guide for information technology management regarding personal data protection of the industrial business sector in Thailand. *International Journal of Instructional Cases, 8*(2), 196–210. https://ijicases.com/menuscript/index.php/ijicases/article/view/159

Turnagöl, H. H., Koşar, Ş. N., Güzel, Y., Aktitiz, S., & Atakan, M. M. (2022). Nutritional considerations for injury prevention and recovery in combat sports. *Nutrients, 14*(1), 53. DOI: 10.3390/nu14010053 PMID: 35010929

Turner, O., Chessor, R., & Mitchell, N. (2025). Fuelling gold medals: Developing a 'periodised nutrition system'for elite athletes and applying it in practice. *Performance Nutrition, 1*(4), 1–23. DOI: 10.1186/s44410-025-00001-x

UNDP & WHO. (2021, November 23). *Prevention and control of noncommunicable diseases in Thailand: The case for investment.* https://www.undp.org/thailand/publications/prevention-and-control-noncommunicable-diseases-thailand-case-investment

Utama, D. N., & Wibowo, A. (2022, February). Virtual plant computational model of green-leaf vegetable plant bok choy (Brassica chinensis L.) for investment decision. In *IOP Conference Series: Earth and Environmental Science* (Vol. 998, No. 1, p. 012049). IOP Publishing. DOI DOI: 10.1088/1755-1315/998/1/012049

van Dijk, J. A. (2006). Digital divide research: Achievements and shortcomings. *Poetics, 34*(4-5), 221–235. DOI: 10.1016/j.poetic.2006.05.004

Via, J., Reid, J., & Oehlert, G. (2024). Pedalling toward a deeper understanding of exercise effects on immune function. *The Journal of Physiology, 602*(19), 4705–4707. Advance online publication. DOI: 10.1113/JP287173 PMID: 39167713

Vitale, K. C., Hueglin, S., & Broad, E. (2017). Tart cherry juice in athletes: A literature review and commentary. *Current Sports Medicine Reports, 16*(4), 230–239. DOI: 10.1249/JSR.0000000000000385 PMID: 28696985

Vitale, K., & Getzin, A. (2019). Nutrition and supplement update for the endurance athlete: Review and recommendations. *Nutrients, 11*(6), 1289. https://www.mdpi.com/2072-6643/11/6/1289. DOI: 10.3390/nu11061289 PMID: 31181616

Wahyudi, N. T., & Yunus, M. (2025). Enhancing athlete performance with mobile health applications: Benefits and challenges. *Health Frontiers: Multidisciplinary Journal for Health Professionals, 3*(1), 1–9. DOI: 10.62255/mjhp.v3i1.141

WAN. Y. (2026). Intelligent Algorithms in Enhancing Sports Performance: Theoretical Reconstruction, Technological Breakthroughs, and Future Challenges. https://www.researchsquare.com/article/rs-8830620/v1

Wang, L., Koh, D., Li, F., Yaakop, N., & Wang, Y. (2026). The Construction of Personalized Sports Health Management System under Generative AI System. *Journal of Mechanics in Medicine and Biology, 2640043*, 2640043. https://www.worldscientific.com/doi/abs/10.1142/S0219519426400439. DOI: 10.1142/S0219519426400439

Wang, L., Meng, Q., & Su, C.-H. (2024). From Food Supplements to Functional Foods: Emerging Perspectives on Post-Exercise Recovery Nutrition. *Nutrients*, *16*(23), 4081. DOI: 10.3390/nu16234081 PMID: 39683475

Wang, P., Wang, A., & Wang, S. (2026). Integrating multimodal AI technologies for sports injury prediction and rehabilitation: Systematic review. *Journal of Human Sport and Exercise*, *21*(1), 22–37. DOI: 10.55860/w6j5wc21

Wang, Q., Su, M., Zhang, M., & Li, R. (2021). Integrating digital technologies and public health to fight COVID-19 pandemic: Key technologies, applications, challenges and outlook of digital healthcare. *International Journal of Environmental Research and Public Health*, *18*(11), 6053. DOI: 10.3390/ijerph18116053 PMID: 34199831

Wang, Y., Wen, Y., Wu, X., Wang, L., & Cai, H. (2025). Assessing the role of adaptive digital platforms in personalized nutrition and chronic disease management. *World Journal of Innovation and Modern Technology*, *8*(1), 24–31. DOI: 10.53469/wjimt.2025.08(01).05

Westerbeek, H., & Schaik, T. V. (2025). Platform power, athlete branding, generative AI, and the future of sport governance—A systematic review. *Frontiers in Sports and Active Living*, *7*, 1642180. DOI: 10.3389/fspor.2025.1642180 PMID: 41031328

Wheatley, V. M., & Spink, J. (2013). Defining the public health threat of dietary supplement fraud. *Comprehensive Reviews in Food Science and Food Safety*, *12*(6), 599–613. https://ift.onlinelibrary.wiley.com/doi/abs/10.1111/1541-4337.12033. DOI: 10.1111/1541-4337.12033 PMID: 33412717

Willett, W., Rockström, J., Loken, B., Springmann, M., Lang, T., Vermeulen, S., & Murray, C. J. (2019). Food in the Anthropocene: The EAT–Lancet Commission on healthy diets from sustainable food systems. *Lancet*, *393*(10170), 447–492. https://www.thelancet.com/journals/lancet/article/PIIS0140-6736(18)31788-4/fulltext. DOI: 10.1016/S0140-6736(18)31788-4 PMID: 30660336

Wingrove, K., Lawrence, M. A., & McNaughton, S. A. (2022). A systematic review of the methods used to assess and report dietary patterns. *Frontiers in Nutrition*, *9*, 892351. DOI: 10.3389/fnut.2022.892351 PMID: 35694166

Witard, O. C., Jackman, S. R., Breen, L., Smith, K., Selby, A., & Tipton, K. D. (2014). Myofibrillar muscle protein synthesis rates subsequent to a meal in response to small and large bolus doses of dairy proteins. *The American Journal of Clinical Nutrition*, *99*(1), 86–95. DOI: 10.3945/ajcn.112.055517 PMID: 24257722

Wolfe, R. R. (2017). Branched-chain amino acids and muscle protein synthesis in humans: Myth or reality? *Journal of the International Society of Sports Nutrition, 14*(1), 30. DOI: 10.1186/s12970-017-0184-9 PMID: 28852372

World Health Organization. (2019). *Meeting report: WHO technical consultation: nutrition-related health products and the World Health Organization model list of essential medicines–practical considerations and feasibility: Geneva, Switzerland, 20–21 September 2018* (No. WHO/NMH/NHD/19.1). World health organization. https://iris.who.int/bitstream/handle/10665/311677/WHO-NMH-NHD-19.1-eng.pdf

Xiao, Y., Deng, Z., Sun, W., Li, J., & Gao, W. (2025). Effects of protein supplementation on body composition, physiological adaptations, and performance during endurance training: A systematic review and meta-analysis. *Frontiers in Nutrition, 12*, 1663860. DOI: 10.3389/fnut.2025.1663860 PMID: 40851900

Xiong, Y.. (2024). Overview of anti-inflammatory diets and their promising effects on chronic disease prevention. *The British Journal of Nutrition, 132*(4), 601–625.

Yang, C. S., & Landau, J. M. (2000). Effects of tea consumption on nutrition and health. *The Journal of Nutrition, 130*(10), 2409–2412. DOI: 10.1093/jn/130.10.2409 PMID: 11015465

Yasul, Y., Yılmaz, B., Yasul, M. E., Şenel, Ö., & Çinar, V. (2024). *Recovery response of coenzyme Q10 to exercise-related physiological muscle damage, inflammation and oxidative stress: A systematic review*. Turkish Journal of Kinesiology., DOI: 10.31459/turkjkin.1429014

Yeo, W. K., Paton, C. D., Garnham, A. P., Burke, L. M., Carey, A. L., & Hawley, J. A. (2008). Skeletal muscle adaptation and performance responses to once a day versus twice every second day endurance training regimens. *Journal of Applied Physiology (Bethesda, Md.), 105*(5), 1462–1470. DOI: 10.1152/japplphysiol.90882.2008 PMID: 18772325

Yeung, A. W. K., Torkamani, A., Butte, A. J., Glicksberg, B. S., Schuller, B., Rodriguez, B., Ting, D. S. W., Bates, D., Schaden, E., Peng, H., Willschke, H., van der Laak, J., Car, J., Rahimi, K., Celi, L. A., Banach, M., Kletecka-Pulker, M., Kimberger, O., Eils, R., & Atanasov, A. G. (2023). The promise of digital healthcare technologies. *Frontiers in Public Health, 11*, 1196596. DOI: 10.3389/fpubh.2023.1196596 PMID: 37822534

Yuduang, N., Ong, A. K. S., Prasetyo, Y. T., Chuenyindee, T., Kusonwattana, P., Limpasart, W., Sittiwatethanasiri, T., Gumasing, M. J. J., German, J. D., & Nadlifatin, R. (2022). Factors influencing the perceived effectiveness of COVID-19 risk assessment mobile application "MorChana" in Thailand: UTAUT2 approach. *International Journal of Environmental Research and Public Health, 19*(9), 5643. DOI: 10.3390/ijerph19095643 PMID: 35565040

Yu, X., Pu, H., & Voss, M. (2024). Overview of anti-inflammatory diets and their promising effects on non-communicable diseases. *The British Journal of Nutrition, 132*(7), 898–918. DOI: 10.1017/S0007114524001405 PMID: 39411832

Yuxin, L., Salih, S. A., & Shaari, N. (2025). Technical functions of digital wearable products (DWPs) in the consumer acceptance model: A systematic review and bibliometric analysis with a biomimetic perspective. *Biomimetics, 10*(8), 483. DOI: 10.3390/biomimetics10080483 PMID: 40862856

Zacharia, A., Thomas, A. C., Mathew, P. C., Cleetus, R. S., John, S. E., & Joseph, J. (2024). Exploring the intersection of e-commerce and healthcare: A visual analysis of research trends. *Cureus, 16*(9), e69865. DOI: 10.7759/cureus.69865 PMID: 39435212

Zawadzki, K. M., Yaspelkis, B. B.III, & Ivy, J. L. (1992). Carbohydrate-protein complex increases the rate of muscle glycogen storage after exercise. *Journal of Applied Physiology (Bethesda, Md.), 72*(5), 1854–1859. https://journals.physiology.org/doi/abs/10.1152/jappl.1992.72.5.1854.DOI: 10.1152/jappl.1992.72.5.1854 PMID: 1601794

Zhan, Z. (2025). *The Distinct Roles of Subjective and Objective Food Knowledge in Fad Diet Preference: A Heuristic-Systematic Perspective* (Doctoral dissertation, University of Guelph). https://atrium.lib.uoguelph.ca/items/aceaac13-ea09-4432-9b98-0acf5b96ca49

Zhao, S., & Huang, H. (2025). The impact of the sports industry on the development of the health industry: An exploration of mediating and threshold effects. *Frontiers in Public Health, 13*, 1691241. DOI: 10.3389/fpubh.2025.1691241 PMID: 41341443

Zhong, X., Wang, J., & Zhong, Z. (2025). Spatial evolution characteristics and influencing factors of sports brand resources in Chinese urban agglomerations. *Scientific Reports, 15*(1), 22138. https://www.nature.com/articles/s41598-025-09706-4. DOI: 10.1038/s41598-025-09706-4 PMID: 40594806

Zion Market Research. (2025, May 15). *Global B2B sports nutrition market revenue estimated around USD 5.25 billion by 2034.* https://www.zionmarketresearch.com/news/global-b2b-sports-nutrition-market

Zouhal, H., Bagheri, R., Triki, R., Saeidi, A., Wong, A., Hackney, A. C., Laher, I., Suzuki, K., & Ben Abderrahman, A. (2020). Effects of Ramadan intermittent fasting on gut hormones and body composition in males with obesity. *International Journal of Environmental Research and Public Health*, *17*(15), 5600. https://www.mdpi.com/1660-4601/17/15/5600. DOI: 10.3390/ijerph17155600 PMID: 32756479

Zovi, A., Vitiello, A., Sabbatucci, M., Musazzi, U. M., Sagratini, G., Cifani, C., & Vittori, S. (2025). Food supplements marketed worldwide: A comparative analysis between the European and the US regulatory frameworks. *Journal of Dietary Supplements*, *22*(1), 25–40. https://www.tandfonline.com/doi/full/10.1080/19390211.2024.2389397. DOI: 10.1080/19390211.2024.2389397 PMID: 39221704

About the Contributors

Supaprawat Siripipatthanakul is working as an Adjunct Professor at Manipal GlobalNxt University, Malaysia, and a Faculty Member at the Faculty of Education at Bangkok Thonburi University, Thailand. He is also a Visiting Professor at the Faculty of Economics and Business at Universitas Terbuka, Indonesia. He has published more than 90 papers and books on Google Scholar. He has a CEFR Level 5 (C1), an English Teacher certificate from AAARYA Business College in Singapore, TEFL & TESOL certificates. 9 certificates in research (Scopus & WOS), and 8 certificates of Ethics in Research. He lectures on research methodology (business/ education/ healthcare) for international universities. He has been invited to review the manuscripts of Q1 and Q2-Scopus, WOS journals/Scopus, and Springer books (205 verified reviews by WOS/ 340 verified reviews by ORCID) since 2022. He is an Editor of IGI Global Scopus Books and PLoS One, Scopus & WOS, SJR Q1 USA.

Astri Andriani was born on April 21 in Cianjur Regency. Completed her undergraduate education in communication science at Universitas Putra Indonesia in 2012, and became the best graduate at that time. Then continued her master's degree in communication science at Bandung Islamic University, and graduated in 2015. In 2022, Communication Science at Padjadjaran University, Bandung with expertise in topical communication. Having been a radio announcer, reporter, editor-in-chief of a magazine, and public relations manager, finally in 2015 Astri anchored her heart in the world of education, by becoming a lecturer at Universitas Putra Indonesia until now. In addition to actively teaching, Astri is also entrusted with additional duties as Chancellor at Universitas Putra Indonesia. In addition to academic activities, Astri is also active in organizational and social activities, including in Next Generation (NXG) Indonesia and the Association of Higher Education Study Programs in Communication Science (ASPIKOM) West Java Regional Coordinator. Astri is also active as a researcher at the Indonesian Poldata Consultant and a human resources expert at several government institutions in the fields of youth studies, health communication, digital media literacy, and public speaking.

***

Saranchana Asanprakit is a researcher at the International College, Pathumthani University. She is actively engaged in academic research and has a growing portfolio of work at the intersection of digital transformation and management. Her primary research interests include digital business, business management, electronic commerce (e-commerce), and social commerce (s-commerce).

Shuvasree Banerjee is a Asst. Professor with over nine years of teaching experience in Tourism and Hotel Management Institutes. She holds a Bachelor of Business Administration (BBA) in Tourism and Hospitality from Burdwan University, West Bengal, followed by a Post Graduate Diploma in Management (PGDM) in Travel & Tourism Management from the Indian Institute of Tourism and Travel Management (IITTM) Bhubaneswar, an autonomous body under the Ministry of Tourism, Government of India. Additionally, she has completed a Master of Business Administration (MBA) in Tourism and Hospitality from the National Institute of Tourism and Hospitality Management (NITHM), Hyderabad, under affiliation with Jawaharlal Nehru Technological University, Hyderabad. She is awarded a PhD degree in Tourism and Hospitality from Chandigarh University. As an active research scholar, she has presented papers at 14 international conferences from 2022 to 2025 and has 16 publications to their credit. Her scholarly contributions include one paper published in a Scopus Q1 journal and 8 book chapters, with 2 paper and 8 chapters indexed in Scopus.

Swapan Banerjee is an academician, researcher, and clinical nutrition expert currently serving as an Assistant Professor in the Department of Hospital and Health Management at Poornima University, Jaipur, India. With more than 25 years of professional experience in nutrition, public health, and healthcare management, he has established himself as a dedicated educator and an active contributor to research in the fields of clinical nutrition and lifestyle disease management. Dr. Banerjee's teaching focuses on nutrition science, public health, hospital management, and wellness education. He is committed to integrating academic knowledge with practical healthcare applications, helping students understand the role of nutrition in disease prevention and health promotion. Through interactive teaching methods, research supervision, and academic mentoring, he encourages students to engage with emerging health challenges and evidence-based nutritional practices. As a researcher, Dr. Banerjee has contributed significantly to the scientific community with numerous publications in the areas of nutrition, metabolic disorders, endocrine health, and preventive medicine. He has authored several research papers, book chapters, and books, and has also been involved in interdisciplinary research addressing lifestyle diseases such as diabetes, obesity, and thyroid disorders. His work often explores the relationship between diet, public health, and disease management, contributing valuable insights to both academic and clinical communities. In addition to his academic responsibilities, Dr. Banerjee actively participates in editorial and scholarly activities. He serves as Editor-in-Chief of the *Journal of Preventive Medicine and Holistic Health* and contributes as a reviewer and editor for various international journals. His engagement in conferences, seminars, and public health initiatives reflects his dedication to spreading awareness about nutrition and healthy lifestyles. Through his combined efforts in teaching, research, and community outreach, Dr. Swapan Banerjee continues to promote scientific knowledge, nutritional awareness, and improved healthcare practices among students, researchers, and the broader society.

Prashant Choudhary hails from Port Blair, Andaman and Nicobar Islands. His sporting journey began on the tennis court, and showing exceptional promise, he relocated in 2005 to the Haryana National Tennis Academy for advanced training, which laid the foundation for his decorated junior tennis career. He went on to be ranked among the top five players nationally in the Under-12, Under-14, Under-16, and Under-18 categories, receiving sponsorship from the All India Tennis Association. Before joining college in 2014, he earned the prestigious ITF Level 1 and Level 2 International Tennis Federation coaching certifications, adding to his technical grounding in the sport. Later, he represented Lakshmibai National Institute of Physical Education (LNIPE), Gwalior in numerous university championships. Dr. Choudhary completed his Bachelor's, Master's, and Doctoral degrees in Physical Education and Sports Sciences at LNIPE, earning his Ph.D. in 2024. He has qualified the UGC-NET JRF and MP SET examinations, further demonstrating his academic merit. In 2024, he joined Lovely Professional University as an Assistant Professor, before moving later that year to LNIPE, Gwalior, where he currently serves as an Assistant Professor in the Department of Physical Education Pedagogy. His research interests include sports sciences, athlete wellbeing, motor learning, sports performance enhancement, talent identification, and coaching science, with multiple research papers published in Scopus.

Denny Dwiwarman is an Associate Professor at Universitas Putra Indonesia with a deep focus on Human Resource Development (HRD) and Strategic Policy. His research explores the synergy between human capital and digital transformation, specifically how soft and hard skills integrate into modern organizational performance. With a doctoral background in Social Sciences, he frequently bridges the gap between public policy—notably his evaluations of Regional Development Plans (RPJMD)—dan private sector efficiency. His work is widely cited, particularly in the areas of digital marketing innovation, organizational commitment, and the impact of distributive justice on professional performance.

Chirapat Kaewnaknaew is an active independent researcher and Scopus book author published with IGI Global (USA), currently collaborating with a research team of professors across Malaysia, Thailand, and Indonesia. She is an alumna of City University, Malaysia, with an Executive Master of Business Administration (EMBA). Chirapat specializes in management and social science research, with key interests in business, education, healthcare, technology, marketing, and Human Resource Management (HRM). In addition to her academic research, she serves as an editorial team assistant for the international journal "Advance Knowledge for Executives" and currently manages management strategies for a private company in Thailand.currently manages management strategies for a private company in Thailand.

Shikha Khullar is an academician and researcher specializing in Artificial Intelligence, computational intelligence, and intelligent systems. She is actively involved in scholarly research, book editing, and academic writing with reputed publishers such as IGI Global and Wiley–Scrivener. Her work focuses on emerging technologies including AI-driven fraud detection, smart city architectures, and next-generation intelligent systems. She has contributed to several research publications and book chapters and is committed to advancing innovation in AI-enabled applications.

Indra Kishor is currently serving as an Assistant Professor in the Department of Computer Science and Engineering at PIET, where he has been contributing for the past three years with his multifaceted expertise and dedication to both teaching and research. With over a decade of impactful experience across teaching, research, and industry, Mr. Kishor has built an extraordinary academic portfolio. He has authored more than 103 research papers, contributed to 30+ book chapters, and published several Tier-1 journal articles in collaboration with international scholars from some of the world's most prestigious universities. He also holds an impressive 15 Indian patents, 2 Canadian copyrights, and a UK design patent in drone technology.

Pongsakorn Limna, also known as Palm, is currently a postdoctoral researcher in the Digital Business program at the International College, Pathumthani University, Thailand. He is an active scholar with numerous publications in leading academic journals, including those indexed in Scopus and the Thai Citation Index (TCI). He also serves as a reviewer for several national and international journals and academic conferences, demonstrating his strong commitment to academic excellence and scholarly contribution. His research interests span a wide range of interdisciplinary fields, including the digital economy, digital business, business administration, management, communication, technology, artificial intelligence (AI), and consumer behavior. In 2012, Dr. Limna was awarded a prestigious scholarship jointly provided by the Office of the Basic Education Commission of Thailand and the Wisconsin Department of Public Instruction, USA, to participate in the Thailand–Wisconsin International Sunrise Program in Wausau, Wisconsin. He holds a Bachelor of Arts (B.A.) degree from the Faculty of Humanities and Social Sciences at Burapha University, Thailand, with a major in English and a minor in tourism management. He later earned an Executive Master of Business Administration (Executive MBA) from the Faculty of Business and Technology at UNITAR International University in Malaysia. He completed his Doctor of Philosophy (Ph.D.) in Digital Economy at Rangsit University, Thailand, with the support of the esteemed Prasit – Khunying Pattana Ourairat Scholarship.

Udit Mamodiya is an accomplished academician, researcher, and innovator currently serving as Associate Professor and Associate Dean (Research) at Poornima University. With more than a decade of experience in teaching, research, and academic administration, he has made notable contributions to engineering and emerging technology research. His primary research interests include renewable energy systems, smart solar photovoltaic technologies, industrial automation, Internet of Things (IoT), artificial intelligence, and machine learning applications. Dr. Mamodiya has an impressive academic record with numerous research publications in SCI, Scopus, and UGC-CARE indexed journals, along with several book chapters and conference papers in the fields of intelligent systems and sustainable technologies. His work has received hundreds of citations, reflecting the growing impact of his research in renewable energy optimization, AI-driven systems, and smart infrastructure. In addition to his research output, Dr. Mamodiya is actively involved in innovation and technology development, holding multiple patents, design registrations, and copyrights. He has also contributed to academia as an editor, reviewer, and technical committee member for various international journals and conferences. Through his teaching, research leadership, and innovation initiatives, Dr. Mamodiya continues to promote sustainable technology solutions and interdisciplinary research, advancing engineering education and technology-driven societal development. If you want, I can also prepare:

Khoiruddin Muchtar is a lecturer and researcher at UIN Sunan Gunung Djati Bandung, specializing in Political Communication, Public Relations, and Organizational Communication. He has published extensively on intercultural communication, political branding, and digital media strategies. His research is characterized by a multidisciplinary approach, often integrating anthropological and technological perspectives into communication studies. He currently holds an h-index of 11 on Google Scholar.

Sohom Saha is a passionate academic and sports psychology professional, currently pursuing his Ph.D. in Physical Education at the Lakshmibai National Institute of Physical Education (LNIPE), Gwalior. He completed his Master of Physical Education (M.P.Ed.) with distinction from LNIPE, following his Bachelor of Physical Education (B.P.Ed.) and Bachelor of Arts (B.A.) in Physical Education from Visva-Bharati University, Shantiniketan, West Bengal. His areas of specialization include Sports Psychology, Volleyball, and Yoga, where he integrates scientific knowledge with practical expertise. Throughout his academic journey, Mr. Saha has actively participated in national-level sports events, including the All-India Inter-University Yoga and Ball Badminton Championships, and has secured championships in NCC Inter-Battalion Football and Badminton tournaments. Alongside his athletic pursuits, he has contributed significantly to sports research, publishing multiple articles in Scopus-indexed, Web of Science, and peer-reviewed journals. His research interests focus on emotional resilience, psychological well-being, performance optimization, and contemporary trends in sports psychology. Beyond research and sports, Mr. Saha has authored several books on sports psychology and technology in sports. He serves as an active reviewer for leading international journals, including PLOS ONE and Frontiers, as well as other reputed platforms, and is a member of the Sports Psychology Association of India. Mr. Saha's work reflects a strong commitment to promoting inclusivity, mental toughness, and holistic development in the field of sports. Through his scholarly contributions, practical experience, and professional engagements, he aspires to inspire future generations of athletes, educators, and researchers in building a more inclusive and psychologically enriched sporting world.

Asep Setiawan is an academic at UIN Sunan Gunung Djati Bandung, specializing in Dakwah Management and Hajj & Umrah Management. His research focuses on the intersection of religion, media, and economic empowerment. With over 600 citations and an h-index of 10, he has published extensively on the methodology of dakwah and the management of Islamic institutions. He is a member of several international researcher databases, including Scopus and ORCID.

Yarnaphat Shaengchart is a lecturer at the International College, Pathumthani University. He is actively engaged in academic research and has a growing portfolio of work at the intersection of digital transformation and management. His primary research interests include information technology, the digital economy, digital business, and business management.

Sachin Shekhawat is an emerging researcher in the field of Physical Education and Sports Sciences. He completed his Bachelor of Physical Education (B.P.Ed.)

from the University of Rajasthan and went on to pursue his Master of Physical Education (M.P.Ed.) from the prestigious Lakshmibai National Institute of Physical Education, Gwalior. He is currently pursuing his Ph.D. at the same institute, focusing on advanced research in sports science. A dedicated sportsperson, Mr. Shekhawat has represented his university multiple times in Handball at the Inter-University level, showcasing both skill and competitive excellence. In addition to his sporting achievements, he has demonstrated strong academic capability by qualifying the UGC NET-JRF examination multiple times, reflecting his commitment to research and higher education. His combined experience in academics and sports performance positions him as a promising contributor to the field of sports science and physical education.

Mahendra Singh is a Professor of Sports Psychology in the Department of Sports Psychology at Lakshmibai National Institute of Physical Education (LNIPE), Gwalior, Madhya Pradesh, under the Ministry of Youth Affairs & Sports, Government of India. He is currently also serving as the Controller of Examinations at LNIPE, Gwalior. He holds B.P.E., M.P.E., M.Phil., and Ph.D. degrees from LNCPE/LNIPE, Gwalior, has qualified UGC NET, and completed various yoga certifications including a Certificate Course in Yoga from Lonavla, Pune, as well as Yoga Pravesh and Yoga Parichaya from LNCPE, Gwalior. He also holds an NCC 'B' Certificate from the 8 MP Battalion, Gwalior. Dr. Singh has been engaged in teaching for over 34 years, including more than 19 years in postgraduate and Ph.D.-level teaching and research. He has extensive administrative experience, having served as Former Incharge Registrar, Former Dean of Academics, Sport Sciences, and Physical Education and Applied Areas, Former Chief Proctor, Former Chairman of the UGC Student Grievance Redressal Cell, Former Nodal Officer for the UGC Grievance Portal, Former HOD of the Department of Sports Psychology at LNIPE, Former Deputy Controller of Examinations, Former HOD of the School of Law at Guru Ghasidas Central University, Bilaspur, Former HOD of the Department of Physical Education at CSJM University, Kanpur, Anti-Ragging Coordinator at GGV, Bilaspur, Warden of various boys' hostels across Engineering, Pharmacy, and other UG/PG courses at CSJM University and Administrative Warden at GGV. He has authored six books on Physical Education, Sports, and Yoga, and published more than 50 research papers in national and international journals, including SCOPUS-indexed journals. Dr. Singh has presented over 35 papers at various national and international conferences/seminars. He is a member of academic bodies of various universities, a continuing member and former Chairperson of the Board of Studies and Departmental Research Committee at LNIPE, and has served as Secretary of the Board of Management at LNIPE. He has frequently been invited as a resource person, chairperson, and keynote speaker at national and international conferences and seminars. Additionally, he has extensive experience as an external examiner, paper setter, and evaluator for UG/PG/Ph.D. courses across various universities and has handled confidential assignments with state public service commissions. Dr. Singh has organized several mega events, sports tournaments, seminars, and conferences, and guided numerous Ph.D. scholars, with several more currently under his supervision. He also serves as the Chief Editor of conference proceedings publications and is on the editorial boards of reputed journals. During his student years, he represented Jiwaji University in Inter-University Tournaments in Basketball and Kho-Kho under AIU, and also participated in M.P. State Inter-University Tournaments in the same sports, along with several other achievements.

Mahendra Singh is a Professor of Sports Psychology in the Department of Sports Psychology at Lakshmibai National Institute of Physical Education (LNIPE), Gwalior, Madhya Pradesh, under the Ministry of Youth Affairs & Sports, Government of India. He is currently also serving as the Controller of Examinations at LNIPE, Gwalior. He holds B.P.E., M.P.E., M.Phil., and Ph.D. degrees from LNCPE/LNIPE, Gwalior, has qualified UGC NET, and completed various yoga certifications including a Certificate Course in Yoga from Lonavla, Pune, as well as Yoga Pravesh and Yoga Parichaya from LNCPE, Gwalior. He also holds an NCC 'B' Certificate from the 8 MP Battalion, Gwalior. Dr. Singh has been engaged in teaching for over 34 years, including more than 19 years in postgraduate and Ph.D.-level teaching and research. He has extensive administrative experience, having served as Former Incharge Registrar, Former Dean of Academics, Sport Sciences, and Physical Education and Applied Areas, Former Chief Proctor, Former Chairman of the UGC Student Grievance Redressal Cell, Former Nodal Officer for the UGC Grievance Portal, Former HOD of the Department of Sports Psychology at LNIPE, Former Deputy Controller of Examinations, Former HOD of the School of Law at Guru Ghasidas Central University, Bilaspur, Former HOD of the Department of Physical Education at CSJM University, Kanpur, Anti-Ragging Coordinator at GGV, Bilaspur, Warden of various boys' hostels across Engineering, Pharmacy, and other UG/PG courses at CSJM University and Administrative Warden at GGV. He has authored six books on Physical Education, Sports, and Yoga, and published more than 50 research papers in national and international journals, including SCOPUS-indexed journals. Dr. Singh has presented over 35 papers at various national and international conferences/seminars. He is a member of academic bodies of various universities, a continuing member and former Chairperson of the Board of Studies and Departmental Research Committee at LNIPE, and has served as Secretary of the Board of Management at LNIPE. He has frequently been invited as a resource person, chairperson, and keynote speaker at national and international conferences and seminars. Additionally, he has extensive experience as an external examiner, paper setter, and evaluator for UG/PG/Ph.D. courses across various universities and has handled confidential assignments with state public service commissions. Dr. Singh has organized several mega events, sports tournaments, seminars, and conferences, and guided numerous Ph.D. scholars, with several more currently under his supervision. He also serves as the Chief Editor of conference proceedings publications and is on the editorial boards of reputed journals. During his student years, he represented Jiwaji University in Inter-University Tournaments in Basketball and Kho-Kho under AIU, and also participated in M.P. State Inter-University Tournaments in the same sports, along with several other achievements.

Prapasri Siri received her Ph.D. in Digital Economy from the Faculty of Economics, Rangsit University, Thailand. She obtained her Master's degree in Economics from Ramkhamhaeng University in 2009 and her Bachelor's degree in Communication Arts (Information) from Phranakhon Rajabhat University. Her research interests include digital economy and health economics.

Tamonwan Sitthipon is a researcher collaborating with professors from Thailand, Malaysia, and Indonesia. Dr. Tamonwan Sitthipon is now a Scopus Book Editor in the topic "Nutrition Balance for Athletic Performance and Recovery" that will be published by IGI Global Scientific Publishing, USA Dr. Tamonwan Sitthipon is now an author in the Scopus Journals database (in review); Scopus Q1 & Q2. Dr. Tamonwan Sitthipon is now a reviewer for Frontiers in Education (Q2-Scopus, WOS & SJR, Switzerland). Dr. Tamonwan Sitthipon is now an intended reviewer for PLOS ONE (Q1-Scopus, WOS & SJR, PLOS ONE). Dr. Tamonwan Sitthipon is now an invited reviewer for Scopus books. Dr. Tamonwan Sitthipon is now a reviewer for a Thai TCI journal (Advance Knowledge for Executives). Her research area of interest is business and management strategies, contemporary research, AI, and Digital Intelligence.

Patcharavadee Sriboonruang (Dr. PLE) is an Associate Professor in the Faculty of Agriculture at Kasetsart University, Thailand, with a strong multidisciplinary academic background, including a PhD in Educational Technology and Communications from Chulalongkorn University and an M.S. in Development Communication. She holds bachelor's degrees from the University of the Thai Chamber of Commerce (Communication Arts, 2nd Honor) and multiple degrees from Sukhothai Thammathirat Open University (Guidance, Educational Technology, and Agricultural Management). Dr. Sriboonruang also serves as an invited reviewer for international publications, including PLOS ONE and IGI Global Scientific Publishing since April 2025.

Mohammad Talukder is an Associate Professor in the College of Tourism and Hospitality Management at IUBAT–International University of Business Agriculture and Technology, Dhaka. He holds a PhD in Hotel Management and has over fifteen years of combined academic, administrative, and industry experience in tourism, hospitality, and hotel management education. Dr. Talukder has served in leadership roles as Head of Department at multiple institutions and has extensive industry exposure in food and beverage management. His research interests include tourism and hospitality service quality, food service management, sustainable tourism, digital marketing, and emerging technologies such as artificial intelligence in hospitality, with numerous publications in Scopus-indexed journals, book chapters, and edited volumes.

Ira Ulfah is a researcher and lecturer in the fields of management, marketing, and entrepreneurship, with a strong focus on strategic marketing, digital marketing, and franchising. She is actively engaged in academic writing and book chapter development, committed to bridging theoretical advancement with practical and contextual business applications. Through her scholarly contributions, Ira strives to generate relevant, adaptive, and impactful ideas that enrich academic literature while also supporting business practice and policy development across various sectors.

Index

A

B

C

D

O

P

R

S

U

www.ingramcontent.com/pod-product-compliance
Lightning Source LLC
LaVergne TN
LVHW080908300926
849162LV00003B/604

* 9 7 9 8 3 3 7 3 9 5 4 4 9 *